CLINICAL VOICE PATHOLOGY

Theory and Management

CLINICAL VOICE PATHOLOGY
Theory and Management

Second Edition

Joseph C. Stemple, Ph.D.
Institute for Voice Analysis and Rehabilitation,
Dayton, Ohio

Leslie E. Glaze, Ph.D.
Otolaryngology and Head and Neck Surgery,
St. Paul, Minnesota
and
ENT Professional Associates
Minneapolis, Minnesota

Bernice K. Gerdeman, Ph.D.
Institute for Voice Analysis and Rehabilitation,
Dayton, Ohio

SINGULAR PUBLISHING GROUP, INC
San Diego, California

Singular Publishing Group, Inc.
4284 41st Street
San Diego, California 92105-1197

©1995 by Singular Publishing Group, Inc.

Typeset by So Cal Graphics in 10/12 Palatino
Medical illustrations by John Barrord, M.D.
Printed in the United States of America by McNaughton & Gunn

Library of Congress Cataloging-in-Publication Data

Stemple, Joseph C.
    Clinical voice pathology: theory and management/Joseph C.
Stemple, Leslie E. Glaze, Bernice K. Gerdeman: medical illustrations by
John Barrord
       p. cm.
    Includes bibliographical references and index.
    ISBN 1-56593-342-7
    1. Voice disorders. I. Glaze, Leslie E. II. Gerdeman, Bernice K.
III. Title
    [DNLM: 1. Voice Disorders. 2. Larynx, Artificial. WV 500 S824c 1994]
RF510.S74 1994
618.85'5—dc20
DNLM/DLC
for Library of Congress   94-27024
                                                  CIP

CONTENTS

PREFACE

Through our many years of clinical work we have discovered the enjoyment and the challenge of working with the voice disordered population. Each patient provides us with questions which must be answered in order to return the voice to an improved condition. To answer these questions, voice pathologists must draw on many areas of knowledge including anatomy, physiology, etiologic correlates, and laryngeal pathologies. Diagnostic skills must be honed which include developing an effective patient interview style, techniques for the perceptual analysis of voice, and more recently, an understanding of voice acoustics, aerodynamics, and evaluation of vocal fold movement patterns. Finally, the voice pathologist must understand and be able to initiate a wide range of therapy techniques which, through the diagnostic procedure, have been determined to be the treatments most likely to effect positive vocal change.

This text was developed as an aid to speech-language pathology students in their study of clinical voice pathology. The ordering of the chapters was designed to slowly build the areas of knowledge necessary to eventually manage the voice disordered patient. Chapter 1 presents a history of voice disorders and describes the manner in which speech-language pathologists became involved with the evaluation and treatment of these disorders. The importance and the advantages of the "team approach" are emphasized. Chapter 2 describes the anatomy and physiology of the laryngeal mechanism including recent information that expands our traditional understanding of the cellular layered microstructure of the vocal fold. Recent advances in our recognition of the self-oscillating mechanism that governs vocal fold vibration are also described.

Chapter 3 offers a presentation of common etiologies associated with the development of voice disorders while Chapter 4 presents a discussion of laryngeal pathologies categorized as congenital laryngeal pathologies, pathologies of the vocal fold cover, neurogenic laryngeal pathologies, and pathologies of muscular dysfunction. With the knowledge of anatomy and physiology, common etiologies, and laryngeal pathologies, the reader is then prepared to learn how to conduct the diagnostic voice evaluation. Chapter 5 details subjective voice evaluation including the patient interview and perceptual voice analysis. Chapter 6 is new to this edition and presents information on the new state-of-the-art in voice analysis, instrumental assessment of vocal function. This chapter provides an introduction to the basic science principles of acoustics, aerodynamics, and laryngeal stroboscopy. This foundation is then bridged to the practical tasks of clinical analysis of vocal function in the voice laboratory.

Following the diagnostic voice evaluation, the voice pathologist is prepared to initiate the treatment plan. Chapters 7 and 8 provide the reader with a large sampling of treatment suggestions and therapy techniques. Chapter 7 introduces the philosophies related to voice treatment including symptomatic, psychogenic, etiologic, physiologic, and eclectic voice therapy orientations. Chapter 8 describes the more medical pathologies of voice and summarizes our understanding of the organic processes, both focal and systemic, that influence vocal fold health and voice production.

Chapter 9 presents some comments on the professional voice. Salespeople, teachers, ministers, actors, singers, and others who are dependent upon a healthy vocal system for their livelihoods are considered professional voice users. Because of their dependence on the vocal mechanism, professional voice users with voice disorders often require special considerations regarding their physical and emotional well-being and their courses of treatment. This chapter discusses these treatment considerations.

The final chapter, Chapter 10, deals with the total rehabilitation of the laryngectomized patient and the patient's family. From pre-operative counseling to the reestablishment of oral communication, the rehabilitative processes are discussed from the perspective of the rehabilitation team. Oral communication methods, including artificial larynges, esophageal voice, and the use of surgical prostheses, are described and illustrated in detail. The newest in-dwelling prosthesis is also described.

Clinical voice pathology has rapidly become a specialty within the field of communication disorders. It is our hope that this text will help to prepare students and clinicians who are interested in treating voice disorders by providing the appropriate science foundation which permits the development of the artistic nature of voice therapy.

Numerous individuals have contributed to the development of this text. We are deeply indebted to Thomas Murry, Ph.D. for encouraging the development of this project and for his strong editorial support. In addition, the guidance of our editors, Marie Linvill and Goretti Fernandes, was instrumental in bringing this text to print. Finally, we are indebted to the production staff, under the direction of Angie Singh, who were responsible for the look of the final product.

ACKNOWLEDGMENTS

A writing project of this kind may occur only with the support of those closest to us, through the teachings and works of those who came before us, and by the experiences gained through working with those around us. With deep gratitude we acknowledge our families who have supported our goals and projects with love, patience, and endurance; our teachers and colleagues, who inspired, encouraged, and challenged our learning; and our patients, whose strength and perseverance make the entire process meaningful, productive, and ultimately worth our every professional effort.

MEDICAL ILLUSTRATIONS
BY JOHN BARRORD, M.D.

Special thanks to Dr. Barrord who is an Otolaryngologist Head and Neck Surgeon in private practice in Middletown, Ohio. He obtained his medical degree in 1982 from the University of Cincinnati College of Medicine where he also completed his residency. As a Chief Resident, Dr. Barrord received the distinguished Alter Peerless Memorial Award in recognition of his leadership, knowledge, and technical skill. He has served as Chairman of the Eye, Ear, Nose, and Throat Department at Middletown Regional Hospital for the past two years and also is on the Board of Directors for a recently established Physician Hospital Organization. His artistic talent combined with his knowledge of the surgical anatomy of the larynx made Dr. Barrord the ideal medical illustrator for this text.

DEDICATION

This book is dedicated to the memory of a special friend and colleague, Michelle Chappelear. Michelle's life provided great enjoyment and love to those who had the privilege of knowing and working with her. It was because of her outstanding professional skills that I was able to take the time to finish this project. There are some people who say that it can't be done and some people who just do it. Michelle's short life symbolized the latter.

JCS

1

VOICE: A HISTORICAL PERSPECTIVE

Voice, articulation and language are the major elements of human speech production. When a disorder is present related to any of these elements, the ability to communicate may be impaired. Voice is the element of speech that provides the speaker with the vibratory signal upon which speech is carried. Regarded as magical and mystical in ancient times, today the production of voice is viewed as a powerful communication and artistic tool. It serves as the melody of our speech and provides expression, feeling, intent, and mood to our articulated thoughts. This text is concerned with voice and voice disorders.

A voice disorder exists when a person's quality, pitch, and loudness differ from those of similar age, sex, cultural background, and geographic locations (Aronson, 1980; Boone, 1977; Greene, 1972; Moore, 1971). In other words, when the acoustic and aerodynamic properties of voice are so deviant that they draw attention to the speaker, a voice disorder may be present. A voice disorder may also be present when the structure and/or function of the laryngeal mechanism no longer meets the voicing requirements established for the mechanism by the speaker. These requirements include vocal difficulties that are not readily recognized by others, such as the negative effects of vocal fatigue, but are reported to be present by the owner of the voice. Successful management of a voice disorder is dependent upon the individual recognizing the problem and accepting the need for improvement. The effects of a voice disorder are relative to the voicing needs of the individual. Those with a great need for normal voice production, such as professional voice users, may be unusually concerned with the presence of even minor vocal difficulties. Those with low vocal needs may not be greatly

1

concerned with even more severe vocal problems. Indeed, Koufman and Isaccson (1991) suggested that identifying the vocal needs of each patient is extremely important in successfully treating voice disorders.

The speech pathologist plays a major role in the evaluation and management of voice disorders. This role focuses on three major goals: (a) evaluation of laryngeal function using perceptual, acoustic, aerodynamic, and visual imaging techniques; (b) identification and modification or elimination of the functional causes that have led to the development of the voice disorder; and (c) evaluation and modification of specific deviant vocal components such as pitch, loudness, and so on when the use of deviant components contributes to the voice disorder. To accomplish these goals, the speech pathologist must have an extensive understanding and knowledge of the normal anatomy and physiology of the laryngeal mechanism as well as knowledge of common laryngeal pathologies. Etiologic factors that lead to the development of voice disorders must also be understood as well as appropriate diagnostic techniques and skills for discovering the causes. Finally, based on the previous knowledge, the speech pathologist must develop a bank of clinical management approaches for remediating the voice disorder.

Only in the recent history of voice disorders have speech pathologists played this evaluation and management role. Indeed, the first persons in the profession who became interested in the remedial aspects of voice did so only about 60 years ago (Moore, 1977; Stemple, 1993). The advent of voice therapy was a unique blend of the knowledge that speech correctionists, as speech pathologists were then called, gained from training in the areas of public speaking, oral interpretation, and theater arts combined with understanding in the areas of anatomy, physiology, psychology and pathologies of the laryngeal mechanism. In more recent history, speech pathologists have been required to also gain knowledge in vocal fold movement patterns, voice acoustics, and the aerodynamics of voice production. These years during which speech pathologists have dealt with the remediation of voice disorders represent only a small component of time when compared to the total history of the evaluation and treatment of voice disorders.

ANCIENT HISTORY

The earliest accounts of voice disorders, like all other medical information, were handed down orally. These accounts were mainly represented by folk remedies for various recognized disorders. Folklore remedies for disorders of the throat included liniment derived from centipedes, the juice of crabs, an owl's brain, and the ashes of a burned swallow. Plant remedies included gargles made from cabbage, garlic, nettles, pennyroyal, and sorrel. The wearing of beads of various kinds or a black silk cord around the throat was also recommended as well as the excommunication of sore throats in the name of God (Stevenson & Guthrie, 1949).

One of the earliest written histories of a voice disorder was presented about 1600 B.C. in the Edwin Smith Papyrus. One of many Egyptian papyri discovered in burial tombs, the Edwin Smith Papyrus contained very early medical writings. It described 50 traumatic surgical cases beginning with injuries to the head and continuing down the body to the thorax. One of these cases was a detailed description of a crushing injury to the neck, which caused the loss of speech. The Egyptian writings contained a hieroglyph portraying the lungs and trachea (Figure 1–1). The larynx was not pictured, because no organ for voice had yet been identified (Fink, 1975).

The ancient Hindu civilization presented much medical information including mention of diseases of the throat. The most notable information was presented in the Sanskrit-Atharva-Veda (700 B.C.). Surgical achievements of the Hindus included tonsillectomy and rhinoplasty. Nose flaps became a necessity in this civilization, for cutting off the nose was the corporal punishment for adultery. Hindu gargles for throat disorders included oils, vinegar, honey, the juices of fruit, and the urine of sacred cows (Wright, 1941).

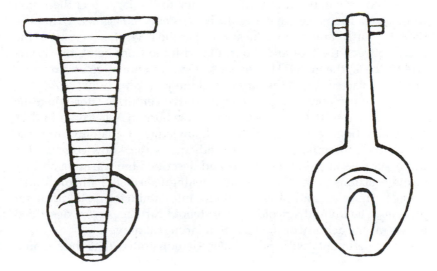

Figure 1–1.   Egyptian hieroglyphs of the trachea and lungs.

In the fifth century B.C., Hippocrates, the "Father of Medicine," was responsible for finally separating medicine from magic. One of Hippocrates' greatest contributions to medicine was his insistence upon the value of observation. Observation remains one of the speech pathologist's most powerful diagnostic tools. Hippocrates made many observations regarding diseases associated with the throat and voice, although he, too, failed to identify the source of voice. Several of these observations, as translated by Chadwick and Mann (1950), include:

Aphorism 58:	Commotion of the brain, from any cause, is inevitably followed by loss of voice.
Coan Prognosis 240:	Aphonia is of the most serious significance if accompanied by weakness.
Coan Prognosis 243:	Aphonia during fever in the manner of that seen in seizure, associated with a quiet delirium, is fatal.
Coan Prognosis 252:	A shrill whining voice and dimness of the eyes denote a spasm.

These examples demonstrate that Hippocrates studied symptoms more than treatments of diseases. Hippocrates was the first person to write that observation of voice quality, whether it be clear or hoarse, is one means by which a physical diagnosis may be reached (Chadwick & Mann, 1950). Observation of voice quality remains a powerful diagnostic tool.

Aristotle was the first writer to refer to the larynx as the organ from which the voice emanates. In his *Historia Animalium*, written in the late fourth century B.C., he stated that the neck was the part of the body between the face and the trunk, with the front being the larynx and the back, the gullet. He further stated that phonation and respiration took place through the larynx and the windpipe (Fink, 1975).

This information lay dormant until five centuries later when the first true anatomist, Claudius Galenus, was born in Asia Minor in A.D. 131. Galen (Figure 1–2) derived his knowledge of anatomy from the dissection of animals. He greatly advanced the knowledge of the upper air passages and the larynx and described the warming and filtering functions of the nose. He also distinguished six pairs of intralaryngeal muscles and divided them into abductor and adductor muscles. The thyroid, cricoid, and arytenoid cartilages were described as well as the activity of the recurrent laryngeal nerves.

In experiments with pigs, Galen demonstrated that they would always cease squealing when the recurrent laryngeal nerve was severed. This led him to conclude that muscles move certain parts of the body on which breathing and voice depend and that these muscle

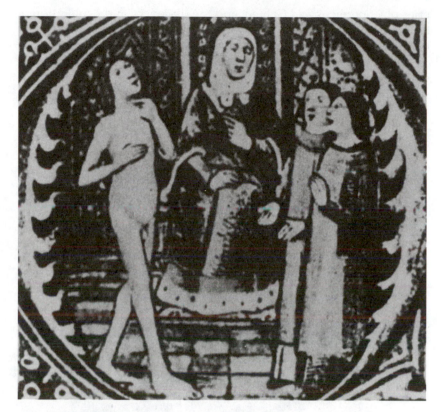

Figure 1–2.   Claudius Galenus (Galen).

movements are dependent on nerves from the brain. Galen, therefore, proved that the larynx was the organ of voice, thus disproving the still popular belief at that time that the "voice was sent forth by the heart" (Stevenson & Guthrie, 1949).

THE RENAISSANCE

Galen did much to further medical progress, but his theories and views, which were by no means totally accurate, were blindly accepted for 1,500 years as the world went through the Dark Ages. The Dark Ages was a historical period of intellectual and artistic stagnation that was finally broken in the late fourteenth and early fifteenth centuries A.D. with the invention of the printing press, the astronomical discoveries of Copernicus and Galileo, and the discovery and exploration of the Western Hemisphere. With these and other discoveries, the world began the great growth period known as the Renaissance.

A genius of the renaissance, the bold artist Leonardo da Vinci (1452–1519) did not hesitate to exchange his painting brush for a dissection scalpel to explore the human anatomy. Andreas Vesalius (1514–1564) reformed the knowledge of anatomy (Figure 1–3). In his 1542 publication *De Humani Corporis Fabrica*, this 29-year-old anatomist and artist corrected many of the age-long errors of Galen. He clarified

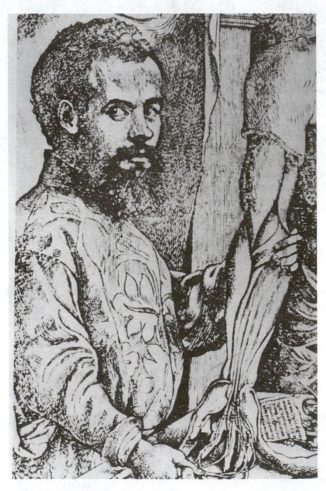

Figure 1–3.   Andreas Vesalius, 1514–1564.

the laryngeal anatomy and presented the function of the epiglottis. Vesalius' work is considered to be the anatomic classic of all time (Stevenson & Guthrie, 1949).

During this same time period, Bartolomeus Eustachias (1520-1574) (Figure 1–4) was one of the first anatomists to accurately describe the structure, course, and relations of the Eustachian tube. More interesting were his descriptions and carvings of the anatomy of the larynx, which were not discovered until the eighteenth century in the Vatican Library, and are even more detailed and accurate than those of

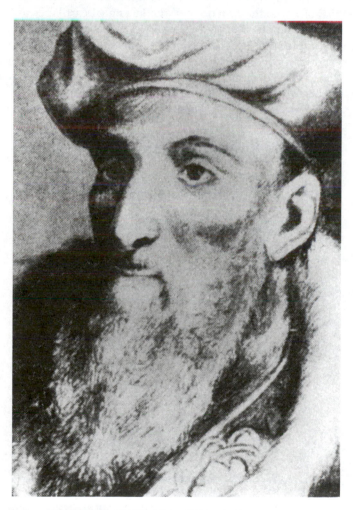

Figure 1–4.   Bartolomeus Eustachius, 1520–1574.

Vesalius. Fabricius, of Padua, authored the first monograph on the larynx (1600), entitled *De Visione Auditu*. In his monograph, Fabricius named the posterior cricoarytenoid muscles and described the action of the other laryngeal muscles.

THE SEVENTEENTH TO NINETEENTH CENTURIES

The discoveries of anatomy, physiology, and pathology of the laryngeal mechanism continued, highlighted by descriptions of the laryngeal ventricles by the Italian anatomist Giovanni Morgagni (1682–1771); further clarification of the purpose of the epiglottis by Francois Magendie (1783–1855) of Paris; the functions of the laryngeal cartilages and muscles in the production of voice by Robert Willis in Cambridge in 1829; and finally in Fredrick Ryland's (1837) publication called *Treatise on the Disease and Injuries of the Larynx and Trachea*. This important publication clearly described the diseases of the larynx (Figure 1–5) as they were understood before the use of the laryngeal mirror.

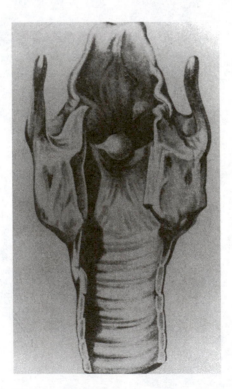

Figure 1–5.   Polyps of the larynx. Plate from Ryland's *Treatise on diseases and injuries of the larynx and trachea*, 1837.

THE LARYNGEAL MIRROR

The idea of examining the larynx in living humans had been in many minds since the time of Aristotle. It was not, however, until 1854, that a Parisian singing teacher named Manuel Garcia (1804–1906) (Figure 1–6) made the discovery that ushered in the modern era of laryngology.

Strolling through the gardens of Palais-Royal on a bright September day, Garcia observed the flashing sun in the window panes of the quadrangle buildings.

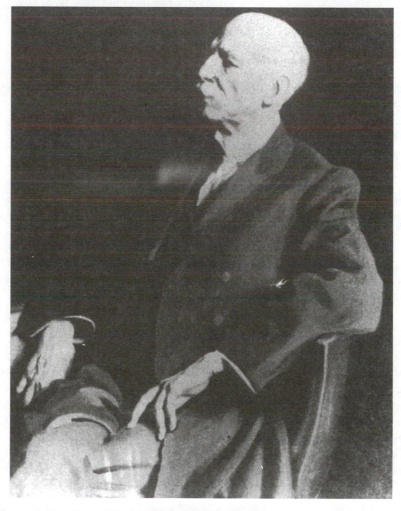

Figure 1–6.   Manuel Garcia at the age of 100.

Suddenly I saw the two mirrors of the laryngoscope in their respective positions, as if actually present before my eyes. I went straight to Charriere, the surgical instrument maker, and asking if he happened to possess a small mirror with a long handle, was informed that he had a little dentist's mirror, which had been one of the failures of the London exhibition of 1851. I bought it for six francs. Having also obtained a hand mirror, I returned home at once, very impatient to begin my experiments. I placed against the uvula the little mirror (which I heated in warm water and carefully dried), then flashing upon its surface with the hand mirror a ray of sunshine, I saw at once, to my great joy, the glottis, wide and open before me, and so fully exposed that I could perceive a portion of the trachea. When my excitement had somewhat subsided, I began to examine what was passing before my eyes. The manner in which the glottis silently opened and shut and moved in the act of phonation, filled me with wonder. (Garcia, 1881)

The use of the laryngeal mirror (Figure 1–7) was taken up quickly in the major medical centers of the world, with the major improvement of artificial illumination made in Budapest by Johann Czermak in 1861. The laryngeal mirror was first introduced in the United States in 1858 by Ernst Krakowizer, but credit for the development of laryngology as a specialty in the United States was given to Louis Elsberg, of New York, and J. Dobs Cohen, of Philadelphia. Elsberg taught laryngoscopy in the University Medical School of New York in the 1860s, and Cohen published the first American textbook on diseases of the throat in 1872. Cohen also performed the first total laryngectomy in the United States.

Other laryngeal examination techniques followed including stroboscopy (1878), direct laryngoscopy (1895), and ultra-high speed photography developed at the Bell Telephone Laboratories in 1937. These techniques are further described in Chapters 5 and 6.

VOICE THERAPY

The evaluation and treatment of voice disorders remained very much the province of the medical profession until about 1930. It was at this time that a few laryngologists as well as singing teachers, instructors in the speech arts, and a fledgling group of speech correctionists became interested in retraining individuals with vocal disorders (Murphy, 1964). Using drills and exercises borrowed from training manuals designed to enhance the normal voice, these specialists attempted to modify the production of the disordered voice. Many of these rehabilitation techniques were created by enterprising teachers and tailored to individual student's needs. The techniques, however, were not based

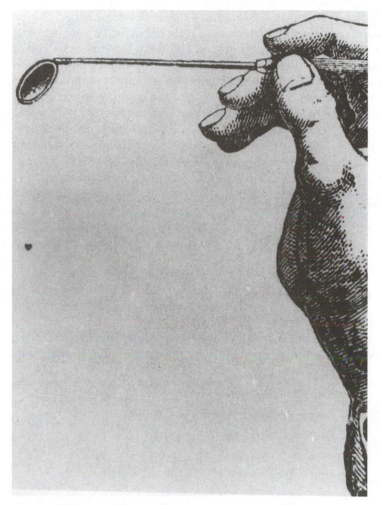

Figure 1–7.   The position of the hand and the laryngeal mirror.

on scientific principles of laryngeal, respiratory, and resonatory physiology. It is, therefore, particularly interesting how many of these techniques remain with us today, testimony to the insight and creativity of
early speech pathologists.

The study and practice of voice therapy were greatly advanced
with the publication of two books, *The Rehabilitation of Speech* by West,
Kennedy, and Carr (1937), and Charles Van Riper's *Speech Correction
Principles and Methods* (1939). In their chapter related to voice disorders, West, Kennedy, and Carr concentrated on the organic problems

of voice and diseases related to laryngeal dysfunction. The authors made the important statement that there is always a reason when the voice is disordered and, if properly studied, the reason will be discovered. Causes of the disorder may be neuropathological, emotional, or the result of improper vocal habits and structural pathology. For rehabilitating the voice, the authors suggested techniques including (a) ear training, (b) breathing exercises, (c) relaxation training, (d) articulatory compensations, (e) emotional retraining, and (f) special drills and exercises to be used with cleft palate and velopharyngeal insufficiency.

Van Riper stressed remedial measures to be used specifically by speech correctionists. He was the first author to suggest that voice disorders could be classified under the major headings of disorders of pitch, intensity, and quality. Voice therapy followed a medical examination, to rule out organic pathology, and a detailed evaluation of pitch, intensity and quality. Van Riper's description of therapy techniques was the most detailed of the time. The general thrust of his therapy approaches included (a) recognition of the problem by the patient; (b) production of a new, more appropriate sound; (c) stabilization of the new vocal behavior in many contexts; and (d) habituation of the new voicing behavior in all situations.

From these early foundations of voice rehabilitation have arisen several general management orientations. These orientations may be classified as

- symptomatic voice therapy
- psychogenic voice therapy
- etiologic voice therapy
- physiologic voice therapy
- eclectic voice therapy

In short, symptomatic voice therapy focuses on modification of the deviant vocal symptoms identified by the voice pathologist—such as breathiness, low pitch, glottal attacks, and so on. The focus of psychogenic voice therapy is on the emotional and psychosocial status of the patient which led to and maintained the voice disorder. Etiologic voice therapy concentrates on discovering the causes of the voice disorder and modification/elimination of these causes. The physiologic orientation of voice therapy focuses on directly modifying and improving the balance of laryngeal muscle effort to the supportive airflow as well as the correct focus of the laryngeal tone. Finally, the eclectic approach to voice therapy is the combination of any and all of the previous voice therapy orientations. Indeed, none of these philosophical orientations is pure. Much overlap is present, often leading, of course, to the use of eclectic voice therapy. (Stemple, 1993, p. 2)

CLINICAL VOICE PATHOLOGY

The role of the speech-language pathologist has expanded significantly in the evaluation and management of voice disorders. Indeed the "voice pathologist" has become an integral part of the **team** responsible for treating these individuals. This team is composed primarily of the laryngologist and voice pathologist, with other team members including other medical specialists, as required, as well as vocal coaches and singing instructors. Never before, in the history of the treatment of voice disorders, have patients had the opportunity for such integrated care. The physician's medical expertise combined with the voice pathologist's knowledge of speech and vocal processes have significantly improved the accuracy of diagnosis and the management care of these individuals.

This text is designed to introduce and integrate the **artistic** nature of voice care with the **scientific** areas of knowledge that are necessary for the development of a **"voice pathologist."** Voice analysis and treatment is, indeed, a unique blend of art and science. The artistic nature of voice care involves sensitive human interactions. The vocal mechanism is really quite strong and resilient physiologically, but very sensitive psychologically. The voice pathologist must develop a caring compassion, empathy, and understanding for the patient and the problems created by the voice disorder.

These interaction skills require that a person have the ability to listen, not only to the characteristics of the voice quality, but also to **what** the patient says. In turn, gathering of appropriate information related to the voice disorder is dependent upon the interview skills of the voice pathologist. Considering all of the parts of a diagnostic voice evaluation, we would suggest to you that the patient interview is the most valuable tool in the evaluation and remediation of a voice disorder.

Considering the strong relationship between voice production and the emotional state of the patient, the voice pathologist must also develop strong counseling skills. It is quite usual for voice-disordered patients to share much personal information regarding their thoughts, feelings, and relationships. Often this information must be discussed in depth as it relates to the voice problem. Counseling by a voice pathologist, however, should also include the awareness of when the problem exceeds those skills and thus requires further referral.

Finally, patient motivation is an art. Motivational skill is the ability to instill action for change. Although many patients come to the voice pathologist already highly motivated to improve voice production, some do not. The voice pathologist must not only have the skills to motivate the somewhat noncompliant patient, but also the ability to maintain motivation in those who proceed through the sometimes arduous tasks of therapy. We would suggest that the ability to monitor progress through objective measures and vocal imaging procedures has significantly improved patient compliance and motivation.

The scientific nature of voice care involves a broad knowledge base. This knowledge base includes:

- normal anatomy and physiology
- laryngeal pathologies
- etiologic correlates
- vocal acoustics
- vocal aerodynamics
- laryngeal imaging techniques

The voice pathologist must possess a complete understanding of the anatomy and physiology of the normal laryngeal mechanism, respiratory system, and supraglottic structures. With this understanding, management approaches based on the specific physiologic needs of the patient may be planned and implemented.

Knowledge of the microscopic anatomy of the vocal folds is also necessary in understanding the many different laryngeal pathologies. The voice pathologist must have knowledge of the various laryngeal pathologies, including their causes, signs, symptoms, and typical management approaches. Laryngeal pathologies may manifest as tissue lining changes of the vocal fold cover or may be neurologically, psychologically, or functionally induced changes in voice production.

The many causes of laryngeal pathologies must also be well understood by the voice pathologist. These causes may be behavioral in origin, medically related, or psychologically induced. The voice pathologist who possesses a large bank of etiologic correlates will likely be very successful in discovering specific causes of voice disorders, which is the first step in successful remediation.

Recently, the ability to objectively measure many aspects of voice production has added an additional useful tool in voice evaluation and management. Along with this tool comes the need to develop additional knowledge bases including knowledge related to the science of voice acoustics, aerodynamics, and laryngeal imaging. Many commercial instruments are now available that provide multitudes of measures related to voice production. It is the responsibility of the voice pathologist to understand the science of the specific measures and to utilize the measures as only one part of the diagnostic voice evaluation.

The practice of clinical voice pathology has a deep, rich, and interesting history that continues to rapidly evolve at this writing. Indeed, because of the greatly expanding bases of knowledge that are required to successfully manage voice disorders, the profession is steadily progressing toward specialty certification. By combining the speech-language pathologist's natural artistic abilities related to human interaction skills with a strong scientific base, the voice pathologist is emerging. Improved patient care will be the ultimate result.

REFERENCES

Aristotle. (1965). *Historia animalium* (A. Peck, Trans.). Cambridge, England: Howard University Press.

Aronson, A. (1980). *Clinical voice disorders: An interdisciplinary approach.* New York: Brian C. Decker.

Boone, D. (1977). *The voice and voice therapy* (2nd ed.). Englewood Cliffs, NJ: Prentice-Hall.

Chadwick, G., & Mann, W. (1950). *The medical works of Hippocrates.* Oxford: Blackwell Scientific Publications.

Czermak, J. (1860). *Du laryngoscope et son emploi en physiologie et en medicine.* Paris.

Fabricius. (1600). *De visiona voce auditu.* Venice.

Fink, R. (1975). *The human larynx: A functional study.* New York: Raven Press.

Galen, C. (1968). *De usa partium corporis humani* (M. May, Trans.). Ithaca, NY: Cornell University Press.

Garcia, M. (1881). *Transaction section of laryngology.* Paper presented at the VII International Congress of Medicine, London.

Greene, M. (1972). *The voice and its disorders* (3rd ed.). Philadelphia: J. B. Lippincott.

Koufman, J., & Isaccson, G. (1991). The spectrum of vocal dysfunction. In J. Koufman & G. Isaccson (Eds.), *The otolaryngologic clinics of North America: Voice disorders.* Philadelphia: W.B. Saunders. 24: 985–8.

Moore, P. (1971). *Organic voice disorders.* Englewood Cliffs, NJ: Prentice-Hall.

Moore, P. (1977). Have the major issues in voice disorders been answered by research in speech science? A 50-year retrospective. *Journal of Speech and Hearing Disorders,* 42: 152–160.

Morgagni, G. (1709). *Adversaria anatomica prima.* Padua.

Murphy, A. (1964). *Functional voice disorders.* Englewood Cliffs, NJ: Prentice-Hall.

Ryland, F. (1837). *Treatise on the diseases and injuries of the larynx.* London: Longmans.

Stemple, J. (1993). *Voice therapy: Clinical studies.* St. Louis: Mosby Year Book.

Stevenson, S., & Guthrie, G. (1949). *A History of otolaryngology.* Edinburgh: E.&S. Livingstone.

Van Riper, C. (1939). *Speech correction principles and methods.* Englewood Cliffs, NJ: Prentice-Hall.

Vesalius, A. (1542). *De humani corporis fabrica.* Basle.

West, R., Kennedy, L., & Carr, A. (1937). *The rehabilitation of speech.* New York: Harper and Brothers.

Wright, J. (1941). *A history of laryngology and rhinology* (2nd ed.). Philadelphia: Lea and Febiger.

2

ANATOMY AND PHYSIOLOGY

Knowledge of the anatomy and physiology of the laryngeal mechanism is paramount to understanding the disorders of voice. This knowledge serves as a foundation for examination of the larynx and evaluation of phonatory function and is essential for recognizing the impact of specific pathologies on voice production. A solid understanding of the normal structure and function of the larynx is the basis for the interpretation of evaluative findings and the development of appropriate voice treatment plans.

The larynx is essentially a cartilaginous tube that connects inferiorly to the respiratory system (trachea and lungs) and superiorly to the vocal tract and oral cavity (Figure 2–1). This cartilage framework houses a complex arrangement of muscles, mucous membranes, and other connective tissue (Figures 2–2 and 2–3). Together, the muscles and cartilage create three levels of "folds," or valves, which serve as sphincters that provide both communicative and vegetative functions in the body (Fink & Demarest, 1978; Kirchner, 1984). The upper rim of the larynx is composed of the aryepiglottic folds, which separate the pharynx from the laryngeal vestibule, and offer the first line of defense for preservation of the airway.

The second sphincter is formed by the ventricular folds, which are not normally active during phonation, but may become hyperfunctional during effortful speech production. Figure 2–4 displays the coronal view of the supraglottic vocal tract. The ventricular folds are directly superior to the ventricle and the true vocal folds, to form a "double layer" of medial closure, if needed. The principle function of the ventricular sphincter is to increase intrathoracic pressure by blocking the outflow of

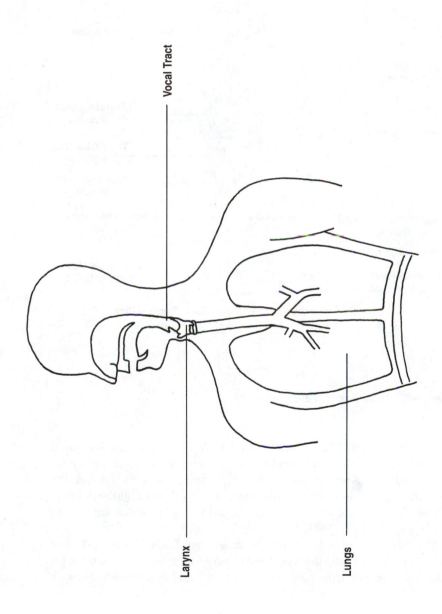

Figure 2–1. Orientation of the larynx in the body.

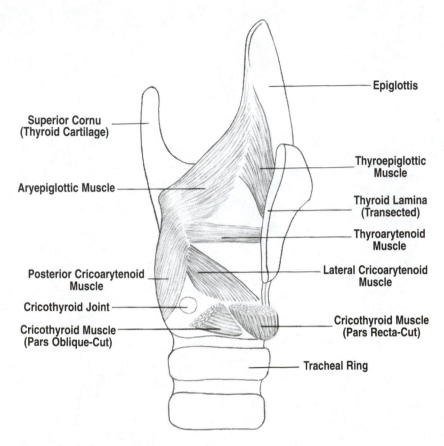

Figure 2–2.   Lateral view of the larynx.

air from the lungs. The ventricular folds compress tightly for rapid contraction of the thoracic muscles (e.g., coughing or sneezing) or for longer durations when building up subglottic pressure to stabilize the thorax during certain physical tasks (e.g., lifting, emesis, childbirth labor, or defecation). The ventricular folds also add airway protection during swallowing (Kirchner, 1984; Tucker, 1987).

The third and final layer are the true vocal folds (Figure 2–4). For speech communication, the vocal folds provide a vibrating source for phonation. They also close tightly for nonspeech and vegetative tasks, such as coughing, throat clearing, and grunting. Thus, in a mechanical sense, the larynx and vocal folds function as a variable valve, modulating airflow passing through the vibrating vocal folds during phonation, closing off the

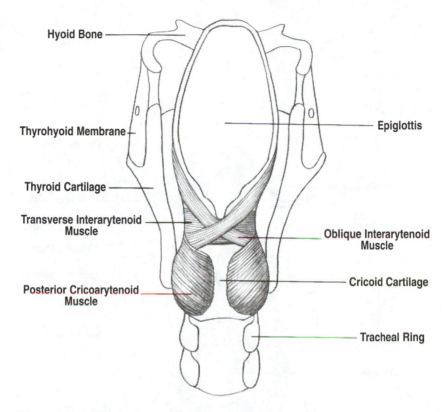

Hyoid Bone

Thyrohyoid Membrane

Thyroid Cartilage

Transverse Interarytenoid
Muscle

Posterior Cricoarytenoid
Muscle

Epiglottis

Oblique Interarytenoid
Muscle

Cricoid Cartilage

Tracheal Ring

Figure 2–3.   Posterior view of the larynx.

trachea and lungs from foods and liquids during swallowing actions, and providing resistance to increased abdominal pressures during straining, lifting, pushing, childbirth, or defecation (Kirchner, 1984; Tucker, 1987).

The communicative function of the larynx relies heavily on the integration of a three-part system: respiration, phonation, and supraglottic resonance. Specifically, the lungs function as the power supply; the larynx provides the vibratory source for phonation, and the vocal tract serves as the resonating cavity. Differential diagnosis of voice disorders requires careful assessment of these three components. Obviously, laryngeal health and overall function will influence the quality of voice production. But respiratory support and supraglottic resonance will also affect the speech product. For example, a patient with weak or inconsistent respiratory support will be unable to generate adequate vocal fold vibration to support normal vocal loudness or quality. Conversely, alteration of the shape and size of the vocal

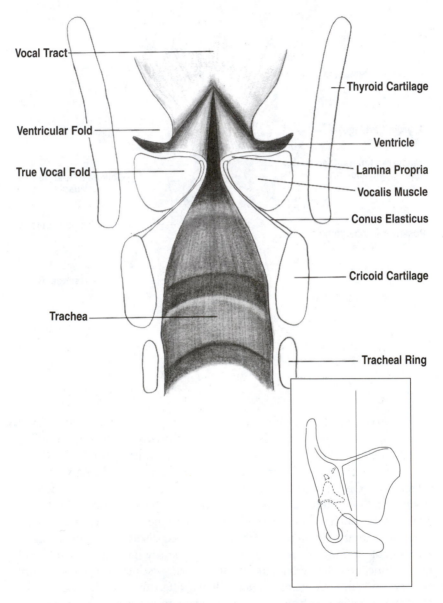

Figure 2–4. Coronal view of the ventricular and true vocal folds (Figure 2–4 insert: Coronal plane of Figure 2–4).

tract can result in improved vocal resonance by enhancing the phonatory sound source generated by the vocal folds (Acker, 1987; Lessac, 1967).

RESPIRATION FOR PHONATION

Vocal fold vibration is the sound source that produces phonation and provides the speech signal. Phonation is dependent on the respiratory power provided by the lungs and the abdominal and thoracic musculature. During inhalation, the diaphragm contracts (flattening downward in the body), compresses the viscera, and expands the lung volume as air is drawn into the lungs. During quiet exhalation, the vocal folds are at rest, and abducted in the paramedian position. For speech exhalation, however, the vocal folds adduct at midline, creating a quasiperiodic constriction of the airflow stream as it exits the lungs. This aerodynamic energy sets the vocal folds into oscillation, creating the vibratory sound source that is phonation (Titze, 1983, 1994). Without this airflow, no sustained phonatory sound source can be achieved. The covarying relationship between the amount and rate of airflow passing through the vibrating vocal fold valve influences the overall pitch, loudness, and quality of phonation (Gauffin & Sundberg, 1989).

VOCAL TRACT RESONANCE

As sound waves generated by the vocal folds travel through the supraglottic air column, into the pharynx, oral and nasal cavities, and across more rigid structures such as the velum, palate, tongue, and teeth, the excitation of air molecules creates a phenomenon called resonance. The model of acoustic energy (phonation) traveling through a filter (vocal tract) modified in variable shape, size, and constriction characteristics (articulatory gestures) is the basis for Fant's Acoustic Theory of Speech Production (Fant, 1983). This theory underlies our understanding of the three components of the acoustic speech product: glottal sound source, vocal tract filtering, and resonating characteristics (Fant, 1983; Kent & Read, 1993).

The shape and size of the vocal tract and its constrictions have a direct influence on the quality and strength of the acoustic product perceived by listeners. Resonance is the reinforcing or prolongation of sound by reflection of waveforms off another structure. The manipulation of the vocal tract shape and oral posturing for maximum vocal resonance has been the study of professional voice users, actors, and singers for a long time (Acker, 1987; Lessac, 1967). Its application to remediation of speech and voice pathologies has also been given attention (Verdolini-Marston, Burke, Lessac, Glaze, & Caldwell, 1993).

BLOOD SUPPLY AND SECRETIONS

The internal fluid balance of the larynx is controlled by the blood supply, while external secretions control the external "hydration" of the vocal folds. The blood supply arises from the superior laryngeal, cricothyroid, and inferior laryngeal arteries (Hirano, 1981; Tucker, 1987). There is virtually no blood supply to the superficial layers and epithelium of the vocal fold to avoid extra mass which would inhibit vibration (Hirano, 1981).

Serous and mucous glands are located in the tissues lateral, superior (ventricle), and inferior to the vocal folds, again avoiding the medial edge (Gracco & Kahane, 1989). Mucous propagation along the margin of the fold is assisted by the texture of the epithelial layer, which has microscopic irregularities that allow increased surface tension and greater affinity of the liquid to the membranous surface (Fukuda et al., 1988; Hirano, 1981, 1991).

INNERVATION AND CENTRAL NERVOUS SYSTEM CONTROL

The larynx is innervated by the **vagus,** which is cranial nerve X. The vagus gives rise to the recurrent and superior laryngeal nerves, which contain all the sensory and motor fibers that supply the larynx (Figure 2–5). Vagus means "wandering," and it is appropriately named because it describes its circuitous and far-reaching route through the body to innervate sites from the skull to the abdomen. The first portion of the vagus that innervates the larynx courses alongside the carotid artery before branching off to form the superior laryngeal nerve (SLN). The second portion branches off from the vagus in the thorax, and forms long loops through the heart, before coursing superiorly back to the larynx. Thus, it is named the recurrent laryngeal nerve (RLN). The right RLN courses under the subclavian artery; the left RLN courses under the aortic arch before it reaches the larynx. Consequently, these nerves (especially on the left) are extremely susceptible to injury, and a patient with an unexplained idiopathic vocal fold paralysis should be evaluated for possible cardiac compromise to rule out this possibility.

The SLN arises from the vagus near the nodose ganglia and forms internal and external branches. The internal branch inserts superior to the vocal folds and provides all the sensory information to the larynx. The external branch provides motor innervation to the cricothyroid muscle only. The RLN supplies all sensory information below vocal folds and all motor innervation to the posterior cricoarytenoid, thyroarytenoid, lateral cricoarytenoid, and interarytenoid muscles.

Two characteristics of the SLN and RLN ensure the ability of the intrinsic laryngeal muscles to move quickly and with a great amount of fine motor control. First, the laryngeal nerves have a high conduction velocity (second only to the eye), which allows rapid contractions.

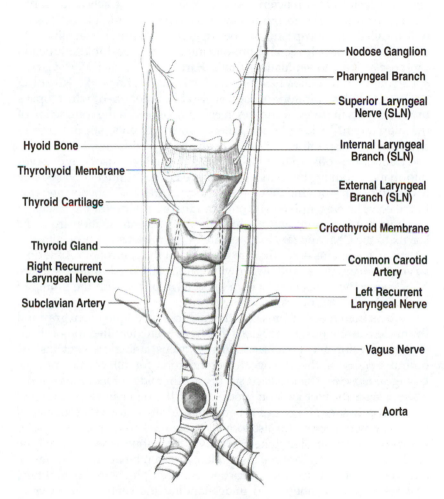

Figure 2–5.   Vagus innervation of the larynx.

Nodose Ganglion

Pharyngeal Branch

Superior Laryngeal Nerve (SLN)

Hyoid Bone

Internal Laryngeal Branch (SLN)

Thyrohyoid Membrane

Thyroid Cartilage

External Laryngeal Branch (SLN)

Cricothyroid Membrane

Thyroid Gland

Common Carotid Artery

Right Recurrent Laryngeal Nerve

Left Recurrent Laryngeal Nerve

Subclavian Artery

Vagus Nerve

Aorta

Second, the innervation ratio per motor unit is low, allowing for very fine control (Garrett & Larson, 1991).

A complex and detailed system of laryngeal reflexes exists for the principle function of airway preservation. Sensory receptors in the larynx respond to touch, vibration, changes in air pressure, and liquid stimuli, and they elicit tight sphincteric closure to close off the trachea and lungs from foreign material in the upper airway. An extreme glottic closure reflex, called laryngospasm, can be triggered by stimuli reaching sites closer to the glottic level, and prolongation of the vocal fold adduction can pose a threat to ventilation (Davis, Bartlett, & Luschei, 1993: Garrett & Larson, 1991; Kirchner, 1984; Suzuki, 1987; Udaka, Kanetake, Kihara, & Koike, 1988). A respiratory reflex has also been identified, which opens the vocal folds in rhythmic timing in coordination with the contraction of the diaphragm. In long-term tracheotomized patients, suppression of this rhythmic respiratory reflex has been observed (Suzuki, 1987).

Central nervous system mechanisms that relay sensory and motor information from the brain to the larynx are not well understood because of difficulties in studying the anatomical structures and function and due to the complex vegetative and communicative activities of the larynx in respiration, phonation, and deglutition. Afferent information from the larynx to the CNS appears to terminate in the nucleus tractus solitarius. This region contains areas that are involved in the control of respiration, laryngeal maneuvers, and swallowing. In anesthetized animal studies, NTS fiber activity has been shown to occur in phase with the timing of evoked swallowing or respiratory events.

Fibers from the NTS project to the midbrain periaqueductal gray and the nucleus ambiguus, two regions that have been identified for localized control of voluntary vocalization. The nucleus ambiguus contains the central origins of the laryngeal motoneurons for all of the intrinsic laryngeal muscles. The localized site of cricothyroid motoneurons is more distinct than the motoneuron groupings of the other intrinsic muscles, which appear to converge in a general area. Motoneurons for esophageal and respiratory control are also located in the nucleus ambiguus. Studies that examine laryngeal motoneuron activity have found that units may be task-specific, for vocalization, inspiration, or a combination of expiration and vocalization. Thus, the interaction between phonation, deglutition, and respiration is inherent to understanding the central pathways of laryngeal control, reflexive activity, and voluntary laryngeal maneuvers for nonspeech gestures and speech production (Garrett & Larson, 1991; Larson, Wilson, & Luschei, 1983).

STRUCTURAL SUPPORT FOR THE LARYNX

The larynx is suspended in the neck from a single bone, the **hyoid.** Six laryngeal cartilages, three unpaired **(epiglottis, thyroid, and cricoid)** and three paired (**arytenoid, corniculate,** and **cuneiform**) provide structural support for the larynx and vocal folds (Figures 2–6 and 2–7).

The **hyoid** bone marks the superior border of the laryngeal complex of muscles and cartilage. It articulates with the superior cornu of the thyroid cartilage and attaches to the thyroid through the thyrohyoid membrane. Although the hyoid serves as the muscular attachment for many extrinsic muscles of the larynx, it is notable as the sole bone in the body that does not articulate with any other bone.

The **epiglottis** cartilage is shaped like a long leaf, with its base attached to the inner portion of the anterior rim of the thyroid cartilage. This attachment allows the blade of the epiglottis cartilage to fold along its midline and move forward and back. It forms the first level of the three tiers of a sphincteric folding mechanism, closing down inferiorly

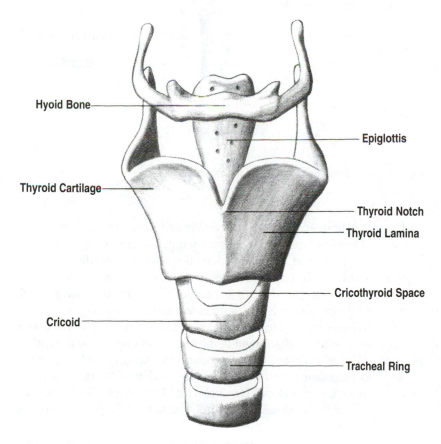

Figure 2–6.   Anterior view of the laryngeal cartilages.

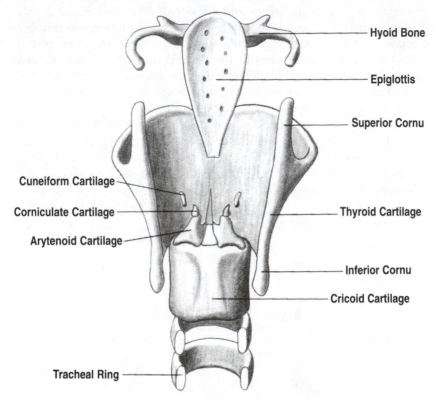

Figure 2–7.   Posterior view of the laryngeal cartilages.

and posteriorly over the laryngeal vestibule to protect the airway from particles of food or liquid during swallowing. The epiglottis is composed of elastic cartilage and, therefore, does not ossify, or harden, with age. This composition is important because this structure must remain flexible throughout life to allow a pliable free edge for closing off the airway and diverting foods and liquids toward the esophagus.

The **thyroid** cartilage forms an angled saddle-shaped curve. The thyroid cartilage is the anterior attachment of the true vocal folds at the internal rim of the anterior curve. Posteriorly are two superior cornu, or horns that extend upward to articulate with the hyoid bone, and two inferior cornu that articulate with the cricoid cartilage below it. The thyroid is composed of hyaline cartilage that does ossify and limit flexibility with age (Kahane, 1983, 1987). The lateral walls form quadrilateral plates, called **laminae,** that attach at the anterior midline in a **notch** or prominence. The angle of these lateral plates is more acute for males than females, resulting in the characteristic

"Adam's apple," or thyroid notch, which can be seen or palpated at the front of the neck. Clinically, the position and movement of the thyroid notch can signal maladaptive laryngeal behaviors, including excessive muscle tension or misuse in voice pathologies (Rammage & Morrison, 1988).

Below the thyroid cartilage is the **cricoid** ring, another hyaline cartilage. Its shape is described as a "signet ring," with a narrow anterior curve and broad posterior rim. The cricoid has two sets of paired facets, or flat surfaces, to allow articulation with adjacent cartilages via synovial joints. The cricothyroid joint connects the cricoid to the inferior cornu of the thyroid cartilage. The cricoarytenoid joints are positioned on the top of the posterior cricoid rim. Figures 2–8 and 2–9 display the articular facets of the cricoid cartilage, which provide the joint attachments for the thyroid cartilage on the lateral edge and the arytenoid cartilages on the superior rim. Inferior to the cricoid cartilage are the tracheal rings, the airway to the lungs.

The three paired cartilages are the **arytenoid, corniculate,** and **cuneiform** cartilages. All are hyaline cartilages. The arytenoid cartilages are pyramid-shaped, with three surfaces, facing anteriorly, laterally, and medially. The anterior angle projects forward at its base, forming the vocal

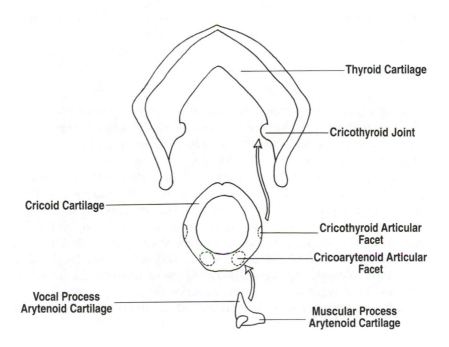

Figure 2–8.   Superior view of the laryngeal joint attachments.

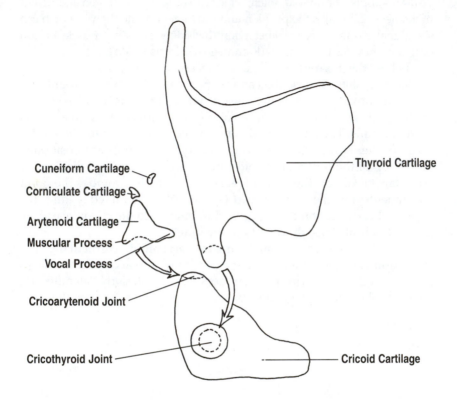

Figure 2–9.   Lateral view of the laryngeal joint attachments.

process, which is the posterior point of attachment of the true vocal folds. The lateral angle is the muscular process, which attaches to the intrinsic laryngeal muscles that abduct and adduct the vocal folds. The medial angle faces its arytenoid pair, forming an even surface for medial movements when the glottis is closed. The bases of the arytenoid cartilages are concave to allow smooth articulation with the humped superior surface of the posterior cricoid cartilage. This cricoarytenoid joint is a crucial mechanical feature of the larynx, allowing both rocking and sliding motions to abduct, adduct, and stabilize the vocal folds (Fink & Dearest, 1978; Hirano et al., 1987; Kahane, 1988; Von Leden & Moore, 1961).

The corniculate cartilages (also called the cartilages of Santorini) are attached by a synovial joint to the superior tips of the arytenoids. The cuneiform cartilages (also known as the cartilages of Wrisberg) are embedded in the muscular complex even superior to the corniculates. These tiny cartilages provide no clear function, but may add stability to the abduction motion for airway preservation.

MUSCLES

There are two logical groupings of the laryngeal muscles: extrinsic and intrinsic. The larynx moves vertically in the neck for lifting, swallowing, or phonating. The function of the extrinsic muscles is to influence laryngeal height or tension as a gross unit. Manipulations of the extrinsic muscles also alter the shape and filtering characteristic of the supraglottic vocal tract (Erickson, Baer, & Harris, 1983). Extrinsic laryngeal muscles attach to a site on the larynx and to an external point (e.g., sternum, mandible). The intrinsic muscles have both ends attached within the laryngeal cartilages and are responsible for discrete movements and position of the larynx and vocal folds.

Extrinsic Laryngeal Muscles

The many extrinsic muscles of the larynx can be divided into two regional groupings: suprahyoid and infrahyoid (above and below the hyoid bone), for easier recall (Figure 2–10; Table 2–1). The location of many of the muscles can be identified based on their names, which describe the anatomical attachment. The infrahyoid muscles pull the hyoid bone and larynx to a lower position in the neck. The suprahyoid muscles raise the larynx generally, by pulling the hyoid bone forward, backward, and upward. This action is particularly important during a swallow, when laryngeal elevation can help protect the airway from aspiration.

Intrinsic Laryngeal Muscles

When contracted, the muscles increase tension and shorten, providing a "pull" between the cartilage attachments. The combination of varying length and tension relationships between these muscle contractions creates two critical effects:

1. altering the shape and configuration of the glottis, the opening between the vocal folds
2. changing the position of the cartilage framework that houses the vocal folds (Hirano, Kiyokawa, & Kurita, 1988).

The five intrinsic muscles of the larynx are also identifiable by their names, which describe the cartilaginous attachments (Table 2–2). The **cricothyroid** tenses and thins the vibrating edge of the vocal folds by pulling the cricoid cartilage up and back, thereby decreasing the cricothyroid space and lengthening the vocal folds (Figure 2–11). Because of its control of the length and tension of the vocal folds, the cricothyroid muscle contributes greatly to vocal pitch control, especially for production of higher tones.

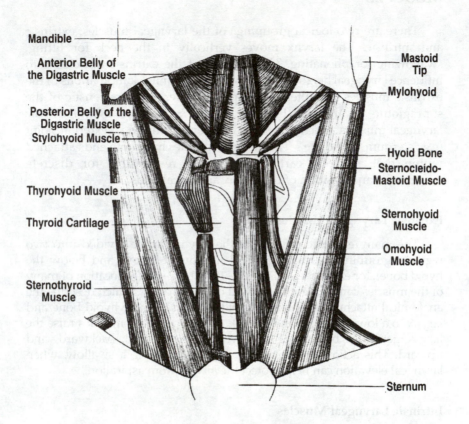

Mandible

Anterior Belly of
the Digastric Muscle

Posterior Belly of the
Digastric Muscle

Stylohyoid Muscle

Thyrohyoid Muscle

Thyroid Cartilage

Sternothyroid
Muscle

Mastoid
Tip

Mylohyoid

Hyoid Bone

Sternocleido-
Mastoid Muscle

Sternohyoid
Muscle

Omohyoid
Muscle

Sternum

Figure 2–10. Extrinsic laryngeal muscles.

The **thyroarytenoid** has been traditionally divided into two separate muscle bellies, a medial portion (thyrovocalis) and lateral portion (thyromuscularis). However, the histologic division between the two is unclear and controversial. When contracted, the thyroarytenoid shortens the vocal fold length by drawing the arytenoid cartilages anteriorly and thickens the vocal fold by increasing the mass of the vibrating medial edge. Thus, the thyroarytenoid contributes greatly to generation of lower pitch and louder productions.

The **lateral cricoarytenoid** is a broad, fan-shaped muscle that extends from the lateral rim of the cricoid to the anterior portion of the arytenoid muscular process. When contracted, it serves as an adductor, pulling the arytenoids laterally, rotating the vocal processes medially on the cricoarytenoid joint, and thus approximating the vocal folds (Figure 2–12).

Table 2–1. Extrinsic Laryngeal Muscles

MUSCLE	ATTACHMENTS	FUNCTION
I. *Infrahyoid Muscles*		
Thyrohyoid	Thyroid to hyoid	Brings thyroid cartilage and hyoid bone closer
Sternothyroid	Sternum to thyroid	Lowers thyroid cartilage
Sternohyoid	Sternum to hyoid	Lowers hyoid bone
Omohyoid	Scapula to hyoid	Lowers hyoid bone
II. *Suprahyoid Muscles*		
Stylohyoid	Temporal bone (styloid process) to hyoid	Raises hyoid bone posteriorly
Mylohyoid	Mandible to hyoid	Raises hyoid bone anteriorly
Digastric	Two bellies, anterior and posterior:	
anterior	Mandible to hyoid	Raises hyoid bone anteriorly
posterior	Temporal bone (mastoid process) to hyoid	Raises hyoid bone posteriorly
Geniohyoid	Mandible to hyoid	Raises hyoid bone anteriorly

The **interarytenoid** muscles are also adductors and especially responsible for forceful closure of the posterior glottis (Figure 2–12). The **transverse** (horizontal) portion brings the medial faces of the arytenoids together, while the **oblique** (crossed) portion closes the arytenoid apices.

The **posterior cricoarytenoid** is the sole abductor of the vocal folds, and it contracts to open the vocal folds for respiration and during quick opening gestures of the glottis during unvoiced sound productions (Figure 2–13). Abductory movement occurs in two stages: lateral rocking of the vocal processes, which separates the membranous portion of the vocal folds, and sliding of the posterior arytenoid facets on the cricoarytenoid joint. To summarize the functional importance of specific muscle contractions along a number of parameters, Table 2–3 indicates the predicted result for each aspect.

There are three "all except" rules that apply to the intrinsic muscles of the larynx to help remember similarities and differences among their functions.

- First, all muscles are paired, having a matched left and right muscle, except the transverse interarytenoid, which functions as a single unit, bringing the arytenoid cartilages closer together.

Table 2–2. Intrinsic Laryngeal Muscles

MUSCLE	ATTACHMENTS AND FUNCTION
Cricothyroid (CT)	Cricoid to thyroid
Pars recta	Cricoid to inferior border of the thyroid lamina; rocks the cricoid anteriorly and superiorly, closer to the thyroid
Pars oblique	Cricoid to inferior cornu of the thyroid; pulls the cricoid posteriorly
Thyroarytenoid/Vocalis (TA)	Thyroid to arytenoid
Lateral cricoarytenoid (LCA)	Lateral cricoid to arytenoid
Interarytenoid (IA)	Joins the left and right muscular processes of the arytenoids; two bellies:
Transverse:	Unpaired muscle sheath, attaching to the lateral laminae of the left and right arytenoids, and running horizontally.
Oblique:	Paired muscles, coursing from the base of one arytenoid upward and across to the apex of the other, forming an X-configuration.
Posterior cricoarytenoid (PCA)	Posterior aspect of the cricoid to arytenoid

- Second, all of the intrinsic muscles serve as adductors (bringing the vocal folds closer) except the posterior cricoarytenoid, the sole abductor, or vocal fold opener.
- Third, all of the muscles are innervated by the recurrent laryngeal nerve except the cricothyroid muscle, which is innervated by the external branch of the superior laryngeal nerve.

VOCAL FOLD MICROSTRUCTURE

The membranous portion of the vocal folds is an intricate layered structure that incorporates five histologically discrete layers that vary in composition and mechanical properties (Figure 2–14). It is this membranous structure which oscillates, or vibrates, to create sound in the larynx. The integrity of the vibrating pattern for phonation relies on a very pliable, elastic structure. Both flexibility and stability are provided by the vocal fold microstructure (Hirano, 1977, 1981).

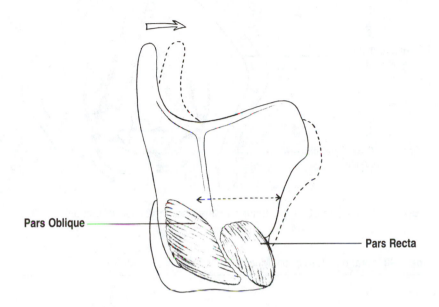

Figure 2–11. Action of the cricothyroid muscle.

Pars Oblique

Pars Recta

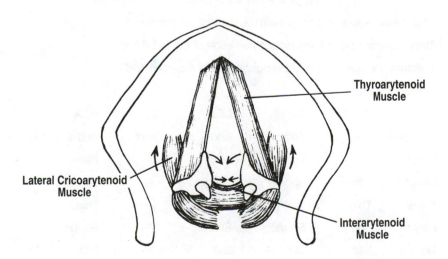

Figure 2–12. Action of the lateral cricoarytenoid and interarytenoid muscles (adduction).

Thyroarytenoid Muscle

Lateral Cricoarytenoid Muscle

Interarytenoid Muscle

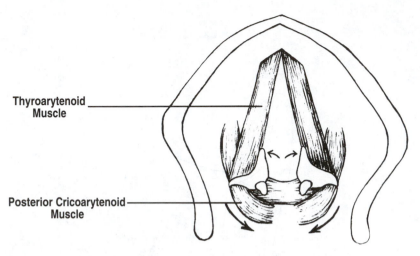

Thyroarytenoid Muscle

Posterior Cricoarytenoid Muscle

Figure 2–13. Action of the posterior cricoarytenoid muscle (abduction).

Table 2–3. Intrinsic Laryngeal Muscle Functions

I. *Parameters*

Function: ad- or abduction of the vocal folds

Glottic level: raise or lower the larynx

Length: shorten or lengthen the true vocal folds

Thickness: thickening or thinning the body of the vocal fold

Edge: sharpening or rounding the free edge of the vocal fold

Tension: increasing or decreasing stiffness of the vocal fold

II. *Muscle Actions*

	CT	TA	LCA	IA	PCA
Function	—	Add	Add	Add	Abd
Level	—	Lower	Lower	—	Raise
Length	Longer	Shorter	Longer	—	Longer
Thick	Thin	Thick	Thin	—	Thin
Edge	Sharp	Round	Sharp	—	Round
Tension	Stiff	Stiff	Stiff	—	Stiff

CT=cricoarytenoid, TA=thyroarytenoid, LCA=lateral cricoarytenoid, IA=interarytenoid, PCA=posterior cricoarytenoid

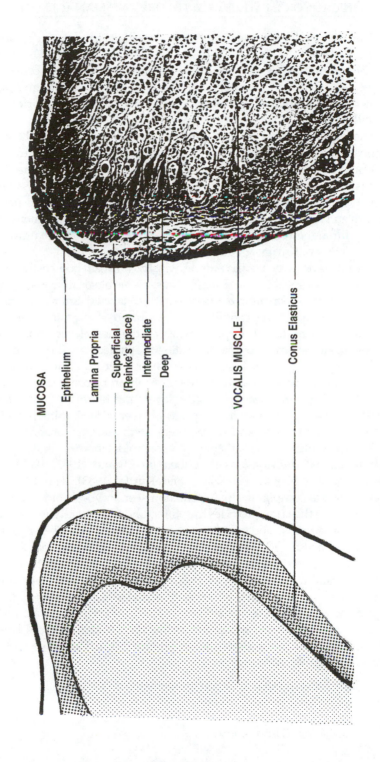

Figure 2–14. Layered microstructure of the vocal fold.

MUCOSA

Epithelium

Lamina Propria

Superficial
(Reinke's space)

Intermediate

Deep

VOCALIS MUSCLE

Conus Elasticus

The five histologic layers, from most superficial to most deep, are as follows:

The **epithelium** is a thin mucosal covering of squamous cells that wraps over the internal contents of the vocal folds. It offers no mass, and is totally compliant, but needs a thin layer of mucous lubrication to oscillate best.

The **lamina propria** consists of three layers. The **superficial layer** is composed of a loose fibrous matrix, known commonly as Reinke's space, and its composition is described as soft gelatin. The **intermediate layer** is composed of elastic fibers and offers slightly more mass. The **deep layer** is denser still, composed of collagenous fibers. The tissues of the third and fourth layers together are known as the vocal ligament and develop throughout childhood until the larynx reaches full maturity at puberty (Hirano, Kurita, & Nakashima, 1983).

The fifth layer is the **vocalis muscle**, which is the main body of the vocal fold and provides stability and mass. Thus, as histological layers change from superficial to deep, from epithelium to three-layered lamina propria to muscle tissue, each level contributes a graduated change in mass and compliance for vibration. The epithelial layer is the most elastic component; subsequent layers form a complex transition to stiff deep muscle tissue.

Although the five histological layers are distinct in their composition, the functional differences for vibratory properties are not as clear. As a general description, the layers are regrouped into three divisions: **cover** (epithelium and superficial layer of the lamina propria), **transition** (intermediate and deep layers of the lamina propria), and **body** (vocalis muscle). The theory of vocal fold vibration is based on these functional divisions, as described by Hirano (1977, 1981) and Hirano, Matsuo, Kakita, Kawasaki, and Kurita (1983). The vibrating cover forms the compliant, fluid oscillation seen in vocal fold vibratory patterns, while the body provides the stiffer, underlying stability of vocal fold mass and tonus. The transition serves as the coupling between the superficial mucosa and the deep muscle tissue of the vocal fold during vibration. Thus, the Body-Cover Theory of Vibration accounts for the mass and stability provided by the vocalis muscle and deep layer of the lamina propria over which the compliant and elastic layers of the lamina propria and epithelium oscillate (Hirano, 1977, 1981; Hirano et al., 1983).

This "undulation" or oscillation of the vocal fold superficial layers creates a ripple of tissue deformation (Figure 2–15). The wave motion occurs in three vibratory phases:

1. horizontal (medial to lateral movements)
2. longitudinal (anterior to posterior "zipper-like" wave), and
3. vertical phase (inferior to superior opening and closing of the vocal folds) (Hirano, 1991).

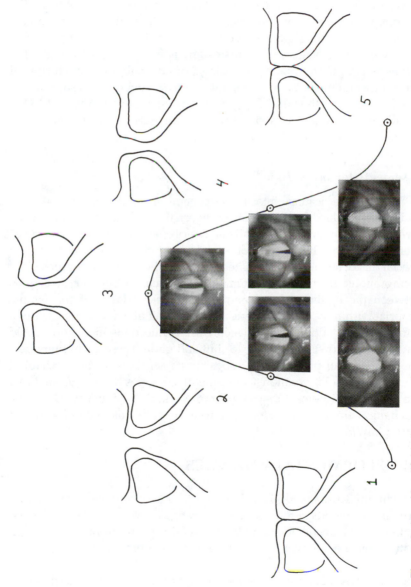

Figure 2–15. Vocal fold vibratory cycle.

Clinically, only horizontal and longitudinal changes can be seen readily from an endoscopic (superior) view. However, experimental observations of a unilateral vocal fold in vibration against a plate of glass have revealed the importance of vertical phase change contributions to the oscillation of vocal folds (Titze, Jiang, & Hsaio, 1992).

Two special connective tissue structures support the vocal folds at points of greatest mechanical stress. The anterior and posterior **macula flava** are small bundles of elastic fibers that provide stability to the endpoints of the membranous vocal folds at their anterior attachments to the thyroid cartilage and posterior attachments to the vocal process of the arytenoid cartilage. The **conus elasticus** is a strong membrane that serves as a supportive shelf, extending from the subglottic tracheal wall superiorly and medially, inserting into the vocal ligament to support the inferior border of the vocal fold. The vocal ligament lies adjacent to the vocalis muscle and lends stability and stiffness to the membranous portion (Hirano, 1981).

Basement Membrane Zone

Recent investigations into the histochemical composition of the vocal folds have identified a transition area between the epithelium and superficial layer of the lamina propria. This region, known as the **basement membrane zone (BMZ)**, was observed using electron microscopy and special histochemical staining techniques. The zone is composed of membranous fibers and proteins that attach to cellular structures between the epithelial layer and the superficial layer of the lamina propria. Within the BMZ is a series of anchoring fibers, which provides a framework for supporting collagen fiber connections in the vocal fold mucosa and allowing the tissue to shift and glide. These anchoring fibers are composed of proteins and appear to be sensitive to the mechanical stress of vocal fold vibration. Consequently, theories have suggested that the BMZ contributes to possible representation of injury sites due mechanical trauma and shearing effects of vocal fold vibration (Gray, 1991; Gray, Hirano, & Sato, 1993).

DEVELOPMENTAL CHANGES

Hirano, Kurita, and Nakashima (1983) have examined the size and structure of the vocal folds across age ranges (Table 2–4) and observed that, while the overall length of the vocal folds grows from birth through maturation, the covarying ratio between the membranous to cartilaginous portions of vocal folds also changes. In newborn infants, the ratio is approximately 1:2. Because the newborn membranous vocal fold has no

Table 2–4.   Length of Vocal Folds

	NEWBORNS	ADULT FEMALES	ADULT MALES
Total	2.5–3 mm	11–15 mm	17–21 mm
Membranous	1.3–2 mm	8.5–12 mm	14.5–18 mm
Cartilage	1–2 mm	2–3 mm	2–3 mm

Source: Adapted from Hirano, M., Kurita, S., & Nakashima, T. (1983). Growth, development, and aging of human vocal folds. In D. M. Bless & J. Abbs (Eds.), *Vocal fold physiology* (pp. 22–43). San Diego: College-Hill Press.

vocal ligament and, therefore, little stability, the greater ratio of cartilage to membrane length provides better mechanical protection of the airway. The vocal ligament emerges between the ages of 1 to 4 years, and is fully developed by maturity. Thus, the cartilaginous to membranous portion changes, reaching a maturation ratio of 1:4 in adult females and 1:6 in adult males.

Geriatric Vocal Folds

Voice pathologists have become increasingly aware of deterioration in voice quality, pitch and loudness range, and endurance with advancing age. In some cases, the vocal folds have appeared thinned (bowed) in geriatric speakers without other explanation of pathology except advanced chronological age (Biever & Bless, 1989; Linville, 1992). Geriatric changes in the larynx may account for this phenomenon, clinically termed "presbylaryngeus," or aging larynx. Hirano, Kurita, and Nakashima (1983) reported morphologic disorganization and breakdown of the collagenous and elastic fibers and fibroblasts in aging vocal folds. Intermediate layers of the vocal folds were observed as looser and thinner, contributing to loss of bulk of the vibratory edge, and having a bowed appearance during glottic closure patterns. They also observed increased thickening of the superficial layer of the lamina propria, which would account for changes in pitch and quality of phonation.

PHYSIOLOGY OF PHONATION

Theory of Vibration

Vocal fold vibration is achieved based on the physical process of flow-induced oscillation (Titze, 1994), where a consistent stream of air flows past the tissues, creating a repeated pattern of opening and closing.

The classical description of the **aerodynamic-myoelastic theory** (Van den Berg, 1958) allows that both airflow (aerodynamic) and muscular (myoelastic) properties account for the passive convergent and divergent motions of the vocal folds during phonation. The theory recognizes the reciprocal role of the aerodynamic properties, subglottal pressure and transglottal flow, as they interact with the myoelastic resistance and elasticity provided by the vocal fold tissues.

The theory holds that at the onset of phonation, subglottal pressure rises as expiratory forces are met by resistance from the adducted vocal folds. When pressure rises to overcome this resistance, the folds are blown apart and subglottal pressure diminishes, creating a momentary drop in air pressure at the glottic level (also known as the Bernoulli effect), thus "sucking" the vocal folds back toward midline and completing a full cycle of vibration. With the vocal folds re-approximated, subglottal pressure builds again to repeat the process. The oscillation is achieved then by both aerodynamic contributions of the covarying pressure and flow and the mechanical properties of tissue deformation and collision posed by the elastic vocal fold tissues (Hirano, 1977; Scherer, 1990).

Titze (1994) has expanded on this theory to describe the vocal folds as a flow-induced oscillating system, sustained across time by aerodynamic force provided by the pulmonary airstream. In this model, respiration is the driving force that sets the vocal folds in motion (oscillation), and the interchange between pressure and flow at three critical sites keeps the vocal folds vibrating as described below.

1. **Subglottal region:** at the area directly beneath the vocal folds, where the "leading edge" is set into motion by the pulmonary airflow
2. **Intraglottal space:** directly between the paired vocal folds, as the convergent and divergent shaping of vocal fold back-and-forth motion is influenced by the exchange of airflow and pressure peaks
3. **Supraglottal air column:** immediately above the vocal folds, where the air molecules in the vocal tract are alternately compressed or rarified in a delayed response to the alternate pressure and flow fluctuations modulated by the vibrating vocal folds. The excitation of the supraglottic air column facilitates a "top down" loading effect that helps sustain vocal fold oscillation, and augments the traditional explanation offered by the aerodynamic-myoelastic theory.

Scherer (1990) and Titze (1994) described a sequence of vocal fold oscillation that explains the interchange between aerodynamic events and mechanical tissue response.

1. **Translaryngeal flow** is positive as the folds are blown open, moving medially and laterally. Flow is negative as folds recoil

(elastic) to midline. During positive flow, the greatest effect is on glottal opening.

2. **Intraglottal pressures** keep vocal folds oscillating and have the greatest effect during glottal closing. Recall that pressure and flow are reciprocal for this system. Thus, as the vocal folds open, intraglottal pressure is positive, but dropping as flow increases. As the vocal folds close, intraglottal pressure is negative, but rising as flow is cut off by the closing glottis.

3. An **oscillation threshold pressure** is defined as the minimal pressure needed to blow vocal folds apart, and it varies with biomechanical properties of the vocal fold tissue, including tissue damping, mucosal wave, flexibility, and mass. Subglottal pressure is needed to set vocal folds in motion and keep them in motion via intraglottic pressure changes.

4. In the **supraglottic vocal tract**, molecules in the air column are pushed and released in response to puffs of pressure and flow released from the oscillating vocal folds. This asymmetrical "top-down" driving force transfers energy from the fluid (air pressure) to the tissue (vocal folds) and assists in sustaining the oscillation.

Control of Fundamental Frequency

Several factors influence the rate of vocal fold vibration, or fundamental frequency. The primary determinants of pitch control are vocal fold length and tension, including passive tension on the vocal fold cover and active stiffness of the vocal fold body. To achieve higher pitch, the vocal folds lengthen and the medial edge thins due to contraction of the cricothyroid muscle. To lower pitch, contraction of the thyroarytenoid shortens vocal fold length, decreasing tension on the cover and rounding the medial edge for greater amplitude of vibration. Two other factors appear to covary with fundamental frequency in predictable ways. Subglottal pressure increases proportionally with increased fundamental frequency. Amplitude motion of the vocal folds is inversely proportional to the rate of vocal fold vibration, increasing with lower pitch (Scherer, 1990).

Control of Intensity

The intensity of the glottal sound source produced increases proportionally with increased subglottal pressure and is achieved mechanically due to a longer vibratory phase closure pattern. Intensity also tends to covary proportionally with fundamental frequency, although this is not a consistent relationship. Finally, the vocal tract tuning or filtering characteristic can influence the loudness of the glottal source, as increased supraglottic resonance can increase the acoustic radiation of sound energy (Scherer, 1990).

Laryngeal Quality

Audio-perceptual judgments of voice quality are highly subjective, but generally, phonatory quality is affected by the integrity of the glottal valving waveform, as defined by regularity, symmetry, and phase shape of tissue deformation across vibratory cycles, and the slope of the glottal flow waveform (Scherer, 1990). Deviations in the cycle-to-cycle slope and shape of the waveform characteristics will impair the resulting acoustic signal. The filtering characteristic of the supraglottic vocal tract will also enhance or detract from the perceived voice quality of the signal. In sum, the quality of voice relies on multiple factors, including compliant and symmetric biomechanic properties of the vocal folds, an adequate and consistent subglottic pressure and flow source, and appropriate vocal tract tuning characteristics.

SUMMARY

The complexity of the larynx is demonstrated well by the many functions that this remarkable organ serves, for both vegetative and communicative purposes. Research continues into the further definition of its anatomic and morphologic structure, central and peripheral control mechanisms, and physiologic function. The underpinnings of laryngeal anatomy and physiology are critical for understanding the relationship between voice pathologies, their consequential effects on voice production, and the recognition of reasonable rehabilitative planning. Additional chapters in this text will describe measurement tools that seek to define our understanding of vocal function and its relationship to voice production.

REFERENCES

Acker, B. F. (1987). Vocal tract adjustments for the projected voice. *Journal of Voice*, 1(1), 77–82.

Biever, D. M., & Bless, D. M. (1989). Vibratory characteristics of the vocal folds in young adult and geriatric women. *Journal of Voice*, 3(2), 120–131.

Davis, P. J., Bartlett, Jr., D., & Luschei, E. S. (1993). Coordination of the respiratory and laryngeal systems in breathing and vocalization (Chapter 5). In I. R. Titze (Ed.), *Vocal fold physiology* (pp. 189–226). San Diego: Singular Publishing Group, Inc.

Erickson, D., Baer, T., & Harris, K. S. (1983). The role of strap muscles in pitch lowering. In D. M. Bless & J. Abbs (Eds.), *Vocal fold physiology* (pp. 279–285). San Diego: College-Hill Press.

Fant, G. (1983). The voice source: Theory and acoustic modeling. In I. R. Titze & R. C. Scherer (Eds.), *Vocal fold physiology* (pp. 453–464). Denver, CO: Denver Center for the Performing Arts.

Fink, B. R., & Demarest, R. J.(1978). *Laryngeal biomechanics*. Cambridge, MA: Harvard University Press.

Fukuda, H., Kawaida, M., Tatehara, T., Ling, E., Kita, K., Ohki, K., Kawasaki, Y., & Saito, S. (1988). A new concept of lubricating mechanisms of the larynx. In O. Fujimura (Ed.), *Vocal fold physiology* (Vol. 2, pp. 83–92). New York: Raven Press.

Garrett, J. D., & Larson, C. R. (1991). Neurology of the laryngeal system. In C. N. Ford & D. M. Bless (Eds.), *Phonosurgery* (pp. 43–76). New York: Raven Press.

Gauffin, J., & Sundberg, J. (1989). Spectral correlates of glottal voice source waveform characteristics. *Journal of Speech and Hearing Research, 32*(3), 556–565.

Gracco, C., & Kahane, J. C. (1989). Age-related changes in the vestibular folds of the human larynx: A histomorphometric study. *Journal of Voice, 3*(3), 204–212.

Gray, S. (1991). Basement membrane zone injury in vocal nodules. In J. Gauffin & B. Hammarberg (Eds.), *Vocal fold physiology* (pp. 21–28). San Diego: Singular Publishing Group, Inc.

Gray, S. D., Hirano, M., & Sato, K. (1993). Molecular and cellular structure of vocal fold tissue (Chapter 1). In I. R. Titze (Ed.), *Vocal fold physiology* (pp. 1–35). San Diego: Singular Publishing Group, Inc.

Hirano, M. (1977). Structure and behavior of the vibratory vocal folds. In T. Sawashima & D. Cooper (Eds.), *Dynamic aspects of speech production* (pp. 13–27), Tokyo: University of Tokyo Press.

Hirano, M. (1981). Structure of the vocal fold in normal and disease states: Anatomical and physical studies. In C. Ludlow & M. Hart (Eds.), *ASHA Reports No.11, Proceedings of the Conference on the Assessment of Vocal Pathology* (pp. 11–30). Rockville, MD: ASHA.

Hirano, M., Kurita, S., & Nakashima, T. (1983) Growth, development, and aging of human vocal folds. In D. M. Bless & J. Abbs (Eds.), *Vocal fold physiology* (pp. 22–43). San Diego, College-Hill Press.

Hirano, M., Matsuo, K., Kakita, Y., Kawasaki, H., & Kurita, S. (1983). Vibratory behavior versus the structure of the vocal fold. In I. R. Titze & R. C. Scherer (Eds.), *Vocal fold physiology* (pp. 26–40). Denver, CO: Denver Center for the Performing Arts.

Hirano, M., Yoshida, T., Kurita, S., Kiyokawa, K., Sato, K., & Tateishi, O. (1987). Anatomy and behavior of the vocal process. In T. Baer, C. Sasaki, & K. Harris (Eds.), *Laryngeal function in phonation and respiration* (pp. 3–13). Boston: Little, Brown and Co.

Hirano, M., Kiyokawa, K., & Kurita, S. (1988). Laryngeal muscles and glottic shaping. In O. Fujimura (Ed.), *Vocal fold physiology* (Vol. 2, pp. 49–66). New York: Raven Press.

Hirano, M. (1991). Phonosurgical anatomy of the larynx. In C. N. Ford & D. M. Bless (Eds.), *Phonosurgery* (pp.25–42). New York: Raven Press.

Hirano, M., Yoshida, T., & Tanaka, S. (1991) Vibratory behavior of human vocal folds viewed from below. In J. Gauffin & B. Hammarberg (Eds.), *Vocal fold physiology* (pp. 1–6), San Diego: Singular Publishing Group, Inc.

Kahane, J. C. (1983). A survey of age-related changes in the connective tissues of the human adult larynx. In D. M. Bless & J. Abbs (Eds.), *Vocal fold physiology* (pp. 44–49). San Diego, College-Hill Press.

Kahane, J. C. (1987). Connective tissue changes in the larynx and their effects on voice. *Journal of Voice, 1*(1), 27–30.

Kahane, J. C. (1988). Age-related changes in the human cricoarytenoid joint. In O. Fujimura (Ed.), *Vocal fold physiology* (Vol. 2, pp. 145–158). New York: Raven Press.

Kent, R. D., & Read, C. (1992). *The acoustic analysis of speech.* San Diego: Singular Publishing Group, Inc.

Kirchner, J. A. (1984). *Physiology of the larynx.* Washington, DC: The American Academy of Otolaryngology-Head and Neck Surgery Foundation, Inc.

Larson, C. R., Wilson, K. E. & Luschei, E. S. (1983). Preliminary observations on cortical and brainstem mechanisms of laryngeal control. In D. M. Bless & J. Abbs (Eds.), *Vocal fold physiology* (pp.82–95). San Diego: College-Hill Press.

Lessac, A. (1967). *The use and training of the human voice.* New York: Drama Book Publishers.

Linville, S. E. (1992). Glottal gap configurations in two age groups of women. *Journal of Speech and Hearing Research, 35*(6), 1209–1215.

Rammage, L. A., & Morrison, M. (1988, November). *Muscle tension dysphonia.* Miniseminar presented at Annual Convention of the American Speech-Hearing Association, Boston.

Scherer, R. C. (1991). Physiology of phonation: A review of basic mechanics. In C. N. Ford & D. M. Bless (Eds.), *Phonosurgery* (pp. 77–94). New York: Raven Press.

Suzuki, M. (1987). Laryngeal reflexes. In M. Hirano, J. A. Kirchner, & D. M. Bless (Eds.), *Neurolaryngology: Recent advances* (pp. 142–155). Boston: Little, Brown, and Company.

Titze, I. R. (1983). Mechanisms of sustained oscillations of the vocal folds. In I. R. Titze & R. C. Scherer (Eds.), *Vocal fold physiology* (pp. 349–357). Denver, CO: Denver Center for the Performing Arts.

Titze, I. R., Jiang, J., & Hsaio, S. (1992). Measurements of mucosal wave propagation and vertical phase difference in vocal fold vibration. In I. R. Titze (Ed.), *Progress report 2* (pp. 83–92). Iowa City, IA: National Center for Voice and Speech.

Titze, I. R. (1994). *Principles of voice production.* Englewood Cliffs, NJ: Prentice Hall.

Tucker, H. M. (1987). *The larynx.* New York: Thieme Medical Publishers, Inc.

Udaka, J., Kanetake, H., Kihara, H., & Koike, Y. (1988). Human laryngeal responses induced by sensory nerve stimuli. In O. Fujimura (Ed.), *Vocal fold physiology* (Vol. 2, pp. 67–74). New York: Raven Press.

Van den Berg, J. (1958). Myoelastic-aerodynamic theory of voice production. *Journal of Speech and Hearing Research, 1,* 227–244.

Verdolini-Marston, K., Burke, K., Lessac, A., Glaze, L. & Caldwell, E. (1993). A preliminary study on two methods of treatment for laryngeal nodules. In I.

R. Titze (Ed.), *Progress report 4* (pp. 209–228). Iowa City, IA: National Center for Voice and Speech.

Von Leden, H., & Moore, P. (1961). The mechanics of the cricoarytenoid joint. *Archives of Otolaryngology, 73,* 541–555.

3

SOME ETIOLOGIC CORRELATES

Since West, Kennedy, and Carr (1937) commented that there is always a reason for a voice disorder, speech pathologists have sought to identify those reasons with each new patient. Sometimes the causes are easily identified, as when vocal nodules are present in the shouting child. At other times, finding the contributing causes of the disorder requires the skill of an experienced diagnostician. To enhance the successful outcome of the search, it is advantageous for those seeking the answers to be familiar with as many points of reference as possible. This chapter seeks to provide these reference points through discussion of some of the more common etiologic factors associated with the development of voice disorders. These factors include the major categories of (a) vocal misuse, (b) medically related etiologies, (c) primary disorder etiologies, and (d) personality-related etiologies.

VOCAL MISUSE

Vocal misuse (Table 3–1) refers to functional voicing behaviors that contribute to the development of laryngeal pathologies. These include behaviors of vocal abuse and the use of inappropriate vocal components.

Vocal Abuse

Vocal abuse occurs whenever the vocal folds are forced to adduct in a too vigorous manner causing a hyperfunctioning of the laryngeal mechanism. This hyperfunctioning, when repeated or habitual, may

Table 3–1.   Etiologies of Vocal Misuse

VOCALLY ABUSIVE BEHAVIORS	INAPPROPRIATE VOCAL COMPONENTS
1. Shouting	1. Respiration
2. Loud talking	2. Phonation
3. Screaming	3. Resonation
4. Vocal noises	4. Pitch
5. Coughing	5. Loudness
6. Throat clearing	6. Rate

contribute to laryngeal tissue change as well as strain of the laryngeal musculature (Koufman & Isaacson, 1991; Stemple, Stanley, & Lee, in press). Brodnitz (1971) suggested that sheer force is one of the main elements in the development of many voice disorders. This force may take the form of sudden and violent adduction of the vocal folds or a more persistent use of a vocally abusive behavior. These behaviors may take the forms of excessive **shouting** and **loud talking,** such as children shouting on a playground or a factory worker talking loudly over machine noise. Vocal abuse is also present during **screaming** and in the production of **vocal noises.** Vocal noises refer to those non-speech laryngeal sounds that children make while playing. The standard sounds may include the roar of car, truck, motorcycle, and spaceship engines; the piercing scream of sirens; and various growls, barks, and howls of animals.

One of the most prevalent forms of vocal abuse is incessant, habitual, nonproductive **throat clearing** (Greene, 1972; Wilson, 1979). In one study of 206 patients who were referred for voice therapy due to hyperfunctional voice disorders, 141, or 68%, presented with this abusive behavior (Stemple & Lehmann, 1981). Vigorous, aperiodic adduction of the vocal folds, during even mild throat clearing, was observed through the classic high speed motion films of vocal fold vibration produced by Timcke, Von Leden, and Moore (1959).

Throat clearing may be either a primary or a secondary etiologic factor. As a primary factor it may take a form similar to Mrs. M.'s:

> Mrs. M.'s voice evaluation revealed that she had never experienced vocal difficulties prior to contracting a cold 6 weeks earlier. Accompanying the cold had been excessive coughing and throat clearing. The cold symptoms and the cough subsided after 10 to 12 days, but Mrs. M. unknowingly continued to clear her throat. This caused a mild persistent dysphonia. Indirect laryngoscopy performed during the sixth week revealed mild bilateral vocal fold edema. The subsequent voice evaluation identified continued throat clearing as the only etiologic factor associated with the maintenance of the hoarseness. Habitual throat clearing was extinguished using a "hard swallow" modification approach (see Chapter 7), and the vocal

folds returned to their normal structure and function producing normal voice.

Throat clearing is often identified as a secondary abusive factor for patients who present with various laryngeal pathologies. This behavior is frequently developed as a response to the various laryngeal sensations perceived by the patient. These laryngeal sensations may be caused by the presence of the pathology. Common sensations reported by patients include dryness, tickling, burning, aching, lump in the throat, or a thickness sensation. Patients often become hypersensitive to the laryngeal area as the result of the pathology. When this is the case, even normal sensations, such as those associated with drainage, become magnified with the common response being that of habitual throat clearing. In such cases, throat clearing serves both as a symptom of the pathology and as a contributor to the maintenance of the disorder.

Coughing is also a vocally abusive behavior. Coughing may be the symptom of many different types of respiratory diseases such as asthma, chronic obstructive pulmonary disease, or malignant lung lesions (Irwin & Curley, 1988; Wilson, 1979). When associated with a disease process, coughing is treated by a physician. Chronic cough, like throat clearing, may be developed as a response to laryngeal pathology and not associated with respiratory disease processes. When this is the case, the speech pathologist is often called upon to extinguish this behavior as a part of the vocal management protocol (Blager, Gay, & Wood, 1988; Stemple, 1993).

Inappropriate Vocal Components

Voice production is dependent upon the interrelationship of many different physiologic components. These voicing components include respiration, phonation, and resonation as well as the psychophysical components of pitch, loudness, and rate. It would be expected that any one or all of these components would be modified by the presence of laryngeal pathology. Contrarily, the functional misuse of any component or combination of components may directly cause a laryngeal pathology.

Respiration

In Chapter 2 we learned that vibration of the vocal folds is activated by the respiratory airstream overcoming the resistance of the approximated vocal folds, thus blowing the folds apart. The static compliance of the folds along with the Bernoulli effect draw the vocal folds back together completing one vibratory cycle. Shipp and McGlone (1971) demonstrated that the subglottic air pressure that was necessary to initiate phonation for normal conversational voice was between 3 and 7 cm of H_2O. Hirano (1981) demonstrated that the normal airflow rate for voice production ranges from 50–200 ml/H_2O. When approximation of the vocal folds is compromised by mass lesion, poor muscular control or weakness, or neural problems, airflow rates may increase while subglottic air pressure is decreased. Hyperadduction of the vocal folds will produce the opposite effects.

Normal control of inspiration and expiration is necessary to support normal phonation. Aronson (1980) suggested, and we would concur, that the vast majority of voice patients use anatomically and physiologically normal respiration for the support of voice. However, certain functional respiratory habits and behaviors may lead directly to the development of a voice disorder. For example, the occasional patient may be seen who habitually uses a shallow, thoracic breathing pattern which is not supportive of normal phonation. The resultant voice quality may be characterized by low intensity and breathiness. Another functional breathing behavior that may contribute to the development of a voice disorder is the habit of speaking on residual air. This behavior occurs when a person continues to speak when the normal tidal expiration has been completed. Speaking on residual air increases laryngeal muscle tension and contributes to vocal hyperfunction.

Phonation

The abusive hyperadduction of the vocal folds has previously been discussed. Inappropriate phonation as a functional etiology may also be present in patients who utilize hard glottal attacks and persistent glottal fry phonation.

Hard glottal attack or glottal coup describes one of three means by which phonation for vowel sounds may be initiated. The hard attack is accomplished by complete and rapid adduction of the vocal folds, buildup of subglottic air pressure, and then explosion of the folds while producing the vowel sound (Jackson & Jackson, 1959). Habitual use of a hard glottal attack usually causes an increase in laryngeal area muscle tension. The increased muscle tension requires a greater build-up of subglottic air pressure, all of which contributes to vocal hyperfunction.

The opposite of the hard glottal attack is the breathy attack. When this mode of attack is used to initiate phonation, the vocal folds are abducted as exhalation for phonation begins, and then only adduct after exhalation has been initiated, creating a moment of breathiness which is heard at the initiation of the vowel. Because of the poor glottic closure, the breathy attack is also a voice misuse which may contribute to a voice disorder.

The third mode of vocal attack is the even or static attack. This is the most efficient means of initiating voice onset. With the static attack the vocal folds are nearly approximated as exhalation begins, permitting the onset of phonation to be smooth and effortless.

Glottal fry or pulse register is one of three vocal registers described by Hollien (1974), with the other two being modal and loft register. Glottal fry is the lowest range of phonation along the frequency continuum and the least flexible. Production of glottal fry is characterized by tightly approximated vocal folds whose free edges appear flaccid (Zemlin, 1988). The closed phase of the vibration cycle is very long when compared to the total vibration cycle. The tighter closure requires a greater increase in subglottic air pressure contributing to laryngeal hyperfunction. Persistent use of glottal fry, which has been described as sounding like a poorly tuned motorboat engine, will often cause vocal fatigue, laryngeal tension, and a "lump in the throat" feeling.

Opposite the pulse register is the loft register, which includes the higher range of the vocal frequencies including the falsetto. The range of frequencies normally used in speaking and singing comprises the modal register.

Resonation

Once sound is generated at the level of the vocal folds, it then passes through a series of filters which dampen and enhance the sound and make each voice unique and distinctive to the owner of the voice. There is a wide range of acceptable voice resonance patterns, with the level of acceptability often determined by geographic location. Certain resonance problems may have an organic basis such as those caused by velopharyngeal incompetence or a submucous cleft, whereas others are caused by functional disturbances. Functional resonance disturbances may be caused by the improper coupling of the pharyngeal, oral, and nasal cavities or the improper placement of the tongue and larynx.

Hypernasality or rhinolalia aperta occurs when vowels and voiced consonants are excessively resonated in the nasal cavity. This behavior occurs when the velopharyngeal port remains open during production of the phonemes other than the nasal consonants /m/, /n/, and /ng/. The increase in nasal resonance may or may not be accompanied by excessive nasal air emission, which is heard as a friction noise that accompanies the phonemes produced.

Denasality or rhinolalia clausa occurs when normal nasal resonance is not present on the phonemes /m/, /n/, and /ng/. The physical basis is an overclosure of the velopharyngeal port or an obstruction of the nasal cavity. The acoustic result sounds as if the speaker has a head cold.

Assimilative nasality occurs when the phonemes adjacent to the three nasal consonants are nasalized along with these sounds. The cause is presumed to be the premature opening of the port prior to the nasal consonant and a lingering opening of the port following the nasal consonant. This form of nasal resonance is often heard for a brief period following removal of large tonsils and adenoids.

Cul-de-sac nasality is a closed nasality in which all the vowels, semivowels, and nasals are produced with a hollow-sounding or dead-end resonance. This form of nasality is thought to be caused by obstruction in the anterior nasal cavity.

Retracted tongue and **elevated larynx** are anatomical postures which often accompany each other and contribute to altered resonance and laryngeal tension. When the larynx is elevated the vocal tract will be shortened, thus raising all the formant frequencies. The increased extrinsic and intrinsic and lingual muscle tension also tends to raise the fundamental frequency. The combination of these effects yields a higher pitched voice with a pinched resonance quality. Patients who exhibit these behaviors often complain of laryngeal aching and fatigue due to the increased muscular activity.

Resonance disturbances affect not only voice quality, but also the production of many phonemes. Because of this, it is debatable whether disturbance of the resonance component is a voice, articulation, or voice and articulation problem.

Pitch

Changes in pitch are a very common symptom of voice disorders, especially those associated with mass lesion or other vocal fold cover changes. Because of this, seldom is it appropriate from a therapeutic point of view to be concerned with direct pitch modification. Indeed, as the tissue lining of the vocal folds improves, so too would the inappropriate pitch. To try to ascertain an "optimum" pitch from the pathologic voice would also be ludicrous. The various methods suggested to accomplish this task would be flawed due to the presence of the pathology. Therefore, direct pitch modification is reserved for selected cases where the use of an inappropriate pitch has been isolated as the *primary* etiologic factor associated with the development of the voice disorder.

Pitch is the perceptual correlate of the fundamental frequency of voice. Misuse refers to pitch levels that are either too high, too low, or those which are lacking in variability. Habitual use of an inappropriate pitch may create laryngeal tension and strain. Patients we have treated who have required direct pitch modification have included young men with psuedoauthoritative voices; speakers who frequently talk and lecture either in noisy locations or to large groups in less than adequate acoustical conditions; patients with other illnesses and emotional conditions; patients undergoing vocal fold surgery who have not automatically made the appropriate pitch adjustments; and in a male with functional falsetto and a female with juvenile voice.

Loudness

Loudness is the perceptual term that relates to vocal intensity. The inappropriate use of loudness is demonstrated in voices that are habitually too soft, too loud, or lack loudness variability. The vocally abusive behaviors of shouting and loud talking have been previously discussed. It is important to note that habitual use of an inadequate loudness level may also be a vocal misuse. Vocal intensity is determined by the lateral excursion of the vocal folds and the speed with which they return to approximate as dictated by the subglottic air pressure and the resultant air flow. When a person speaks very softly, the balance between the airflow and the muscular activity is disturbed. The decreased airflow causes more demands to be placed on the intrinsic muscle system, thus leading to possible vocal muscle strain and fatigue. Thus, talking softly may be abusive if not well supported by the airstream.

Rate

As an etiologic factor, rate may contribute to laryngeal pathologies when speech is produced too rapidly. Faulty use of the laryngeal mechanism related to vocal hyperfunction is evident when speech is produced in too rapid a manner (Wilson, 1979). The patient who talks too fast typically does not use proper breath support , often talking on residual air. Increased rate may lead to vocal hyperfunction.

Rarely will a voice pathologist be presented with a voice disorder in which a *single* vocal component is isolated as the primary etiology. If inappropriate components are found to be the cause, a combination of components will usually be identified, with misuse of one being the *predominant* factor contributing to the voice disorder.

Inappropriate components may also be the *result* of laryngeal pathologies that were caused by other etiologic factors. When this is the case, the components are recognized as the *symptoms* of the disorder (such as low pitch, glottal fry, breathiness, and so on).

Vocal misuse represents the most common etiologic factor identified in patients with voice disorders. Cooper (1973) found that of 1,406 patients, 36.6% had disorders associated with vocal misuse. Brodnitz (1971) reported a figure of 25.8%. Voice therapy is particularly effective in the remediation of voice disorders caused by vocal misuse.

MEDICALLY RELATED ETIOLOGIES

This category of etiologic correlates refers to medical/surgical interventions that directly cause voice disorders and medical/health conditions and treatments that may indirectly contribute to the development of voice disorders (see Table 3–2). Your base of knowledge regarding these etiologic factors will aid you during the diagnostic process especially when discussing the patient's medical history.

Table 3–2.   Medically Related Etiologies

SURGICAL TRAUMA	CHRONIC ILLNESSES AND DISORDERS

1. Direct surgery
   a. Laryngectomy (total, hemi, supraglottic)
   b. Glossectomy
   c. Mandibulectomy
   d. Palatal
   e. Other head and neck
2. Indirect surgery
   a. Thyroid
   b. Heart
   c. Carotid
   d. Lung
   e. Hysterectomy
3. Intubation
	1. Sinusitis
	2. Respiratory illnesses
	3. Allergies
	4. Medications
	5. Stomach disorder
	6. Nervous disorder
	7. Endocrine disorder
	8. Cardiac disease
	9. Arthritis
	10. Alcohol/drug abuse
	11. Smoking

Direct Surgery

Direct surgical procedures are those that cause an insult to the anatomical structures directly responsible for phonation and resonation. These surgeries would include *total laryngectomy, hemi-laryngectomy, supraglottic laryngectomy, glossectomy, mandibulectomy, palatal surgery,* and other head and neck excisions such as radical neck dissection and pharyngeal surgeries. Vocal rehabilitation is essential following these surgeries and is described in Chapter 10.

Indirect Surgery

Surgery for other disorders may indirectly contribute to the development of voice disorders. Because of the anatomical relationships of the *thyroid, heart, lungs,* and *carotid arteries* to the recurrent laryngeal nerves, the superior laryngeal nerves, and the branches of the vagus nerve, surgical procedures involving these structures may involve some trauma to the nervous supply of the larynx. Possible consequences may be a vocal fold paresis or paralysis and a loss of sensory innervation to the mucosal lining of the larynx (Ballenger, 1985).

Women who have undergone a complete *hysterectomy*, including the uterus and both ovaries, may also experience vocal difficulties. A temporary or permanent lowering of the vocal pitch may be caused by hormonal changes. Some patients, in an attempt to maintain the "normal" higher pitch, place increased muscle strain on the laryngeal mechanism, thus setting the stage for the development of a voice disorder.

Finally, any surgery that requires general anesthesia and the place-ment of an endotracheal tube has the potential for causing mechanical trauma to the vocal folds (Balestrieri & Watson, 1982; Peppard & Dickens, 1983; Whited, 1979). Friedmann (1980) suggested two differ-ent types of laryngeal injuries caused by intubation. These injuries were trauma to the mucosa over the vocal processes of the arytenoid cartilages in the posterior larynx or trauma caused by constant pres-sure of the tube on the vocal process resulting in tissue necrosis. The result in either case is injury to the mucosa which covers the cartilage with concomitant injury to the perichondrium. In an attempt to repair the damaged area, granulomatous tissue develops (Doyle & Martin, 1991). Treatment for this disorder will often involve a combination of medical, surgical, and voice therapy treatments.

Chronic Illnesses and Disorders

Many chronic illnesses and disorders and their treatments may contribute to the development of laryngeal pathologies. Because of the importance of these etiologic factors, Chapter 8 of this text deals with issues related to changes in vocal function associated with each of these disorders and illnesses in much greater detail. As you see in Table 3–2, voice disorders may develop secondary to other systemic, cardiac, respiratory, immunologic, gastrointestinal, endocrine, inflam-matory, and pharmacological influences.

For example, chronic *sinusitis* and other *upper respiratory infections*, though often limited to the supraglottic structures, may contribute to the development of hoarseness. Since the sinus drainage does not touch the vocal folds, this cause, which is often opined by the patient, cannot be blamed for the hoarseness. However, coughing and throat clearing which often accompany these illnesses are often implicated in voice abuse and may be the direct cause of the voice problem. Medications used to treat these illnesses and their symptoms may also be implicated as a cause. *Antihistamines* are commonly used to dry the secretions but will also cause a reduction in the secretions of the sali-vary and mucous glands, thus contributing to dehydration of the vocal folds. *Anti-cough* medications such as codeine and dextromethorphan are also drying agents (Martin, 1988).

Other, more chronic respiratory illnesses such as *asthma, chronic obstructive pulmonary disease,* and *lung cancer* may directly or indirectly contribute to voice disorders. The increased responsiveness and hyperactivity of the trachea and bronchi of the asthmatic may lead to transitory or prolonged episodes of wheezing, coughing , and dysp-nea. Hoarseness may therefore result from vocal fold tissue lining abuse, poor respiratory support, and the medications used to treat the condition. *Bronchodilators*, such as albuterol (Proventil and Ventolin) may have the side effects of tremor and nervousness. *Corticosteroid* inhalants may contribute to vocal fold bowing and an elevation of fundamental frequency (Watkin & Ewanowski, 1979; Williams, Baghat, DeStableforth, Shenoi, & Skinner, 1983).

Chronic obstructive pulmonary disease (COPD) is a clinical term used to describe a group of diseases characterized by persistent slowing of airflow during exhalation. The most common of these diseases are emphysema and chronic bronchitis both of which may cause the vocally abusive wheezing, coughing, dyspnea, and sputum expectoration. Again, medications used to treat these diseases may have a negative effect on the mucous membrane and the fluid secretion to the vocal folds.

Lung cancer may have a more direct effect on the functioning of the vocal folds. Indeed, one of the symptoms of lung cancer is left vocal fold paralysis caused by damage to the vagus nerve. Radiation treatments, chemotherapy, and direct lung surgery may also violate the nervous supply to the vocal fold.

About one in every five persons in the United States has an *allergy* caused by something inhaled, ingested, touched, or injected. Severity may range from very mild to very severe to fatal. When an airborne allergen (substance that elicits the allergic response) enters the body, it reacts with an antibody that is fixed to the surface of mast cells found in the nose, lungs, and skin. The allergen-antibody binding triggers the release of histamines, which are responsible for the allergic symptoms. The histamine causes contraction of smooth muscles, dilation of blood vessels, and stimulation of mucous glands to produce increased quantities of mucus (Spiegel, Hawkshaw, & Sataloff, 1991).

Allergies may cause congestion and edema of the vocal folds, thus negatively affecting voice production. Treatments for allergies may include medicines such as antihistamines and topical steroids, with the side effects as previously described. Decongestants may also be utilized to decrease the edema of the mucous membrane. Long-term use of a vasoconstrictor, however, may show a diminished drug effect with the return of edema and congestion being greater than was previously present (Colton & Casper, 1990). Persistent allergies may be best treated through injections of the allergen designed to desensitize the patient to that allergen.

Gastrointestinal disorders may also negatively affect voice production. One of the most common disorders in this category is gastroesophageal reflux disease (GERD) (Olson, 1991). Reflux of the acidic stomach contents to the posterior larynx has been implicated in the symptoms of chronic hoarseness, voice fatigue, cough, chronic throat clearing, globus sensation (lump in the throat), and a sensation of choking. The burning of the posterior larynx may cause edema, ulceration, and granulation of the laryngeal mucosa and, when left untreated, may cause hyperkeratosis and even carcinoma of the larynx. We have been very impressed in our own practice with the numbers of patients who have been identified with GERD symptoms. A complete treatment regimen is described in Chapters 8 and 9.

The presence of lower intestinal disorders such as spastic colon, irritable bowel syndrome, and diarrhea may also be implicated in the development of voice disorders. Antispasmodic medications used for these disorders such as atropine, scopolamine, and diphenoxylate hydrochloride reduce glandular secretions and are therefore drying agents (Martin, 1988).

Patients who suffer with *emotional disorders* such as emotional tension, depression, and anxiety may also experience voice disorders from a number of reasons. These reasons may include simple laryngeal area tension, poor respiratory support, whole body fatigue from poor sleep habits to name a few. Psychotropic medications often prescribed for nervous tension, depression, psychotic disorders, and sleep disorders may have a negative effect on voice production because of drying and sedation. Some of these common drugs include Elavil, Lithane, and Lithobid (antidepressants); Thorazine and Haldol (antipsychotics); and antihistamines that are often used for sleep disorders.

Endocrine dysfunction, such as hypothyroidism, hyperthyroidism, hyperpituitarism, amyloidosis, virilization, and minor hormonal changes associated with menstruation has also been implicated as a cause of voice disorders (see Chapter 8). Hoarseness, vocal fatigue, pitch changes, loss of range, breathiness, reduced loudness, and pitch breaks have all been observed in individuals with endocrine disorders (Aronson, 1990; Damste, 1967; Gould, 1972; Sataloff, 1991).

Cardiac and *circulatory problems* may also contribute to the development of voice disorders. We previously discussed the potential negative surgical affects on the recurrent laryngeal nerve. Medications used to control high blood pressure such as methyldopa, reserpine, and captopril are drying agents and their diuretic effect could potentially result in dryness and irritation of the mucous membrane of the vocal folds (Martin, 1988).

Arthritis, an inflammatory disease of the body's synovial joints, has also been implicated in the development of voice disorders. The symptoms of cricoarytenoid joint arthritis are hoarseness, a laryngeal fullness feeling, and pain associated with the inflammation of the joint. In more severe cases the joint may be fixed (cricoarytenoid ankylosis) and imitate the appearance of a vocal fold paralysis. The severity of the symptoms is dependent upon the severity of the arthritis.

Finally, the negative effects of *smoking, alcohol abuse,* and *illicit drug use* on the vocal mechanism cannot be denied. At best, the heat and chemicals from tobacco smoke cause erythema, edema, and generalized inflammation of the vocal tract. The worse case scenario is the contribution tobacco smoke makes to the development of laryngeal carcinoma. In between are polypoid mucosal changes and the precancerous conditions of leukoplakia and hyperkeratosis (Chapter 4) (Wynder & Stellman, 1977). Sataloff (1991b) reported that marijuana smoke is particularly irritating, causing considerable vocal fold mucosal response. He further stated that cocaine can be extremely irritating to the nasal mucosa, causing increased vasoconstriction, altering mucosal sensation, resulting in decreased voice control, and a tendency toward vocal abuse.

Alcohol is a vasodilator and thus may cause drying of the mucous membrane of the vocal folds. In addition, alcohol is a central nervous system depressant, which, when abused, results in symptoms of incoordination, dysarthria, and impaired judgment.

One final note regarding drugs. Caffeine is a drug. It is a central nervous system stimulant which has the potential to cause hyperactivity and tremor. In addition it decreases laryngeal secretions causing laryngeal dehydration. Finally, because of the relaxation effect caffeine has on the upper esophageal sphincter, this drug promotes gastroesophageal reflux.

Smoking and drug and alcohol abuse may directly cause laryngeal pathologies. These chronic external and internal irritants are extremely abusive to the vocal mechanism and have been implicated as causes of many pathologies from chronic laryngitis to laryngeal neoplasms. In addition to the direct abuse of inhaled chemicals, many smokers also have a "smoker's cough," which adds additional vocal abuse to compound the problem.

When dealing with medically related etiologies it is important that the primary medical condition has been identified and is being treated by the appropriate physician specialist. The voice pathologist often proves helpful in identifying for the physician behaviors that may or may not be associated with the medical condition, thus adding to the diagnostic process. Improvement of the medical condition does not automatically improve the concomitant voice disorder. Voice evaluation and therapy proves to be a valuable asset to many patients exhibiting other surgical or medical conditions.

PRIMARY DISORDER ETIOLOGIES

This major etiologic category includes embryological, physiologic, neurologic, and anatomical disorders (see Table 3–3) that have vocal changes as secondary symptoms of the primary disorder. Included in this category are *cleft palate* and *organic velopharyngeal insufficiency*, with their characteristic hypernasal vocal components. The vocal compo-

TABLE 3–3. Primary Disorder Etiologies

Cleft palate
Organic velopharyngeal insufficiency
Deafness
Cerebral palsy
Neurological disorders
Trauma

nents of people who are *deaf* are frequently characterized by an inappropriate high pitch and a pharyngeal resonatory focus. Boone (1966) found that 17- and 18-year-old males who were deaf had a mean fundamental frequency 54 Hz higher than the same measure for normal hearing males of the same age. Individuals with a severe-profound sensorineural hearing loss often speak with the tongue retracted toward the pharyngeal wall, creating a disturbance in normal voice resonance.

The voices of individuals with *cerebral palsy* will vary widely because the neurologic damage is not related to one form of neurologic lesion (Greene & Mathieson, 1989). Individuals presenting with cerebral palsy often speak with a labored, monotonous, and strained phonation with a limited frequency range. Control of intensity, due to positioning and respiratory support limitations, may also be problematic.

Many voice symptoms are present in a wide range of neurologic disorders. In his exceptional review of dysphonias associated with neurological disease, Aronson (1980) reported that, technically, neurologic voice disorders are dysarthrias and are most often imbedded "in a complex of respiratory, resonatory, and articulatory dysarthric signs" (p. 77). The neurological disorders with associated voice symptoms (which are discussed in detail in Chapter 8) may be organized by lesion site, including lesions of:

1. the upper motor neurons,
2. the extrapyramidal system,
3. the cerebellum,
4. the lower motor neurons, and
5. the peripheral nervous system and myoneural junction.

(The reader is also referred to Aronson, Brown, Litin, and Pearson [1968] and Darley, Aronson, and Brown [1975] for excellent references regarding neurological speech and voice disorders.)

Accidental *trauma* is the final cause of a voice disorder listed in the primary disorder category of etiologies. Blunt or penetrating injuries to the larynx often cause edema, fractured laryngeal cartilages, joint dislocations, and lacerations. These injuries may be caused by automobile accidents and sports-related injuries, stabbing and gunshot wounds, strangulation, and, on rare occasions, intubation injuries. Inhalation of flames, gasses, and fumes and swallowing of caustic substances may also cause serious traumatic injury to the larynx. The primary concern related to severe trauma of the larynx is the establishment and maintenance of an adequate airway. Voice therapy will follow recovery from the acute stage of the injury.

As primary disorders, these conditions require appropriate medical, surgical, educational, and rehabilitative interventions. The voice pathologist will most often serve as a part of a team attempting to modify the voice, swallowing, articulation, and language components of these various disorders.

PERSONALITY-RELATED ETIOLOGIES

The final major etiologic category is that of personality-related causes of voice disorders (see Table 3–4). Voice is a very sensitive indicator of emotions, attitudes, and role assumptions (Morrison & Rammage, 1994). Indeed, the way a person feels physically and emotionally is often directly reflected in the quality of voice. The resultant vocal symptoms may simply be the result of a whole body tension causing a more specific hypertonicity of the intrinsic and extrinsic laryngeal muscles causing a tension dysphonia. Or, the symptoms may be a sign of a much more serious underlying psychological disorientation (Kinzl, Bierl, & Rauchegger, 1988). In either case, the tensions and stresses of everyday life may contribute directly to the abnormal functioning of the sensitive vocal instrument.

Environmental Stress

Environmental stress represents the many occurrences in human life that can cause emotional and physical stresses that may provoke vocal disorders in some individuals. For example:

> Mrs. S., an attractive 60-year-old woman, was referred by the laryngologist with the diagnosis of mild bilateral vocal fold edema. She complained of a chronic "hoarseness" and "tiredness" in her voice after only minimal use. Her general voice quality was described as mildly dysphonic, characterized by habitual use of low pitch, breath-

TABLE 3–4.   Personality-related etiologies

Environmental stress
Conversion behaviors
Identity conflict

iness, and intermittent glottal fry phonation. During the voice evaluation, no *vocally abusive behaviors, medically-related causes,* or *primary disorders* were identified. Without further interview, we may have surmised that the cause of this disorder was the use of the inappropriate vocal components of pitch and respiration.

The social history, however, revealed that Mrs. S's husband had died just two months prior to the evaluation. She was in the process of trying to close his affairs and sell the house they had shared for 36 years. As you would now expect, this patient was experiencing what may be called an *emotional dysphonia* due to the depression and stress she was experiencing. The laryngeal muscular tension caused by her generalized hypertonicity led to the use of inappropriate vocal components which physically contributed to the development of vocal fold edema. However, the major cause of this disorder was the environmental stress.

Conversion Behaviors

At times, environmental stress may become so severe that avoidance behaviors may be developed to counteract stressful situations. These avoidance behaviors become an unconscious substitution of a somatic symptom, involving the sensory or motor nervous systems, for the unpleasant or intolerable emotional event or conflict (Morrison & Rammage, 1994). In the psychiatric literature, these behaviors are referred to as psychological conversion disorders (Aronson, Peterson, & Litin, 1966). As a cause of voice disorders, the conversion behavior may manifest as whispering, muteness, or unusual dysphonias. For example:

> Mrs. P. was a 36-year-old homemaker and mother of two sons ages 14 and 16 years. She was referred by the laryngologist with the diagnosis of normal appearing vocal folds. Her voice quality, which she had experienced for 6 weeks, was aphonic with intermittent periods of phonation in the form of a high-pitched squeak.
>
> The social history, gathered during the evaluation, revealed that Mrs. P.'s 16-year-old son had recently been arrested for theft. Until this unfortunate occurrence, he had been a model youth making good grades in school and had participated in sports, drama, and other positive social activities. About the time of his arrest, Mrs. P.'s vocal difficulties began. This was obviously her psychological reaction to this intolerable, stressful situation. Voice therapy was successful in returning the patient's voice to normal within the first session (see Chapter 7).

Identity Conflict

The final personality-related etiology is that of identity conflict. Aronson (1980) stated that psychosexual conflicts are neither signs of environmental stress nor conversion reactions to stressful life problems. Identity problems are embedded in the fabric of the personality. Persons who experience difficulties in establishing their own personalities may present with voice problems as a result. These may include the maintenance of the high-pitched falsetto in the post-adolescent male, or the weak, thin juvenile sounding voice of an adult female, or the desire of the male-to-female transsexual to raise the pitch of her voice. We would strongly caution the reader that while some individuals with these vocal disorders may present with psychological conflicts, the majority do not. Indeed, the voice problem may simply be a learned response or the conscious desire to project a particular image. (The pathologies associated with the etiology of identity conflict are discussed in Chapter 4.)

Voice disorders that are the result of personality-related etiologies are particularly amenable to voice therapy. At times, psychological referral and family counseling may be necessary and appropriate. The voice pathologist must realize the limitations of direct voice therapy and make referrals as necessary. It has been our experience that, in the majority of cases, patients with personality-related voice disorders are well managed by the voice pathologist.

SUMMARY

This chapter has presented some of the etiologic correlates of voice disorders in a categorical manner. It should be well understood, however, that most voice disorders have more than one contributing etiologic factor. One of the enjoyments of working with patients with voice disorders is the challenge of discovering the pertinent parts of the etiologic puzzle. The perceptual symptoms of many voice pathologies are similar, but the causes for those symptoms are many. Success is in finding the causes and then modifying or eliminating those that maintain the condition, thus resolving the pathology and improving the voice. Chapter 4 discusses the various laryngeal pathologies that develop as a result of these etiologic factors, and Chapters 5 and 6 present ways of discovering these etiologic correlates.

REFERENCES

Aronson, A. (1980). *Clinical voice disorders: An interdisciplinary approach.* New York: Brian C. Decker.

Aronson, A., Brown, J., Litin, E., & Pearson, J. (1968). Spastic dysphonia 1. Voice, neurologic, and psychiatric aspects. *Journal of Speech and Hearing Disorders, 33,* 203–218.

Aronson, A., Peterson, H., & Litin, E. (1966). Psychiatric symptomatology in functional dysphonia and aphonia. *Journal of Speech and HearingDisorders*, *31*, 115–127.

Balestrieri, F., & Watson, C. (1982). Intubation granuloma. *Otolaryngologic Clinics of North America, 15,* 567–579.

Ballenger, J. (1985). *Diseases of the nose, throat, ear, head and neck* (13th ed.). Philadelphia: Lea and Febiger.

Blager, F., Gay, M., & Wood, R. (1988). Voice therapy techniques adapted to treatment of habit cough: A pilot study. *Journal of Communication Disorders, 21,* 393–400.

Boone, D. (1966). Modification of the voices of deaf children. *Volta Review, 68*: 686–692.

Brodnitz, F. (1971). *Vocal rehabilitation* (4th ed.). Rochester, NY: American Academy of Ophthalmology and Otolaryngology.

Colton, R. and Casper, L. (1990). *Understanding voice problems: A physiological perspective for diagnosis and treatment.* Baltimore: Williams and Wilkins.

Cooper, M. (1973). *Modern techniques of vocal rehabilitation.* Springfield, IL: Charles C. Thomas.

Damste, P. (1967). Voice changes in adult women caused by virilizing agents. *Journal of Speech and HearingDisorders, 32,*126–132.

Darley, F., Aronson, A., & Brown, J. (1975). *Motor speech disorders.* Philadelphia: W.B. Saunders.

Doyle, P., & Martin, G. (1991). Paradoxical glottal closure mechanism associated with postintubation granuloma. *Journal of Voice, 5,* 247–251.

Friedmann, I. (1980). Granulomas of the larynx. In M. Paparella & D. Shumrick (Eds.), *Otolaryngology, vol. III, head and neck* (2nd ed.). Philadelphia: W.B. Saunders, 2449–2469.

Gould, W. (1972). Vocal cords can speak of hormonal dysfunction. *Consultant, 12,* 101–102.

Greene, M. (1972). *The voice and its disorders* (3rd ed.). Philadelphia: J.P. Lippincott.

Greene, M., & Mathieson, L. (1989). *The voice and its disorders* (5th ed.). London: Whurr Publishers.

Hirano, M. (1981). *The clinical examination of voice.* Vienna: Springer-Verlag.

Hollien, H. (1974). On vocal registers. *Journal of Phonetics, 2,* 125–143.

Irwin, R., & Curley, F. (1988). The diagnosis of chronic cough. *Hospital Practice, 23,* 82–96.

Jackson, C., & Jackson, C. (1959). *Diseases of the nose, throat and ear.* Philadelphia: W.B. Saunders.

Kinzl, J., Bierl, W., & Rauchegger, H. (1988). Functional aphonia. A conversion symptom as a defensive mechanism against anxiety. *Psychotherapy and Psychosomatics, 49,* 31–36.

Koufman, J., & Isaccson, G. (1991). The spectrum of vocal dysfunction. In J. Koufman & G. Isaccson (Eds.), *The otolaryngologic clinics of North America: Voice disorders.* Philadelphia: W.B. Saunders.

Martin, F. (1988). Tutorial: Drugs and vocal function. *Journal of Voice, 2,* 338–344.

Morrison, M., & Rammage, L. (1994). *The management of voice disorders*. San Diego: Singular Publishing Group, Inc.

Olson, N. (1991). Laryngopharyngeal manifestations of gastroesophageal reflux disease. In J. Koufman & G. Isaccson (Eds.), *The otolaryngologic clinics of North America: Voice disorders*. W.B. Saunders.

Peppard, S., & Dickens, J. (1983). Laryngeal injury following short-term intubation. *Annals of Otology Rhinology and Laryngology, 92*, 327–330.

Sataloff, R. (1991a). Endocrine dysfunction. In R. Sataloff (Ed.), *Professional voice: The science and art of clinical care* (pp. 201–205). New York: Raven Press.

Sataloff, R. (1991b). Patient history. In R. Sataloff (Ed.), *Professional voice: The science and art of clinical care* (pp. 69–83). New York: Raven Press.

Shipp, T., & McGlone, R. (1971). Laryngeal dynamics associated with voice frequency change. *Journal of Speech and Hearing Research, 14*, 761–768.

Spiegel, J., Hawkshaw, M., & Sataloff, R. (1991). Allergy. In R. Sataloff (Ed.), *Professional voice: The science and art of clinical care* (pp. 153–157). New York: Raven Press.

Stemple, J., & Lehmann, D. (1980, November). *Throat clearing: The unconscious habit of vocal hyperfunction*. Paper presented at the American Speech-Language-Hearing Association National Convention, Detroit.

Stemple, J. (1993). *Voice therapy: clinical studies*. St. Louis: Mosby Year Book.

Stemple, J., Stanley, J., & Lee, L. (in press). Objective measures of voice production following prolonged voice use. *Journal of Voice*.

Timcke, R., Von Leden, H., & Moore, P. (1959). Laryngeal vibrations: Measurements of the glottic wave. Part 2. Physiologic variations. *Archives of Otolaryngology, 69*, 438–444.

Watkin, K., & Ewanowski, S. (1979). Effects of triamcinolone acetonide on the voice. *Journal of Speech and Hearing Research, 22*, 446–455.

West, R., Kennedy, L., & Carr, A. (1937). *The rehabilitation of speech*. New York: Harper and Brothers.

Whited, R. (1979). Laryngeal dysfunction following prolonged intubation. *Annals of Otology Rhinology and Laryngology, 88*, 474–478.

Williams, A., Baghat, M., DeStableforth, C., Shenoi, P., & Skinner, C. (1983). Dysphonia caused by inhaled steroids. Recognition of a characteristic laryngeal abnormality. *Thorax, 38*, 813–21.

Wilson, D. (1979). *Voice problems of children*. Baltimore: Williams and Wilkins.

Wynder, E., & Stellmann, S. (1977). Comparative epidemiology of tobacco-related cancers. *Cancer Research, 37*, 4608–4622.

Zemlin, W. (1988). *Speech and hearing science: anatomy and physiology* (3rd ed.). Englewood Cliffs, NJ: Prentice-Hall.

4

PATHOLOGIES OF THE LARYNGEAL MECHANISM

Our definition in Chapter 1 suggested that a voice disorder existed when an individual's quality, pitch, and loudness differed from those of persons of similar age, sex, cultural background, and geographic location. These differences in quality, pitch, and loudness may be the result of structural, physical, or neurologic alterations of the larynx and vocal folds, as well as the respiratory and resonatory systems or may result from use of the mechanism in a functionally inappropriate manner.

INCIDENCE

The incidence of voice disorders has proved difficult to establish with figures ranging from 6% (Senturia & Wilson, 1968) to 23.4% (Silverman & Zimmer, 1975) in the school- age population, with the generally accepted number being closer to the 6% figure (Moore, 1982). In a study describing laryngeal disorders in children evaluated by otolaryngologists, Dobres et al. (1990) found the top five pathologies presented by children in these medical practices to be subglottic stenosis, vocal nodules, laryngomalacia, dysphonia with normal folds, and vocal fold paralysis. It should be noted that much of these data were collected from physicians located within a major children's medical center where more extreme medical conditions would be expected.

Even fewer studies have examined the incidence of voice disorders in adults. LaGuaite (1972) studied 428 patients, aged 18 to 82 years, and found that 7.2% of the males and 5% of the females had various types of laryngeal pathologies. Herrington-Hall et al. (1988) studied the prevalence of pathologies in a group of 1,262 patients who sought evaluation from several otolaryngologists. The pathology types were then investigated as they related to the age, sex, and occupations of the patients.

Results of the Herrington-Hall (1988) study found that the most common pathologies were:

vocal nodules	21.6%
edema	14.1%
polyps	11.4%
cancer	9.7%
vocal fold paralysis	8.1%
no visible pathology	7.9%
laryngitis	4.2%
leukoplakia	4.1%
psychogenic	2.6%

Laryngeal pathologies occurred most often in the middle to advanced age groups with 57% of the patients over age 45 years and 22.4% over the age of 64 years. The remaining 20.6% of the patients were between the ages of 0 and 44 years. The pathologies most common in the younger age group (22–44) were vocal nodules and edema. Polyps and no visible pathology were most common during middle age (45–64), while vocal fold paralysis was the most common pathology associated with more advanced age (> 64). Interestingly, cancer of the larynx was evenly distributed between the middle and advanced aged patients.

Sex differences were also seen related to the prevalence of laryngeal pathologies. Overall, laryngeal pathologies were significantly more common in females than in males (perhaps females sought treatment more often than males). Pathologies that were more common to females were nodules and psychogenic disorders. Males presented with cancer, leukoplakia, and hyperkeratosis in far greater numbers than did females. In males, vocal nodules were most common between 0 and 14 years, edema between 25 and 44 years, polyps between 45 and 64 years, and vocal fold paralysis after 64 years. Females presented with edema, polyps, and nodules most frequently during young (22–44) and middle (45–64) adulthood.

Seventy-three occupations were identified in this study. Of these occupations, laryngeal pathologies occurred most often in the following:

1. retired persons
2. homemakers
3. factory workers
4. unemployed persons
5. executive or managers
6. teachers

7. students   9. singers
8. secretaries   10. nurses

PATHOLOGY CLASSIFICATIONS

We have divided our discussion of laryngeal pathologies into four classifications. These classifications include: (1) **congenital laryngeal pathologies**, (2) **pathologies of the vocal fold cover**, (3) **neurogenic laryngeal pathologies**, and (4) **pathologies of muscular dysfunction**.

Congenital laryngeal pathologies (see Figure 4–1) comprise laryngeal abnormalities that are present at birth. The incidence of these disorders is not well known. Dobres et al. (1990), studied the number and types of laryngeal pathologies in children evaluated by otolaryngologists. Surprisingly, in this study, subglottic stenosis was found to comprise 31.2% of the population of children studied. Laryngomalacia was found in 11.9% of the children. Overall, the incidence of congenital laryngeal pathologies is thought to be small.

Pathologies of the vocal fold cover include those that cause any alteration in the histological structure of the vocal fold mucosal lining. Changes in the mucosal lining will affect the mass, size, stiffness, flexi-

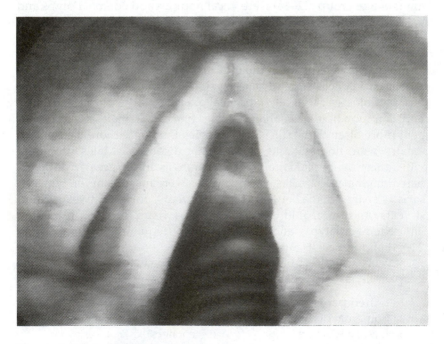

Figure 4–1.   Laryngeal web.

bility, and tension of the vocal folds, as well as the adequate approximation of the folds for phonation. Any one of these vocal fold effects has the potential of changing the quality, pitch, and loudness of the voice.

Neurogenic voice pathologies are represented by those voice disturbances that are caused directly by an interruption in the nervous signal supplied to the larynx. In our discussion of primary disorder etiologies (Chapter 2), voice changes associated with other neurologic disease processes were described. Under the neurogenic pathology classification, our discussion will focus on the few pathologies that are more or less isolated to vocal function.

Pathologies associated with muscular dysfunction include those that occur in the presence of a normal vocal fold cover and without neurologic involvement. These pathologies include the various psychogenic voice disorders as well as those associated with the functional misuse of the laryngeal musculature in the production of voice. Let us examine the various laryngeal pathologies, their causes, and typical treatment modalities.

CONGENITAL LARYNGEAL PATHOLOGIES

The congenital laryngeal pathologies discussed below are listed in Table 4–1.

Congenital Web

A congenital laryngeal web (Figure 4–1) occurs when the vocal folds fail to separate during the 10th week of embryonic development. Webbing may occur anywhere from the anterior to the posterior glottis. When the web is complete at birth, the normal airway is compromised. Without emergency procedures to establish an airway, the infant will asphyxiate. Webbing of the anterior glottis only, will cause various degrees of dyspnea and stridor depending upon the extent of the web (Hollinger, 1979).

The voice qualities of children with congenital webs will range from normal voice to a severe dysphonia, again depending on the extent of the web. The placement and exact attachments of even larger

TABLE 4–1. Congenital Laryngeal Pathologies

Congenital web
Congenital subglottic stenosis
Congenital cyst
Laryngomalacia
Laryngotracheal cyst

webs may be such that breathing and voice may not be negatively affected. Occasionally, the presence of this type of web will go undetected until puberty when the young boy's voice will fail to change and the young girl's pitch will remain childishly high due to the reduced vibratory length of the folds.

Treatment of the disorder is surgical division of the web. The raw margins of the surgical defect are kept apart by the placement of a surgical keel which is removed after several weeks. During the healing period, the airway is maintained via a tracheostomy (Ballantyne & Groves,1982). Greene (1972) suggested that training appropriate pitch levels following surgical repair may be necessary.

Congenital Subglottic Stenosis

Maldevelopment of the cricoid cartilage or arrested embryonic development of the conus will produce a narrowing of the larynx below the glottis. The narrowing will produce an obstruction of the airway causing the voice to be potentially stridorous from birth. In some cases, as the cricoid cartilage continues to develop after birth, the problem is alleviated in infancy or early childhood. In more severe cases, surgical repair of the subglottic region is required (Cotton, 1985)). Voice therapy is often required following surgery to aid the child in establishing normal phonation.

Congenital Cyst

These fluid-filled, sessile cysts normally appear in the laryngeal ventricle between the ventricular folds and the true vocal folds causing both glottic and supraglottic obstruction (Figure 4–2). The cause for the development of congenital cysts is not well known (Kleinsasser, 1968), but they are thought to result from blocked fluid ducts. The position of the cyst may render the voice weak or even aphonic. Treatment is surgical excision.

Laryngomalacia

Another congenital abnormality of the larynx which is of theoretical interest to the voice pathologist is laryngomalacia (congenital laryngeal stridor) (Figure 4–3). This pathology occurs when the epiglottis fails to develop normally, remaining very soft and pliable. As the child breathes, the increased inspiratory and expiratory movements of the epiglottis offer considerable resistance to the air stream, causing stridor. Following diagnosis, no treatment is required for this condition, as the epiglottis will continue to develop and the condition will spontaneously clear by the third year with normal maturation.

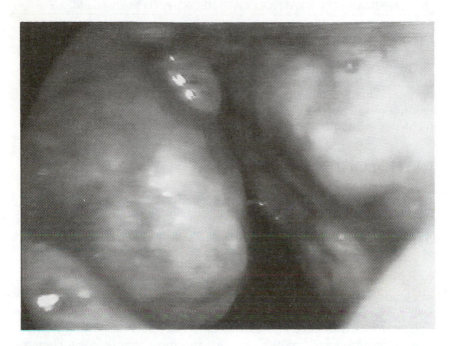

Figure 4–2. Congenital cyst.

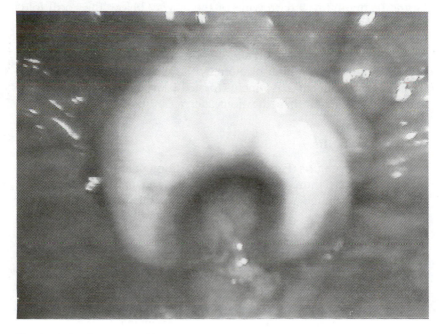

Figure 4–3. Laryngomalacia.

Laryngotracheal Cleft

An interarytenoid cleft will occur causing an open posterior larynx when the dorsal cricoid lamina fails to fuse during embryonic development. This is a most unusual type of cleft that tends to cause more feeding problems than voice concerns. The infants' cry may be weak, feeble, or even aphonic (Aronson, 1990).

PATHOLOGIES OF THE VOCAL FOLD COVER

The pathologies of the vocal fold cover discussed below are listed in Table 4–2.

Acute Laryngitis

The term laryngitis is used to describe an inflammation of the vocal fold mucosa causing mild to severe dysphonia with lowered pitch and pitch and phonation breaks. In severe cases, aphonia may result. The causes of acute laryngitis may be the common cold virus, adenoviruses, influenza viruses, and bacterial infections with the latter two being implicated as the cause of the most severe voice change (Morrison & Rammage, 1994).

Children may experience an even more serious response to acute laryngitis involving a narrowing of the airway below the vocal folds causing a sharp cough, hoarseness, and inspiratory stridor. Parents who have experienced these sudden and somewhat frightening symptoms know that this illness is *croup*. Croup attacks last a variable period from 30 minutes to an hour or more, with repeated attacks being common. The most effective treatments for acute laryngitis include external and internal hydration, medications such as antibiotics, and rest.

Chronic Laryngitis

Chronic laryngitis (Figure 4–4) is a condition of long standing laryngeal mucosal inflammation, viscous mucus, and epithelial thickening and is not associated with infection. Voice quality is mild to severely

TABLE 4–2. Pathologies of the Vocal Fold Cover

Acute laryngitis	Papilloma
Chronic laryngitis	Leukoplakia
Nodules	Hyperkeratosis
Polyp	Carcinoma
Reinke's edema	Hemorrhage
Cyst	Varix
Granuloma	Sulcus vocalis

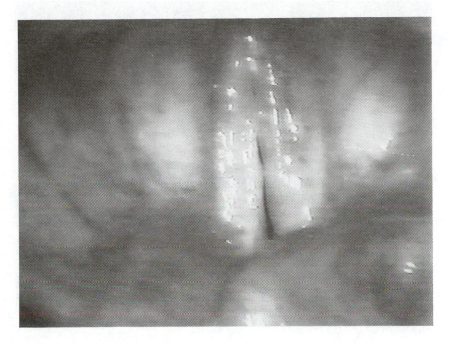

Figure 4–4. Chronic laryngitis.

dysphonic depending upon the severity of the mucosal and epithelial change. Other symptoms include laryngeal fatigue and non-productive coughing and throat clearing, but local pain is seldom present.

The causes of chronic laryngitis include repeated episodes of acute laryngitis, vocal misuse including both abusive behaviors and the use of inappropriate vocal components, smoking, and excessive alcohol consumption. Air pollutants, laryngeal dehydration, both external and internal, airborne allergies, the use of drying medications, gastroesophageal reflux disease, and repeated vomiting associated with bulimia have also been implicated as etiologic factors.

The typical treatment for chronic laryngitis is to attempt to remove the cause. Voice therapy is often very helpful in identification of the specific etiologic factors and in their modification or elimination.

Vocal Nodules

Vocal fold nodules (Figures 4–5 and 4–6) represent a further inflammatory degeneration of the superficial layer of the lamina propria with associated fibrosis and edema. Varying in size from as small as a pinhead to as large as a pea, nodules are located on the medial edge between the anterior one-third and posterior two-thirds of the

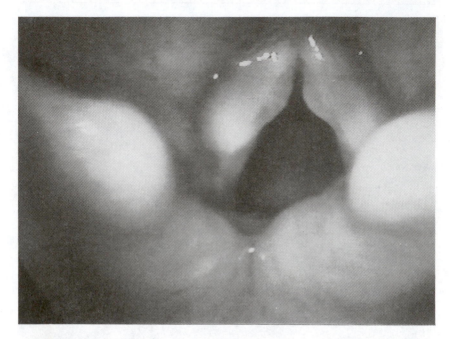

Figure 4–5. Vocal nodules (abduction).

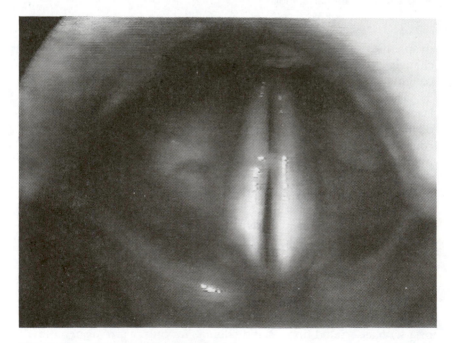

Figure 4–6. Vocal nodules (adduction).

true vocal folds, or the point of maximum lateral excursion and therefore maximum compression during vibration. At least two types of nodules have been described, acute and chronic. Acute nodules appear rather gelatinous and floppy as the overlying squamous epithelium is normal. Chronic nodules appear harder and more fixed to the underlying mass of the mucosa due to increased fibrosis and a thickened epithelium (Vaughn, 1982). During vibration, the mass and stiffness of the vocal fold cover are increased, but the mechanical properties of the transition and body are not affected (Hirano, 1981).

Nodules frequently occur in both male and female children, in female adults, but only occasionally in the adult male. The symptoms of vocal nodules include a mild to moderate dysphonia, characterized by hoarseness, breathiness (due to the common anterior and posterior glottal chinks caused by the approximating nodules) and increased laryngeal area muscle tension.

Nodules are the direct result of vocal misuse including abusive behaviors and the use of inappropriate vocal components. It is also rather common for nodules to occur in untrained singers or singers using inappropriate technique. Aronson (1990) asserted that most individuals with nodules are talkative, socially aggressive, and tense. Further, these individuals have acute or chronic interpersonal conflicts that generate tension, anxiety, anger, or depression. Though the majority of patients are vocally aggressive in some manner, our experience with patients exhibiting vocal nodules has not been as strongly rooted in this psychogenic orientation.

The first line of management for vocal nodules is voice therapy. Removing nodules surgically prior to identification and modification or elimination of the causes would simply be an invitation for the nodules to quickly recur. We would stress that even the chronic type nodule may resolve when the appropriate management program is followed. When nodules do not respond to therapy in the compliant patient, then surgical management may be required followed by postsurgical voice rehabilitation.

Vocal Fold Polyp and Reinke's Edema

A vocal fold polyp is a fluid-filled lesion that develops in the superficial layer of the lamina propria usually in the middle one-third of the membranous vocal fold (Hirano, 1982). Although they usually occur unilaterally, polyps may also occur bilaterally and may be present in sessile or pedunculated forms (Figures 4–7 and 4–8).

The cause of vocal fold polyps is thought to be acute vocal trauma or some form of voice abuse. Vocal symptoms will vary significantly from mild to severe dysphonias depending upon the type and location

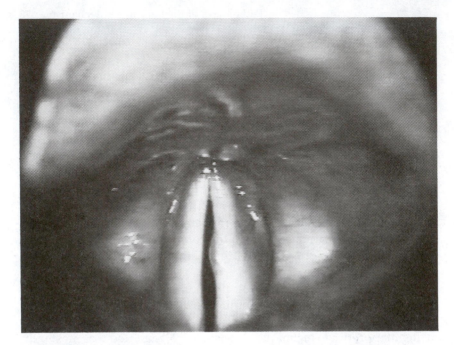

Figure 4–7. Sessile polyp.

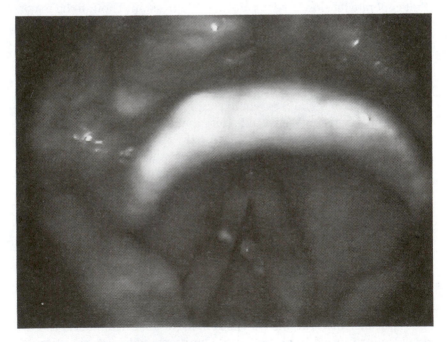

Figure 4–8. Pedunculated polyp.

of the polyp and their interference with glottic closure. For example, a pedunculated polyp may cause an intermittent dysphonia as the polyp, which is attached to a stalk, may at times fall below the vibrating edge of the vocal folds, whereas at other times flip up and interfere with the closure and vibration of the folds. A polyp will cause the mass of the vocal fold cover to increase, but the stiffness of the cover will vary. Stiffness is decreased when edema is the primary cause and increased when a prominent blood vessel is feeding the lesion and when a proliferation of collagenous fibers occurs.

When edema of the superficial layer of the lamina propria becomes more diffuse, filling Reinke's space along the entire length of the fold, **Reinke's edema** is the diagnosis (Figure 4–9). Reinke's edema, sometimes called polypoid degeneration, is caused by chronic misuse of the laryngeal mechanism including vocal abuse, misuse of vocal components, smoking , and alcohol abuse. In our clinic we have seen very few patients with this diagnosis who were not smokers. Because of the water balloon appearance of this typically unilateral lesion, glottic closure is usually complete. Obviously the mass of the cover is increased. The stiffness of the cover is usually decreased causing voice quality to

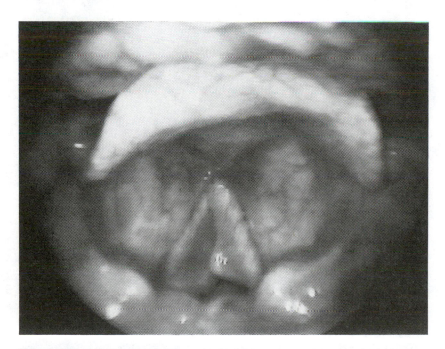

Figure 4–9.   Reinke's edema.

be mild to moderately dysphonic, characterized by low pitch and a husky hoarseness. The voice of Reinke's edema has traditionally been described as a "whiskey" voice. The mechanical properties of the transition and the body of the vocal fold are not affected by the lesion.

Treatment for vocal fold polyps and Reinke's edema is usually surgical excision. Voice therapy is valuable both preoperatively in identifying the causes for the pathology and postoperatively for reestablishing good vocal hygiene and improved voice production.

Vocal Fold Cyst

Cysts of the true vocal folds arise in the superficial layer of the lamina propria of the fold as the result of a blocked mucosal gland duct (Figure 4–10), with occasional extension into the intermediate and deep layers of the fold (Hirano, 1982). These fluid-filled epithelial sacs may occur anywhere in the membranous portion of the vocal fold. Although a cyst usually occurs unilaterally, bilateral cysts may be present. It is not unusual, when a cyst involves the medial edge of a fold, for contralateral tissue thickening to occur as a result of vibratory

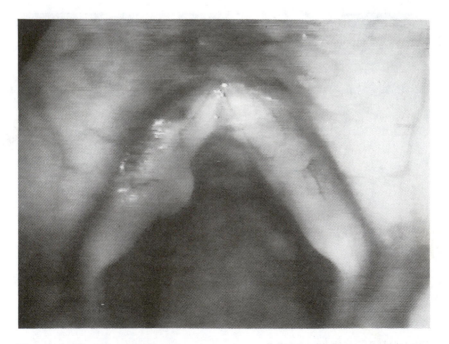

Figure 4–10. Vocal fold cyst.

interference. When this is the case, a unilateral vocal fold cyst may often be diagnosed as bilateral vocal fold nodules. Stroboscopic observation of vocal fold vibration is often very helpful as the mass and stiffness of the vocal fold cover will be increased with the cyst often to a much greater extent than will the thickness of the contralateral side.

Voice qualities that result from the presence of a cyst may be mild to moderate dysphonias depending upon the size and location of the cyst. Even a very small cyst may have a significant negative effect on the singing voice. Treatment for this type of mass lesion is surgical, followed by rehabilitative voice therapy.

Granuloma

Granulomas (Figure 4–11) are mass lesions that develop on the vocal process of the arytenoid cartilage in the posterior larynx. Unless the size is quite large, the presence of a granuloma does not affect the membranous vibrating body of the vocal folds although many patients complain of "throat" pain, restricted pitch ranges, and voice fatigue.

A granuloma is a highly vascular lesion that develops as the result of tissue irritation in the posterior larynx. This irritation may

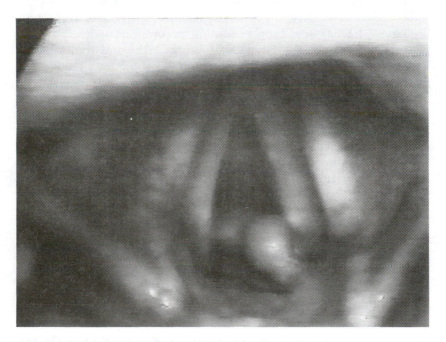

Figure 4–11. Contact granuloma.

be caused by persistent voice misuse, especially the use of a pressed, low pitched voice quality. In this case, the granuloma may be classified a contact granuloma. Intubation granulomas may occur as the result of laryngeal intubation during surgery or long term intubation following surgery or due to a serious illness. Granulomas have also been found to be the result of gastroesophageal reflux. Indeed, Sataloff (1991) suggests that reflux most likely contributes to the development of all forms of granulomas and that the first line of treatment should be an antireflux regimen (see Chapter 7). When this proves unsuccessful in the resolution of the granuloma, then surgery is the treatment of choice. It has been our clinical experience that granulomas are persistent lesions that often recur. The location of the lesion is in an area of constant movement and potential irritation. Patients very often must be supported by the voice pathologist as they struggle through the management process for these lesions.

Papilloma

Papillomas are multiple lesions, wart-like in appearance, that develop in the epithelium and invade deeper into the lamina propria and vocalis muscle affecting the mass and stiffness of the cover, transition, and body of the vocal fold (Hirano, 1981) (Figure 4–12). Thought to be caused by viruses, these persistent tumors may spread through the larynx, trachea, and bronchi leading to compromised respiration. Because of the diffuse locations of these growths and the speed at which they tend to proliferate, tracheostomy is sometimes required to guarantee the patient a functional airway.

Though usually found equally in both sexes of children (Hollinger, Schild, & Maurizi, 1968), the incidence of papilloma has also increased in adults. In children, the development of papilloma usually is retarded with age and often disappears during puberty. Unfortunately, the multiple laser surgeries that are often required for control of these tumors in both children and adults often cause vocal fold scarring. The resultant voice quality may be a mild to severe dysphonia and even aphonia depending upon the extent of the disease and the aggressiveness of the required treatment. Voice therapy is helpful only to the extent of maximizing the most appropriate phonation available to the patient.

Leukoplakia and Hyperkeratosis

Two vocal fold pathologies, typically classified as precancerous lesions, are leukoplakia and hyperkeratosis (Figures 4–13 and 4–14).

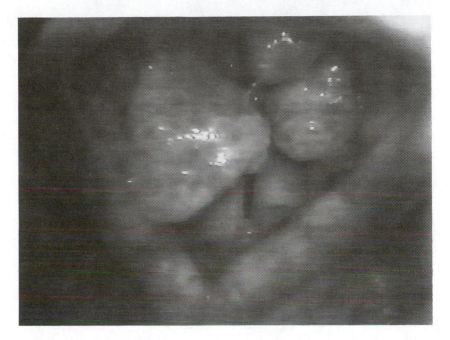

Figure 4–12.   Papilloma.

These lesions arise as asymmetrical, hyperplastic thickenings of the epithelium and may enter and involve the superficial layer of the lamina propria of the vocal fold. Should the lesion invade the intermediate and deep layers of the lamina propria, an early carcinoma is most likely present (Hirano, 1981). The lesions are usually bilateral but can occur unilaterally as well causing an increase in the mass and stiffness of the of the cover of the fold while leaving the transition and the body unaffected. Leukoplakia appears as a patchy, white membrane and is usually located on the anterior one-third of the true vocal folds. Hyperkeratosis is a layered buildup of keratinized cell tissue and is distinctive for its leaf-like appearance.

Etiologic factors associated with the development of these premalignant lesions include the chronic irritations of the chemicals and heat from tobacco smoke, the irritation from alcohol ingestion, incessant coughing and throat clearing, and general voice abuse and misuse. Treatment for both lesions is surgery. It has been our clinical experience that presurgical voice therapy is helpful in identifying the causes for the lesions, modifying the behaviors that contributed to the causes, and initiation of general vocal hygiene. Having gone through these

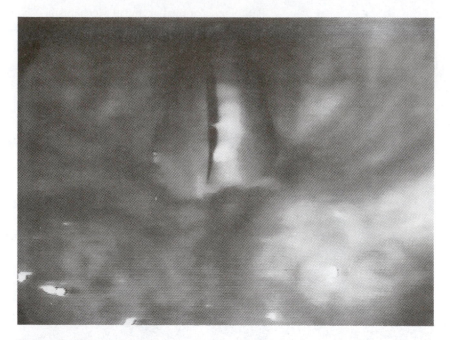

Figure 4–13. Leukoplakia.

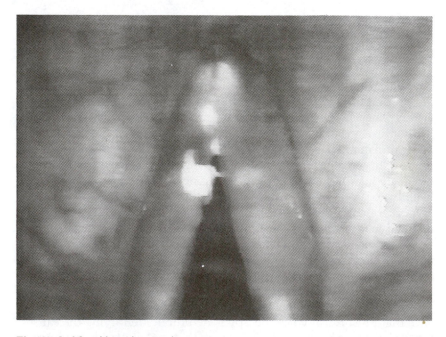

Figure 4–14. Hyperkeratosis.

therapy procedures, the patients' vocal folds are in the best possible condition prior to the surgery. Postsurgical voice rehabilitation is advanced as a result of this presurgical intervention.

Carcinoma

Cancer of the larynx (Figure 4–15) is potentially the most devastating of all laryngeal pathologies due to the life threatening implications of the disease and the initial devastating effect on vocal communication. The most common symptom of this pathology is persistent hoarseness. There is little if any laryngeal area pain or soreness, although either may occur at later stages in the development of the disease and even may be referred to the ears. In advanced disease, the patient may experience both swallowing and respiratory problems.

Most laryngeal carcinomas are of the squamous cell type that originate from the epithelium. When identified at this stage the lesion is called carcinoma in situ. As the lesion develops, it will invade the deeper layers of the vocal fold including the vocalis muscle affecting the mass and stiffness of all affected mechanical layers (Hirano, 1981).

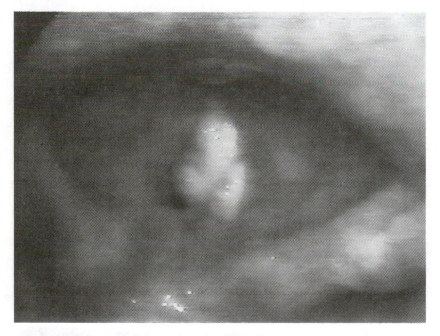

Figure 4–15.   Laryngeal cancer.

Vocal symptoms will therefore vary from a very mild to severe dysphonia depending upon the location and the extent of the lesion.

Laryngeal carcinoma is thought to be caused by chronic irritation of the laryngeal epithelium and mucosa by such agents as tobacco smoke and alcohol. Treatment modalities include radiation therapy or surgical excision, or both. The voice pathologist plays a very important role in preparing the patient and the family for the consequences of the various forms of surgery and in the subsequent voice rehabilitation (see Chapter 10).

Vocal Hemorrhage and Varix

On occasion, a varicose vein on the superior surface of the vocal fold will rupture causing a bleed into Reinke's space (Figure 4–16). The resultant mucosal disruption of stiffness and, in more severe cases, scarring of the vocal fold cover, causes significant acute dysphonia at the time of the bleed and continued hoarseness for some time to follow. While a vocal fold hemorrhage can occur in anyone, Sataloff (1991) suggests that it may be commonly seen in premen-

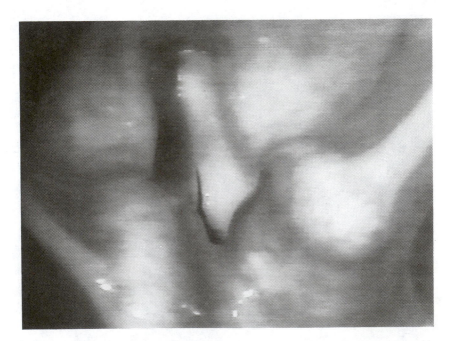

Figure 4–16. Hemorrhage.

strual women using aspirin products. The treatment of choice is strict voice rest which, in most cases, results in spontaneous resolution of the hematoma.

At times, the blunt end of the varicose vein may be seen on the surface of the vocal fold when the hemorrhage resolves. This **varix** (Figure 4–17) may cause an asymmetry in the amplitude of vibration and the mucosal wave, as seen stroboscopically, causing a voice disturbance even though resolution of the hemorrhage is complete. A varix in the nonprofessional voice is usually not cause for concern. However, even this slight disruption in normal vocal fold function may be significant for those who depend on their voices professionally. When treatment of the offending varix is required, laser vaporization is accomplished with care taken to protect the lamina propria of the vocal fold. Without care, the treatment may yield a worse result than the original problem.

Voice therapy following resolution of the hemorrhage may be helpful in rebuilding the strength and balance of the laryngeal muscle system (which has been on voice rest) through appropriate exercise. Some patients also demonstrate an understandable fear in reentering their normal vocal activities. The voice pathologist's support and guidance can be instrumental in directing the patient to full voice use.

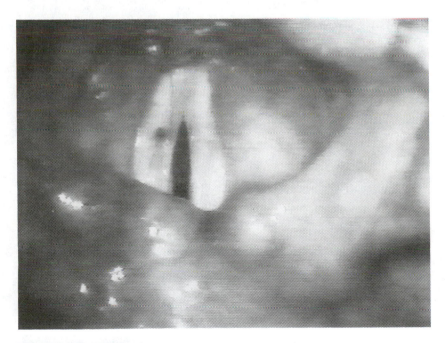

Figure 4–17. Varix.

Sulcus Vocalis

A vocal fold sulcus is a ridge or furrow that runs the entire length of the superior surface of the membranous portion of the vocal fold usually causing the vocal fold edge to bow (Figure 4–18). A sulcus usually occurs bilaterally, though unilateral sulci can occur, and involves the superficial layer of the lamina propria. When a sulcus is present, the mass of the vocal fold cover is reduced while the stiffness of the cover is significantly increased. The deeper structures of the vocal fold are not involved.

According to Bouchayer, Cornut, and Witzig (1985), the presence of a vocal fold sulcus is related to embryological development where maldevelopment of the mucosal lining of the vocal fold results in the furrow. Until the use of stroboscopy, sulcus vocalis was not commonly diagnosed. Even with the advantage of this observational technique, the sulcus may be missed due to a loosely tethered overlying flap of mucous membrane.

Voice quality that results from a vocal fold sulcus may be mild to severely dysphonic depending on the stiffness of the fold and the size of the glottal chink caused by the vocal fold bowing. Treatment attempts

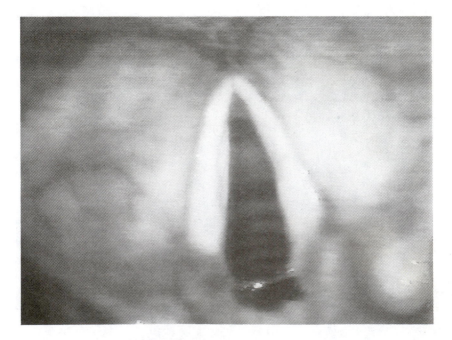

Figure 4–18. Vocal fold sulcus.

involving surgical techniques for removing the sulcus have been attempted with mixed results. Direct voice therapy focused on strengthening the laryngeal musculature in the presence of the sulcus has yielded voice improvement for patients in our clinic.

NEUROGENIC LARYNGEAL PATHOLOGIES

The neurogenic laryngeal pathologies discussed below are listed in Table 4–3.

Spasmodic Dysphonia

One of the more curious and serious voice disorders is that of spasmodic dysphonia. Spasmodic dysphonia is a descriptive term for a family of strained, strangled voices. The cause of this disorder has been debated for many years. Although early descriptions linked the disorder to a psychoneurosis (Arnold, 1959; Brodnitz, 1976), more recent evidence has demonstrated a neurologic origin (Aminoff et al., 1978; Aronson et al., 1968). Dedo et al. (1978) reported information from 12 spasmodic dysphonia patients who underwent examination by a neurologist. Of these patients, 6 showed signs of neurologic disturbances including postural tremor, blepharospasm, idiopathic torsion dystonia, and buccolingual dyskinesia. Blitzer et al. (1986) offered strong evidence that spasmodic dysphonia should be considered a focal dystonia specific to the larynx and similar to other dystonias such as blepharospasm and torticollis.

The incidence of spasmodic dysphonia is unknown, but is thought to be relatively low. The disorder is said to occur equally in men and women with the most common onset in middle age (Aronson et al., 1968; Brodnitz, 1976). We have evaluated patients with onset of the disorder occurring as early as their middle teens. Some patients experience a rapid onset associated with the occurrence of a traumatic event. Others report a more gradual onset following hoarseness associated with an upper respiratory infection. Still others appear to present with an idiopathic spasmodic dysphonia. The severity of the vocal symptoms appears to peak within the first year following the onset of the disorder.

TABLE 4–3. Neurogenic Laryngeal Pathologies

Spasmodic dysphonia
Essential laryngeal tremor
Vocal fold paralysis

Spasmodic dysphonia is classified in two primary groups: adductor and abductor spasmodic dysphonia. Adductor spasmodic dysphonia is the most common type. The laryngeal behavior is characterized by an intermittent, tight adduction of the vocal folds creating a strained, forced voicing behavior. When examined through indirect laryngoscopy, the vocal folds appear normal in structure and function. Intermittent periods of normal phonation may occur during speech production, during both laughter and angry outbursts of speech, and while singing. Some patients are able to reduce the frequency and severity of the spasms when talking at a pitch level that is slightly higher than normal. The majority of patients with adductor spasmodic dysphonia find it difficult to shout.

Many patients with this disorder complain of physical fatigue, tightness of the neck, back, and shoulder muscles and shortness of breath due to their efforts to phonate through the closed glottis. The severity of the symptoms of adductor spasmodic dysphonia vary within and among individuals. Some patients experience only a very mild interruption in normal phonation, while others may be rendered voiceless by the severity of the spasms. In the more severe cases, patients may compensate by whispering or phonating on inspired air. Secondary behaviors similar to those observed in stutterers, such as head jerking, eye blinking, and vocalized starters, may also develop.

Abductor spasmodic dysphonia is a mirror image of the adductor type. Phonation is interrupted by a sudden, involuntary period of aphonia, which is accompanied by a burst of air, as the vocal folds spasm in the abducted position. The vocal fold spasms appear to occur primarily during the production of unvoiced consonants (Aronson, 1980), although Hartman (1980) reported that breathy moments occurred during all positions within words, on whole words, and on several words in succession. Of 13 patients studied by Hartman (1980), 8 reported that their voices improved when they were angry, increased their intensity, or altered their pitch. Voice quality worsened when they were anxious or fatigued.

Spasmodic dysphonia is an insidious disorder causing many psychosocial problems for those who display the symptoms of the disorder. We have seen patients who have searched many years, first for a diagnosis of the disorder and then for a treatment to cure or reduce the symptoms. To this end patients often have seen several otolaryngologists, neurologists, psychologists, and speech pathologists. They have gone through voice therapy, psychotherapy, psychological counseling, drug therapies, EMG and thermal biofeedback, relaxation training, acupuncture, hypnosis, and faith healing. Unfortunately, none of these approaches has proved to be consistently effective in relieving the vocal symptoms. Chapter 8 of this text details the current treatments for both adductor and abductor spasmodic dysphonia.

Organic (Essential) Tremor

Essential tremor is a central nervous system disorder that is characterized by rhythmic tremors (4 to 7 cycles/seconds) of various body parts including the larynx. Tremor may involve the head, arms, neck, tongue, palate, face, and larynx in isolation or in combinations. In some patients, the tremor may only be observed when the affected body part is being used (intentional tremor), whereas other patients will exhibit the tremor behavior even at rest. The onset of essential tremor is usually gradual occurring in middle to late middle age. The disorder occurs most frequently in males, is often hereditary, and is often accompanied by other neurological signs. (Aronson & Hartman, 1981; Brown & Simonson, 1963; Larsson & Sjogren, 1960).

Laryngeal tremor is most noticeable during prolonged vowels as the rhythm of the tremor is easily discerned. Connected speech may be negatively affected as well. In some cases the tremor is so severe that it causes voice stoppages similar to those of spasmodic dysphonia. Indeed, these two disorders, which may accompany each other, are often mistaken for one another. When in doubt regarding the diagnosis, the clinician is reminded to ask the patient to sustain vowels. Treatment for essential tremor is discussed in Chapter 8.

Vocal Fold Paralysis

Vocal fold paralysis is the most common of the neurogenic voice disorders. The symptoms of vocal fold paralysis may vary from no dysphonia (when the paralyzed fold or folds are located at the midline) to a severe dysphonia (when glottic closure has been significantly compromised). Vocal fold paralysis may be bilateral or unilateral and is typically caused by peripheral involvement of the recurrent laryngeal and, less commonly, the superior laryngeal nerves. More superior involvement of the 10th cranial nerve would affect the muscles supplied by both the recurrent and superior laryngeal nerves. Location of the lesion along the nerve pathway will determine the type of paralysis and the resultant voice quality.

There are many possible etiologies of vocal fold paralysis including surgical trauma, cardiovascular disease, neurological diseases, and accidental trauma. It is also important to note that the cause of approximately 30 to 35% of all vocal fold paralysis is idiopathic (Willatt & Stell, 1991).

Recurrent Laryngeal Nerve Paralysis

Four types of vocal fold paralysis are possible with involvement of the recurrent laryngeal nerves including abductor and adductor paralyses, both of which may be unilateral or bilateral.

Bilateral abductor paralysis is the most serious form of vocal fold paralysis in its relation to respiratory function. With this pathology, both folds are positioned near the midline and are unable to abduct, requiring that an adequate airway be established. This may involve a tracheostomy or a surgical procedure in which one of the arytenoid cartilages is either removed or tied off laterally in an effort to open the airway. Voice quality may not be significantly impaired for contextual speech except by the presence of stridor prior to surgical intervention. The voice, of course, will be impaired following lateralization of the fold.

Unilateral abductor paralysis is much less serious, as the paralyzed fold remains at the midline while the other fold abducts and adducts normally. Although this positioning of the paralyzed fold will reduce the size of the airway, it does not typically cause a negative affect to the patient's respiratory status. Voice quality for contextual speech will remain near normal; however, the patient will experience difficulty in building the necessary subglottic pressure to increase intensity due to the laxness of the paralyzed fold.

Bilateral adductor paralysis results in both vocal folds resting in a paramedian position, not able to adduct to close the glottis. Individuals with this form of paralysis will obviously be aphonic, but the primary concern is aspiration. Patients with this form of paralysis often must be fed through a G-tube and aided in communication with an artificial larynx. Six to 9 months following the onset, contracture and fibrosis of the folds may occur causing the folds to be drawn closer to the midline permitting a harsh whisper to be produced and improving the prospects for swallowing. The problem of a limited airway may, however, develop.

Unilateral adductor paralysis (Figures 4–19 and 4–20) is the most common type of vocal fold paralysis with the paralyzed fold resting in an abducted or paramedian position while the other fold adducts and abducts normally. As might be expected, the effect of the paralysis on phonation is determined by the size of the glottal gap. Voice quality is usually characterized by breathiness and diplophonia. The ability to build subglottic air pressure is also impaired resulting in a decrease in vocal intensity and the inability to shout or compete with background noise. Patients with this pathology often complain of physical fatigue resulting from the increased effort to approximate the folds and the breathlessness associated with phonation. Treatment approaches, including voice therapy and surgical intervention, are discussed in Chapter 8.

Superior Laryngeal Nerve Paralysis

Paralysis of the superior laryngeal nerves occurs much less frequently than does paralysis of the recurrent laryngeal nerves due to their much shorter course and their location away from other major areas of potential damage. The diagnosis of superior laryngeal nerve paralysis is often difficult to ascertain. Bilateral paralysis of the cricothy-

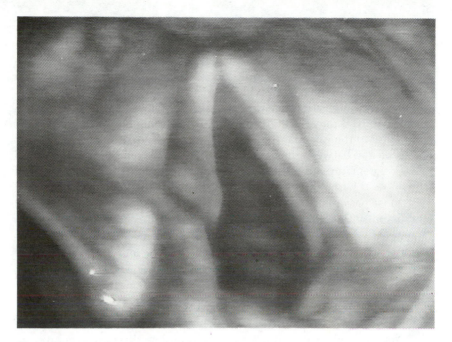

Figure 4–19.   Unilateral vocal fold paralysis (abduction).

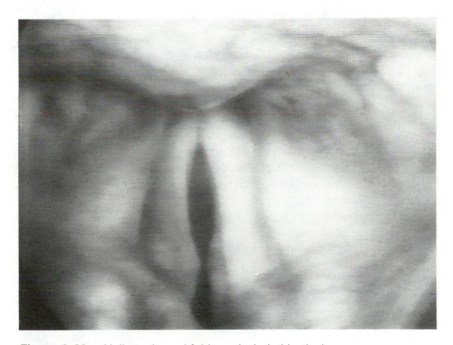

Figure 4–20.   Unilateral vocal fold paralysis (adduction).

roid muscles is rare and often must be confirmed through the use of EMG studies. If paralysis should occur, the vocal folds will lack their normal tone and the patient will experience a voice that is limited in frequency and intensity range and stability. Unilateral superior laryngeal nerve paralysis may result in an oblique positioning or an overlap of the folds due to the unequal rocking of the cricothyroid joint. The overlap creates a gap between the folds causing a decrease in the ability to build subglottic air pressure, thus decreasing vocal intensity. The laxness of the affected fold reduces the ability to increase and control pitch.

Most patients with this pathology complain of vocal fatigue and the inability to sing. While there is no medical treatment for superior laryngeal nerve paralysis, voice therapy may be utilized for educational and voice conservation purposes (see Chapter 8).

PATHOLOGIES OF MUSCULAR DYSFUNCTION

The pathologies of muscular dysfunction discussed below are listed in Table 4–4.

Ventricular Phonation (Plica Ventricularis)

Occasionally during phonation a great amount of supraglottic muscle tension is created in the laryngeal area causing a pull of the ventricular ligaments and approximation of the ventricular folds or false vocal folds as they are sometimes called (Figure 4–21). In the extreme case, the ventricular folds may actually be the source of vibration for voice production. As discussed in Chapter 2, the ventricular folds lie just superior and lateral to the true vocal folds and, although used during effort closure of the laryngeal port, they should rest quietly during phonation. False vocal fold phonation, as a functional behavior, may be caused by physical and emotional tension. In addition, it has been used as a compensatory voice when other serious pathologies make it difficult or impossible to phonate using the true vocal folds.

The voice quality of ventricular phonation is typically a moderate to severe dysphonia characterized by harshness and hoarseness.

TABLE 4–4. Pathologies of Muscular Dysfunction

Ventricular phonation
Conversion aphonia/dysphonia
Functional falsetto
Juvenile voice
Laryngeal myasthenia

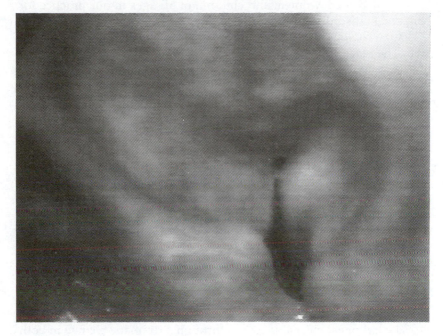

Figure 4–21.   Ventricular phonation.

Treatment of the functional variety involves counseling and vocal reeducation through direct voice therapy (see Chapter 7). Many patients are referred to the voice pathologist with the diagnosis of plica ventricularis. It should be noted that this diagnosis is often made when the false folds compress during the laryngeal exam obstructing the view of the true vocal folds. Many times the vibratory source continues to be the true vocal folds, but because of the medial compression of the false folds, the diagnosis of ventricular phonation is made. The reader is cautioned to be wary of this diagnosis and encouraged to become familiar with the vocal quality of this pathology.

Conversion Aphonia and Dysphonia

The patient who whispers (aphonia) or presents with an unusual voice quality despite having a neurologically and anatomically normal laryngeal mechanism (dysphonia) may have the pathology of conversion aphonia or dysphonia. Onset is normally quite sudden with many patients relating the disorder to symptoms of a cold or flu and often accompanied by a "sore throat." The majority of conversion voice disorders occur in women (Herrington-Hall et al., 1988). However, we have treated men, women, and children of all ages in our practice for conversion disorders of the voice.

A psychological conversion reaction is induced by stress and tension. The reaction behavior, in this case whispering or the production of a dysphonic voice, is the patient's attempt to draw attention away from the real problem. It permits the individual to focus on the voice instead of the true source of the stress or emotional conflict. These voicing behaviors are unconscious methods of avoiding the strong interpersonal conflicts that cause the stress, depression, or anxiety. Often, by the time patients seek help from the laryngologist or voice pathologist, the need for the conversion reaction has diminished significantly and they are ready for the voice problem to be resolved. It must be understood by these professionals that these patients are not malingering. They are not aware that they have the capability of producing normal voice. Although some patients continue to receive secondary gain from the disorder and resist all therapy modifications, the majority will respond quickly to direct voice therapy (see Chapter 7).

Functional Falsetto and Juvenile Voice

The laryngeal mechanism goes through a dramatic change in both male and female children during puberty. The male voice lowers about one octave during mutation and the female voice lowers two to three semitones. When this acoustic change does not take place following the normal physical maturation, the male is said to have a functional falsetto and the female a juvenile or child-like voice.

Many causes for functional falsetto have been suggested. They include attempts to resist the natural growth into adulthood; a strong feminine self-identification; the desire to maintain a competent childhood soprano singing voice; and embarrassment when the voice lowers dramatically, perhaps earlier than those of their peers (Aronson, 1980). We would also suggest that the falsetto voice may also be the result of muscular incoordination and dysfunction without other underlying etiology. The juvenile voice of the post-adolescent female is recognized less commonly than mutational falsetto as the vocal symptoms of this disorder are less dramatic for the female. Women who demonstrate a juvenile voice may have resisted the transition into adulthood or also may have developed a muscular dysfunction.

The voice qualities associated with these pathologies are typically mild dysphonias characterized by high pitch, low intensity, cul de sac nasality, and breathiness. Physiologically, this is caused by persistent hyperfunction of the cricothyroid muscles with a pronounced elevation of the entire larynx (Arnold, 1966). Because of the inability to compress the vocal folds well, patients with these disorders often are not able to build appropriate subglottic air pressure to increase intensity. Common complaints are associated with the inability to shout, to compete with background noise, and voice fatigue. Young males may also demonstrate raspy voice qualities as they attempt to lower the pitch level in the presence of the muscular positioning of the folds and larynx for the falsetto.

Functional falsetto and juvenile voice are most often identified during the first few postadolescent years, with the social consequences being more negative for the male. Effeminacy and weakness are projected by the falsetto voice quality. Occasionally these pathologies are not identified until later adult life. It has been our experience that it has been more difficult to attain and maintain normal voicing in the older patient.

Voice therapy is the treatment of choice with these disorders, with the development of normal voice as the goal of the first therapy session. It must be understood that the pathological voice is the only voice with which the patient is familiar. Subsequent sessions are used to familiarize and stabilize the "new" voice as the patient's own.

Laryngeal Myasthenia

The system responsible for phonation is comprised of muscle, cartilage, and connective tissue and is similar to other jointed systems in the body. Indeed, like other muscles in the body, the laryngeal muscle system may become strained, weakened, and imbalanced in its function leading to impaired phonation (i.e., loss of frequency range and intensity), dysphonia, and laryngeal fatigue. The causes of laryngeal myasthenia are many and may include muscle dysfunction resulting from voice misuse and abuse; muscular adjustments that result from the laryngeal mechanism attempting to compensate for the presence of edema or mass lesions; or simply overuse of the voice. It is not unusual, following acute injuries of the larynx, for patients to present with the symptoms of laryngeal fatigue following resolution of the acute symptomatology.

Laryngeal myasthenia is characterized by complaints of voice fatigue, decrease in frequency and intensity ranges, and a lack of control in voice production. In many cases, the vocal folds will appear normal under indirect laryngoscopy. When observed stroboscopically, the folds often demonstrate an anterior glottal chink, a decrease in the amplitude of vibration, and a phase asymmetry (Stemple et al., in press). Since the disorder is difficult to diagnose without stroboscopic observation of vocal fold vibration, the ultimate diagnosis is one of exclusion of other pathologies. Patients often become very frustrated when they are told that their vocal folds look normal when indeed they are experiencing negative vocal symptoms.

The treatment for the pathology laryngeal myasthenia is direct, physiologic voice therapy. Physiologic voice therapy is described in detail in Chapter 7. It is our opinion that one component of most voice disorders will be the component of laryngeal muscle weakness. Voice pathologists are encouraged to think in terms of muscle dysfunction when evaluating all forms of voice disorders.

SUMMARY

This chapter reviewed the congenital laryngeal pathologies, pathologies of the vocal fold cover, neurologic pathologies, and pathologies of laryngeal muscle dysfunction which may all change the quality, pitch, and loudness of voice production. By being familiar with the nuances of these pathologies and the common etiologic factors that may lead to their development, voice pathologists may plan appropriate management programs. Diagnosis of the laryngeal pathology is the responsibility of the otolaryngologist and has been provided to the voice pathologist prior to the diagnostic voice evaluation. The diagnostic voice evaluation is designed to identify the specific causes of the voice disorder, describe and measure vocal function, and outline the plan of treatment to remediate the disorder. Chapters 5 and 6 describe diagnostic methods designed to meet these goals. Following the diagnostic methods, Chapters 7 and 8 detail specific management philosophies and approaches.

REFERENCES

Aminoff, M., Dedo, H., & Izdebski, K. (1978). Clinical aspects of spasmodic dysphonia. *Journal of Neurology, Neurosurgery and Psychiatry, 41,* 361–365.

Arnold, G. (1959). Spastic dysphonia I: Changing interpretation of a persistent affliction. *Logos, 2,* 3–14.

Aronson, A. (1990). *Clinical voice disorders: An interdisciplinary approach* (3rd ed.). New York: Brian C. Decker.

Aronson, A., Brown, J., Litin, E., & Pearson, J. (1968). Spastic dysphonia. 1. Voice, neurologic, and psychiatric aspects. *Journal of Speech and Hearing Disorders, 33,* 203–218.

Aronson, A., & Hartman, D. (1981). Adductor spastic dysphonia as a sign of essential (voice) tremor. *Journal of Speech and Hearing Disorders, 33,* 52–58.

Ballantyne, J., & Groves, J. (1982). *A synopsis of otolaryngology,* (3rd ed.). Bristol, England: John Wright and Sons.

Blitzer, A., Brin, M., Fahn, S., & Lovelace, R. (1988). Localized injections of botulinum toxin for the treatment of focal laryngeal dystonia (spastic dysphonia). *Laryngoscope, 98,* 193–197.

Bouchayer, M., Cornut, G., Witzig, E., Loire, R., Roch, J., & Bastian, R. (1985). Epidermoid cysts, sulci and mucosal bridges of the true vocal cord: A report of 157 cases. *Laryngoscope, 95*, 1087–1094.

Brodnitz, F. (1976). Spastic dysphonia. *Annals of Otology, Rhinology, and Laryngology, 85*, 210–214.

Brown, J., & Simonson, J. (1963). Organic voice tremor. *Neurology, 13*, 520–525.

Cotton, R. (1985). Prevention and management of laryngeal stenosis in infants and children. *Journal of Pediatric Surgery, 20*, 845–851.

Dedo, H., Townsend, J., & Izdebski, K. (1978). Current evidence for the organic etiology of spastic dysphonia. *Transactions of Otolaryngology, 86*, 875–880.

Dobres, R., Lee, L., Stemple, J., Kummer, A., & Kretchmer, L. (1990). Description of laryngeal pathologies in children evaluated by otolaryngologists. *Journal of Speech and Hearing Disorders, 55*, 526–533.

Greene, M. (1972). *The voice and its disorders*, (3rd ed.). Philadelphia: J. B. Lippincott.

Hartman, D. (1980). *Clinical investigations of abductor spastic dysphonia (intermittent breathy dysphonia)*. Paper presented at the American Speech-Language-Hearing Association Convention, Detroit.

Herrington-Hall, B., Lee, L., Stemple, J., Niemi, K., & McHone, M. (1988). Description of laryngeal pathologies by age, sex, and occupation in a treatment seeking sample. *Journal of Speech and Hearing Disorders, 53*, 57–65.

Hirano, M. (1981). Structure of the vocal fold in normal and disease states: Anatomical and physical studies. In C. Ludlow & M. Hart (Eds.), Proceedings of the conference on the assessment of vocal pathology (pp. 11–30), Rockville: ASHA.

Holinger, L. (1979). Congenital anomalies of the larynx. In G. English (Ed.), *Otolaryngology* (Vol. 3. pp. 1–15). Philadelphia: Harper and Row.

Holinger, P., Schild, J., & Mauriz, D. (1968). Laryngeal papilloma. Review of etiology and therapy. *Laryngoscope, 78*, pp. 14–62.

Kleinsasser, O. (1968). *Microlaryngoscopy and endolaryngeal microsurgery*. Philadelphia: W. B. Saunders.

LaGuaite, J. (1972). Adult voice screening. *Journal of Speech and Hearing Disorders, 37*, 147–151.

Larsson, T. and Sjogren, T. (1960). Essential tremor: A clinical and genetic population study. *Acta Psychiatry and Neurology (Scandinavia), 36* (Suppl. 144), 1–176.

Moore, P. (1982). Voice Disorders. In G. Shames & E. Wiig, (Eds.), *Human communication disorder: An introduction* (pp. 141–186). Columbus, OH: Charles E. Merrill.

Morrison, M. & Rammage, L. (1994). *The management of voice disorders*. San Diego: Singular Publishing Group, Inc.

Sataloff, R. (1991). *Professional voice: The science and art of clinical care*. New York: Raven Press.

Senturia B., & Wilson, F. (1968). Otorhinolaryngologic findings in children with voice deviations. Preliminary report. *Annals of Otology, Rhinology, and Laryngology, 77*, 1027–1042.

Silverman, E., & Zimmer, C. (1975). Incidence of chronic hoarseness among school-age children. *Journal of Speech and Hearing Disorders, 40*, 211–215.

Stemple, J., Stanley, J., & Lee, L. (in press). Objective measures of voice production in normal subjects following prolonged voice use. *Journal of Voice*.

Willatt, D. & Stell, P. (1991). Vocal cord paralysis. In M. Paparella & D. Shumrick, (Eds.), *Otolaryngology*, (3rd ed., pp. 2289–2307). Philadelphia: W. B. Saunders.

5

THE DIAGNOSTIC
VOICE EVALUATION

The previous chapters of this text have described the academic areas of knowledge from a clinical perspective, which are a necessary preparation for the evaluation and treatment of voice disorders. This chapter begins our concentration on the more human skills that are necessary when we assume the responsibility of guiding and helping others. These skills include listening, hearing, feeling, connecting, empathizing, motivating, encouraging, reinforcing, and rewarding. Although academic information may be studied and learned and turned into personal knowledge, human interaction skills develop over a lifetime of observation and interaction. The successful voice pathologist must possess an inherent "feel" for other people and combine vast academic knowledge with the ability to communicate at both a professional and personal human level.

The primary objectives of the diagnostic voice evaluation are to discover the etiologic factors associated with the development of the voice disorder and to describe the deviant vocal symptoms. Voice pathologists use their knowledge of laryngeal anatomy, physiology, pathologies of the laryngeal mechanism, and common etiologic factors in a systematic evaluation designed to determine these specific causes. Once the causes are known and the symptoms are described, a vocal management plan tailored to the individual problems and needs of each patient may be developed.

Diagnosis is the process of discovering the cause of certain symptoms. Diagnosis of voice disorders ordinarily encompasses the recognition and description of individual vocal deviations and a systematic search for the factors that cause these deviations. (Moore, 1971, p. 108)

The voice evaluation may also be used as a tool for patient education and motivation. Most individuals have little knowledge or understanding of voice production. Indeed, the majority of patients who present with voice disorders have little understanding of the problem. During the diagnostic evaluation, the voice pathologist will find it beneficial to explain in simple terms how voice is produced and the effect that their specific pathology plays on the deviant voice production. With a better understanding of voice production, patients are able to be more helpful in answering diagnostic questions specific to discovering the etiologies of the problem.

The patient who is well-informed will also generally be more highly motivated to follow the necessary therapy regimen required to resolve the pathology. Patients who understand the causes of the disorder, are presented with a systematic management approach, and a reasonable estimate of the time needed for completion of the program usually develop a positive therapeutic attitude.

THE PLAYERS

Many components comprise the diagnostic voice evaluation. These components include (1) the medical examination, (2) the patient interview, (3) the psychoacoustic evaluation of voice, (4) the instrumental analysis of voice including acoustic and aerodynamic analyses, (5) and the functional evaluation of vocal fold movement. Use of these diagnostic components has increasingly been accomplished through the teamwork of otolaryngologists, voice pathologists, and when occasion dictates, other professionals such as vocal coaches, voice teachers, and other medical professionals. The otolaryngologist is trained to examine the laryngeal mechanism for pathology and to diagnose the voice disorder. Through the diagnosis, determination will be made whether to treat the disorder medically, surgically, or through referral for functional management. The voice pathologist is trained to identify the causes of the voice disorders, evaluate the vocal symptoms, and to establish improved vocal function through various therapeutic methods. The vocal coach or singing instructor evaluates the efficiency and correctness of performance technique and suggests modifications as needed. Other medical professionals, such as neurologists, allergists, and endocrinologists may be called upon in selected cases to aid in the evaluation process. These complementary professional relationships have significantly improved the care of the voice disordered population (Stemple, 1993).

The teamwork model of evaluation and management of voice disorders has led to the development of formal clinical voice laboratories. In these clinical settings, patients have the opportunity to be evaluated by each of these core professionals during one visit. In addition, instrumentation is now available which permits measures of vocal function to be reported as well as visual studies of vocal function. These more advanced laryngeal function studies are described in Chapter 6.

PATIENT PROFILE

Who are voice patients? They may be anyone of any age, sex, race, or occupation. They may be professional voice users or Sunday morning choir members. Herrington-Hall et al. (1988) demonstrated this fact well in their review of patients who sought evaluation for voice disorders. The top 10 occupations were retired people, homemaker, factory worker, unemployed, executive/manager, teacher, student, secretary, singer, and nurse. Cooper's (1973) most frequently occurring occupations included housewives, teachers, students, salespeople, owners/managers, executives, singers, clerks, lawyers, and engineers. Koufmann and Isaacson (1991) suggested a useful four level scale of vocal usage (see Table 5–1).

In reviewing this scale, however, the voice pathologist must not assume that a voice disorder experienced by a Level IV patient is any less important or has any less of a functional or emotional impact on the patient as those classified as Level I. Although the financial implications of the voice disorder may not be as great, each patient dictates his or her own level of concern related to the effects of the voice problem.

REFERRAL

The majority of voice referrals are received by voice pathologists from the otolaryngologist. When the referral is from elsewhere, the voice pathologist must refer the patient for an otolaryngologic examination. The importance of this medical examination, for both adults and children cannot be overstated. Although Sander (1989) argued against aggressively pursuing voice treatment for children, we have,

TABLE 5–1.   Levels of Vocal Usage.

	Description	Examples
Level I	Elite vocal performer	Singer, actor
Level II	Professional voice user	Clergyman, lecturer
Level III	Nonvocal professional	Teacher, lawyer
Level IV	Nonvocal nonprofessional	Laborer, clerk

unfortunately, seen children who were treated unsuccessfully for "hoarseness" for long periods of time prior to medical evaluation. Subsequent indirect laryngoscopy revealed a small anterior web in one child and papilloma in another. Even more dramatic was the 12-year-old girl who was discovered to have a squamous cell laryngeal carcinoma. This unfortunate young lady required a total laryngectomy. Certainly, the possibility of a life-threatening pathology is greater in the adult population, but these examples demonstrate the need and value of conducting the medical examination prior to the onset of voice therapy.

In more recent years, with the development of managed-care insurance plans, referrals to all medical specialists and therapy services are managed through the patient's primary care physician. The voice pathologist must become educated in issues related to insurance and referral protocols in order to guarantee appropriate coverage for services provided to the patient. If the referral protocols are not followed, then payment will be denied.

Initial identification of the voice problem may have occurred in several ways. From a management standpoint it is most positive when the patient identifies the problem. Our definition from Chapter 1 established that a voice disorder may exist if the structure and/or function of the laryngeal mechanism no longer met the voicing requirements established for it by the owner of the voice. Self-discovery and awareness of the problem yield more highly motivated patients.

Initial identification of vocal symptoms may also have been made by friends or family members, during a speech pathology screening in the schools or during a medical examination conducted by the family physician. When identification of the problem is made by someone other than the patient, the owner of the voice may not consider it to be a problem. When this is the case, it becomes the responsibility of the voice pathologist to educate the patient regarding the disorder and to point out potential problems associated with the disorder (Blood, Mahan, & Hyman, 1979). The ultimate choice for treatment or management remains with the owner of the voice.

The voice pathologist must also remember that the owner of the voice is also the owner of the voice problem and is ultimately responsible for resolving the problem. The history of the medical profession has traditionally placed the responsibility of our illness and wellness squarely on the shoulders of the physician. Too often we hear statements such as "The doctor will take care of it. The doctor will make me better." Successful voice therapy is predicated on a motivated patient taking charge of a well-planned management program and following that program to the desired result, improved voice. The voice pathologist must not permit the patient to transfer ownership of the problem.

MEDICAL EXAMINATION

A complete otolaryngologic examination involves taking a detailed history of the problem and examination of the entire head and neck region. Pertinent medical history is also discussed. The examination includes otoscopic observation of the ears; examination of the oral and nasal cavities; palpation of the salivary glands, lymph nodes, and thyroid gland; and a visual examination of the larynx. The larynx is typically viewed utilizing indirect laryngoscopy (Figure 5–1). To perform this examination, the laryngologist grasps the tongue and gently pulls it forward and down while placing the laryngeal mirror in the pharynx. Artificial light is directed by the head mirror to reflect off the laryngeal mirror, illuminating the pharynx. The larynx is then viewed

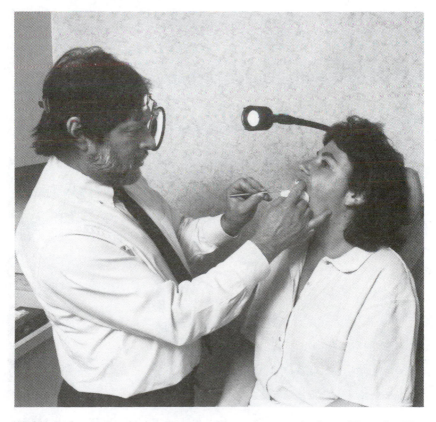

Figure 5–1.   Indirect laryngoscopy using a laryngeal mirror. (Photo by Rick Berkey, St. Elizabeth Medical Center, Dayton, Ohio.)

on the laryngeal mirror with the image of the right and left vocal folds reversed. Patients are typically asked to produce the phoneme /i/ so that the vocal fold approximation may be easily viewed. The attempt to say /i/ draws the epiglottis forward to expose the interior of the larynx. Patients with a sensitive gag reflex may have the tongue and pharynx sprayed with a topical anesthesia to suppress the reflex.

Fiberoptic laryngoscopy is also available as a simple office procedure for examining the larynx directly. When using this technique, the physician introduces a fiberoptic laryngoscope into the patient's pharynx via the nasal cavity (Figure 5–2). This device is a long flexible tube that contains fiberoptic light bundles and a lens. A small hand control permits the flexible end of the scope to be manipulated. When the scope is attached to a light source, the larynx and surrounding struc-

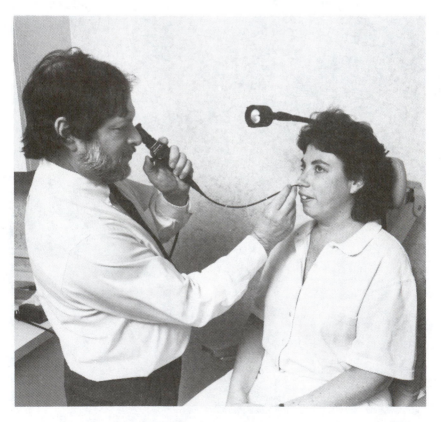

Figure 5–2. Flexible endoscopy. (Photo by Rick Berkey, St. Elizabeth Medical Center, Dayton, Ohio.)

tures may be viewed either through an eyepiece or the larynx may be observed on a video monitor when the eyepiece is attached to a video camera (Yanagasawa & Yanagasawa, 1991). Fiberoptic laryngoscopy is often performed on patients who cannot tolerate indirect mirror laryngoscopy. A topical anesthesia may be used with this procedure.

The larynx may also be viewed through direct laryngoscopy. With this surgical procedure, the patient undergoes a general anesthesia, most often in outpatient surgery. A magnifying laryngoscope is then placed in the pharynx via the oral cavity. A direct microscopic view of the larynx is obtained. Biopsies and surgical excisions may also be performed through the laryngoscope.

The medical examination may also include special radiographs of the head, chest, and neck as well as blood analyses and swallowing studies. The final result of the medical examination and studies is a diagnosis of the problem and recommendations for treatment. Treatment choices may include medical, surgical, voice evaluation and therapy, or any combination of these choices.

VOICE PATHOLOGY EVALUATION

As previously stated, the three major objectives of the diagnostic voice evaluation are (1) to identify the causes of the voice disorder, (2) to describe the present vocal components, and (3) to develop an individualized management plan. Following referral from the otolaryngologist, the voice pathologist will begin this diagnostic process with the patient interview.

The patient interview is the most important component of the voice evaluation. It is during the interview that the voice pathologist will develop an understanding of the causes of the disorder and develop a rapport with the patient that permits the therapeutic process to proceed. Several formats may be utilized to interview the patient. Some voice pathologists choose a questionnaire format that requires the patient to respond to prepared questions either prior to or during the evaluation. The answers to the prepared questions are then used to stimulate further understanding of the problem. Though helpful for the beginning clinician, we find prepared forms to be somewhat restrictive and prefer to use a less formal, yet systematic patient interview format. (This format is described in detail in Stemple, 1993, and is expanded upon here.) Goals have been established for each section of this format and every attempt is made during the interview to accomplish each goal. The suggested format that follows relates to the sample report (**SR**) located at the end of this chapter.

DIAGNOSTIC VOICE EVALUATION

Referral

Goals: Establish the identity of the referral source.

The referral source should be clearly understood at the beginning of the evaluation. The major referral sources will be the otolaryngologist, other speech pathologists, physicians, voice teachers, vocal coaches, the patient's relatives and friends, or the patient may be self referred. **(See SR #1.)**

Reason for the Referral

Goals: (1) Establish exact reason for the patient referral; (2) establish patient's understanding for the referral; (3) develop patient knowledge of the voice disorder; (4) establish credibility of the examiner.

It is important that the voice pathologist have accurate information regarding the exact reason the patient was referred. When a patient is referred by a physician, the specific medical diagnosis should be reported along with the physician's expectations related to your contact with the patient. There are many reasons for patient referrals. These may include simply preoperative tape recording of the voice, laryngeal function studies (see Chapter 6), evaluation without management, preoperative trial voice therapy, postoperative evaluation and treatment, or a complete diagnostic voice evaluation with the appropriate management plan. In our practice, it is not unusual for patients to be referred only for a laryngeal videostroboscopic evaluation. Understanding the physician's expectations will avoid confusion and will help to maintain the necessary cooperative working relationships. **(See SR #2.)**

It is also desirable as you initiate the evaluation that the patient's understanding of the referral for "speech therapy" be established. Quite often the patient is confused about the purpose of being evaluated by a "speech therapist." This confusion may be addressed by simply asking the patient, "Do you understand why Dr. A. referred you here?" When confusion is evident, explanation of the voice pathologist's role is given along with the three major goals you intend to accomplish during the evaluation. As patients better understand the process and procedures, the more reliable they become in communicating pertinent information throughout the evaluation.

It is also helpful to develop the patient's knowledge of the voice disorder before proceeding. This knowledge base may be developed by offering a brief description of how the normal laryngeal mechanism works and how it is affected by the specific pathology. With this information, patients will better understand where certain questions are leading and may be able to give more reliable information. Some patients even volunteer pertinent information following this discussion and before questions are asked. A typical dialogue between a patient (Pt) and voice pathologist (VP) might be:

VP: Do you understand what vocal nodules are and how they might develop?

Pt: Dr. A. said that they're like bumps on my vocal cords and that I got them cause I holler too much.

VP: That may be, but there are many reasons why nodules may develop. Let's talk about it. When Dr. A. looked down your throat with his mirror, he was essentially looking at two solid shelves of muscle tissue, one on each side. (It is helpful to schematically draw the vocal folds or to show a picture so that patients may be able to visualize the anatomy. Use of the patient's own stroboscopic video is extremely helpful if available.) These shelves are the vocal cords, or folds, and we're looking straight down on top of them in this picture. The point where the two folds meet is inside the V of your Adam's Apple. Can you feel yours? Now, the space between the vocal folds is called the glottis and the tube below the folds is the windpipe or trachea. This, of course, is the airway where air travels to the lungs as we breathe.

Attached to the back of each vocal fold we have two cartilages, one here and one here. These cartilages serve as the points of attachment for the vocal folds and for other muscles responsible for approximating and separating the vocal folds. When the vocal folds are approximated, air pressure from the lungs may build beneath the folds. When the pressure is great enough, the air will blow the folds apart and begin the vibration which we hear as voice.

If the muscles pull too hard and the air pressure is too great, such as when we shout, talk loudly over noise, or even when we cough, this excessive tension and pressure will cause the vocal folds to bang and rub together. (Demonstrate with hand clapping movements.) If this banging and rubbing occurs frequently, the impact will eventually cause some swelling or edema of the vocal folds that will usually cause a temporary hoarseness. We have all experienced this kind of hoarseness, maybe at a party or a sporting event. In a day or two this hoarseness goes away. But, if whatever caused the hoarseness persists, the folds may remain edematous and will eventually begin to try to protect themselves from further damage. In your case, they've done this by developing layer by layer small callous-like structures on the point of the vocal folds where they hit the hardest. These growths are called vocal nodules.

As you've experienced, the nodules have caused change in your voice. Because of the edema and the presence of the nodules, your voice may have dropped in pitch; and because the nodules cause gaps to occur on either side of them when the vocal folds approximate to vibrate, a greater amount of air escapes causing you to sound breathy. You've also probably noticed that when you do a lot of talking that your voice weakens, and it becomes quite an effort just to talk. By the end of the day, some people report being worn out from the effort, and simply don't feel like talking anymore.

One final point. Vocal nodules are not a cancerous type of growth and do not eventually lead to cancer. Many people do not understand this, so I think it's important to mention. Does this information help you to better understand what vocal nodules are and how they affect voice?

Pt: Yes, now I do. I am glad that you mentioned the part about cancer. I have to admit that I was worried about that. But, what do you think caused my nodules? I really don't raise my voice that much.

VP: That's what we're here today to try and find out. I'm going to ask you many questions. I need to get to know who you are and how you use your voice in all situations. From that information, we will try to determine specifically what caused your nodules and then develop a plan to attempt to resolve them. Any questions?

It should also be noted that this type of discussion goes far in developing your credibility as the person who is qualified to help resolve this disorder. The voice pathologist will have managed to develop a high level of trust before the actual diagnostic questioning regarding the history of the problem begins.

History of the Problem

Goals: (1) Establish the chronological history of the problem; (2) seek etiologic factors associated with the history; (3) determine patient motivation for resolving the problem.

This section of the evaluation is designed to yield an exact history of the disorder from the onset of vocal difficulties, through the development of the problem over time, and ending with the patient's current vocal experiences. All questions are designed to yield information regarding the causes of vocal difficulties. Finally, the patient's motivation for seeking vocal improvement is determined. (The reader is asked to read **SR#3**.) A list of appropriate questions might include:

- Let's go way back. When did you first begin to notice some change or difficulty in your voice?
- Was that the first time that you ever experienced vocal difficulties?
- How did the problem progress from there?
- What finally made you decide to see your doctor about it?
- What did the doctor tell you?
- How did the doctor treat the problem?
- Did your family doctor refer you to the ear, nose, and throat doctor?
- Has anyone else in your family ever experienced a voice problem?
- Does your voice follow a pattern? For example, is it better in the morning than in the evening or vice versa?
- Do you get more hoarse simply by talking normally?
- Have you ever lost your voice totally?
- Do you have any occasion to raise your voice, to talk over noise, or to shout?
- Are you required to talk to anyone who is hard of hearing?
- Do you have a pet?
- Since I have never heard your voice before, I don't know what your normal voice sounds like. I have a five point scale where 1 represents perfectly normal voice and 5 represents as hoarse as you have ever been with this current problem. Where are you on that scale today?
- How much does this problem actually bother you? Is it causing any daily problems at home or on your job?
- What is your interest in pursuing voice therapy?

Questions similar to these will lead the voice pathologist along the trail of the development of the voice disorder. The answers will also provide the examiner with an idea of the severity level of the problem as perceived by the patient and the motivation to follow the course of treatment necessary for improvement. On rare occasions, patients have at this point expressed a disinterest in continuing with the diagnostic process. Indeed, the problem is not of sufficient concern to them to proceed. We have been referred patients who, once they understood that they did not have cancer, were not interested in the consequences of their dysphonia. While it is the voice pathologist's responsibility to inform the patient and attempt to motivate the patient to seek positive change, the ultimate decision of following through with treatment rests with the patient.

Medical History

Goals: (1) Seek medically-related etiologic factors; (2) establish awareness of patient's basic personality.

The medical history seeks out any medically-related factors that may have contributed to the development of the present voice disorder. Utilizing our knowledge of medically related etiologies, questions are asked regarding past surgeries and hospitalizations. Chronic disorders are probed along with the use of medications. Smoking, alcohol, and drug use histories are also explored and the patient's current hydration habits are discussed.

The medical history is also used to help the voice pathologist establish how patients "feel" about their physical and emotional well-being. This may be accomplished by asking the patient whether, on a day-to-day basis, they feel "excellent, good, fair, or poor." The response to this question will often offer this insight. For example, some patients report lengthy medical histories with many chronic disorders that would give them the right to feel "poor." They indicate, however, that, on a day-to-day basis, they feel "good." Other patients, with unremarkable medical histories, may report feeling only "fair" or "poor."

The answer to this simple question is helpful in learning the basic personality of the patient. A negative response provides the voice pathologist with an excellent opportunity to pursue the line of questioning further. For example, your response may be, " Oh, why just Fair?" This is often a pivotal moment in the evaluation process and, more often than not, patients share many important details related to their emotional well-being. These details may be related to marriage, family, job, or friends. Patients with voice disorders often share their emotions and concerns with voice pathologists because, frankly, we are the first people to ask and show an interest. Handling this information and guiding the patient appropriately becomes a major responsibility. **(See SR#4.)**

Social History

Goals: (1) Develop knowledge of the patient's work, home, social, and recreational environments; (2) discover emotional, social, and family difficulties; (3) seek additional etiologic factors.

The social history is the final opportunity to gather further information about the patient and the patient's work, home, recreational and social environments and lifestyles that may contribute to the development of the voice disorder. All questions probe for answers to possible etiologic factors. For example:

- Are you married, single, divorced, widowed?
- How long have you been married, single, divorced?
- Do you live alone or with other people?
- Do you have children? What are their ages? How many are still at home?
- Does anyone else live in your home? Parents, aunts, friends?
- Do you work outside of the home? Where? How long?
- What kind of work do you do? Specifically, what do you do in your job?
- How much talking is required and how much is social?
- Does your husband/wife work? Where? How long? What shift?
- When you are not working, what do you enjoy doing: clubs, hobbies, groups, organizations, sports, other social activities and so on?
- Are you involved in any hobbies or activities where you are in contact with dust, fumes, chemicals or paints?
- Sometimes stress and tension may contribute to the development of voice problems. In all of these activities and relationships that we've discussed, are their any issues that you think might contribute to this type of tension or stress?

As you begin the questioning related to the social history, you may find it helpful to explain to patients that you need to get to know who they are and what they do in order to find the causes for their vocal difficulties. You want the patient to excuse you if some of the questions seem personal. This questioning is necessary when trying to discover all possible causes. You should not be surprised when patients open up to you with many personal, family, social, marital, or work problems. Because you have developed your credibility and gained the patient's trust, you will most often be given this important information. **(See SR#5.)**

Oral-Peripheral Examination

Goals : (1) Determine the physical condition of the oral mechanism; (2) observe laryngeal area tension; (3) check for swallowing difficulties; (4) check for laryngeal sensations.

A routine oral-peripheral examination should be conducted to determine the condition of the oral mechanism in its relation to the patient's speech and voice production. Also included is observation of the patient's laryngeal area and whole body tension. This is accomplished by utilizing visual observation of posture and neck muscle tension as well as careful digital manipulation of the thyroid cartilage. When tension is not present, the thyroid cartilage may be gently rocked back and forth in the neck. Laryngeal hyperfunction often contributes to laryngeal strap muscle tension precluding this rocking motion, with the muscle tension often causing laryngeal area muscle aching or discomfort. Indeed, patients should be asked about laryngeal sensations as common sensations associated with voice disorders include throat dryness, tickling, burning, aching, lump-in-the-throat, or thickness sensations. Finally, patients should also be asked whether any swallowing difficulties are present. This information will determine whether the swallowing function has been affected by or is affecting vocal production. **(See SR#6.)**

Evaluation of Voice Components

Goals: (1) Describe the present vocal components; (2) examine inappropriate use of vocal components.

The direct evaluation of voice is conducted to describe the present condition of voice production and to determine whether any vocal components are being utilized in a habitual inappropriate manner to the degree of contributing to the development or maintenance of the pathology. Each vocal component is examined separately following a general subjective description of voice quality.

Through the patient interview, the examiner has had an adequate sample of conversational voice in which to make a subjective description of the patient's voice quality. Several formal voice rating scales have been developed and utilized for perceptually judging voice quality (Gelfer, 1988; Hirano, 1981; Wilson, 1979; Wilson, 1970). It has been our experience that most physicians to whom we report diagnostic information are not familiar with these formal scales. We have, therefore, chosen to report the degree of baseline dysphonia on a five point scale with (1) mild, (2) mild to moderate, (3) moderate, (4) moderate to severe, (5) severe dysphonia. This scaled description is followed, for the future reference of the examiner, by a descriptive characterization of the voice including descriptive terms such as hoarseness, harshness, breathiness, raspiness, glottal fry, low pitch and so on. **(See SR#7.)** The vocal properties are then individually reviewed including:

> *Respiration:* This includes a description of conversational breathing patterns including supportive or nonsupportive thoracic or diaphragmatic breathing patterns. We have

not observed the oft used term clavicular breathing in our patients. Use of residual air for phonation is determined through observation. The s/z ratio is formally tested (Eckel & Boone, 1981). The presence of laryngeal mass lesions will yield a longer voiceless /s/ than the voiced /z/ because of the inability of the folds to adequately approximate. Generally, ratios greater than 1.4 are considered abnormal. Several trials of each phoneme are conducted with the patient encouraged each time to give maximum effort in sustaining for as long as possible. In addition, they are coached to produce their maximum inhalation. **(See SR#8.)**

Phonation: Subjective observations regarding the actual voice onset, phonatory register, and strength of phonatory adduction may be made through critical listening. These observations may include the presence of hard glottal attacks, glottal fry, breathiness, or overly compressed adduction. These phonatory symptoms may be observed conversationally throughout the evaluation. The symptoms may also be rechecked simply by having the patient say the ABC's slowly and more rapidly. **(See SR#9.)**

Resonation: Observation regarding the type of resonance quality is made. When abnormal the consistency and stimulability for normal production will be further tested. **(See SR#10.)**

Pitch: The patient's present pitch range is tested by singing up and down the scale from mid-range voice in whole notes until the highest and lowest attainable notes ave been identified. Conversational inflection and pitch variability are also described. **(See SR#11.)**

Loudness: The appropriateness of the patient's speaking loudness level and the variability of loudness, as observed during the interview, is described. It is also important to test the patient's ability to increase subglottic air pressure. This may be done by simply asking the patient to shout *"Hey!"* We have found that the ability to produce a solid phonation during a shout, in the presence of a dysphonic conversational voice, is a positive prognostic sign. When the patient is able to override the dysphonia with increased intensity (which is determined by the ability of the folds to approximate tightly to increase subglottic air pressure), the disorder appears to respond more quickly to remediation methods. **(See SR#12.)**

Rate: The rate of a patient's speech may contribute to the development of laryngeal pathology. This is especially true for the individual who speaks with an exceptionally fast rate of speech. As observed during the diagnostic work-up, the speech rate may be described as normal, fast, or slow. The rate may also be judged to be monotonous, and like pitch and loudness, rate may contribute to a lack of speech and voice variability. **(See SR#13.)**

Impressions

Goal: To summarize the etiologic factors associated with the development and maintenance of the individual's voice disorder.

The impressions section of the diagnostic evaluation is utilized to summarize the causes of the voice disorder discovered throughout the evaluation. These causes are listed in order of perceived importance as they relate first to the initiation of the problem and second to the maintenance of the problem. Remember, the precipitating factor may not be the maintenance factor. **(See SR#14.)**

Prognosis

Goal: To analyze the probability of improvement through voice therapy.

The prognosis for improving many voice disorders through voice therapy is generally good. However, many factors influence prognosis including the patient's motivation, interest, time available, ability to follow instructions, and physical and emotional status, to name a few. The prognosis statement permits the voice pathologist to give a subjective opinion regarding the chances for improved voice production based on the diagnostic information. A reasonable time frame for expected completion of the management program should also be stated. **(See SR#15.)**

Recommendations

Goal: Outline the management plan.

The management plan is then briefly outlined based on the etiologic factors discovered during the evaluation and the medical examination. The outline will include the therapy approaches to be utilized and additional referrals to be made. **(See SR#16.)**

ADDITIONAL CONSIDERATIONS

The evaluation format we have presented may be classified as semistructured. The basic questions remain the same from patient to patient, but the answers given by individual patients dictate the direction in which the questions will proceed and the order in which each diagnostic section is reviewed. The format favors the more experienced voice pathologist. The beginning clinician may feel the need for a more structured format such as the questionnaire format previously mentioned. As experience is gained, the structured formats may prove limiting, with the semistructured method often becoming the method of choice.

The diagnostic report should include only the information pertinent to the development and maintenance of the voice disorder as well as the projected plan of care. Referring physicians are not interested in the patient's life history. Indeed, most physicians turn directly to the sections on impressions and recommendations, thus the need for a detailed explanation of the problem and the plan of care.

Some voice pathologists also feel most comfortable tape recording the entire diagnostic session for later review. This review may help in determining the exact vocal components produced during the evaluation and serves as a record of the baseline voice quality. Even when the entire diagnostic session is not recorded, recording of a standard speech sample is necessary for later reference. It is not unusual for the voice pathologist and the patient to forget the actual severity of the baseline voice quality. Tape recordings serve as an objective reminder and should be used liberally throughout the treatment of the patient.

Finally, the American Speech-Language-Hearing Association mandates that patients who undergo speech, language, and voice evaluations must have a current hearing screening. Audiometric evaluation is important for the patient with a voice disorder. The inability to monitor voice well may result in the use of inappropriate vocal components. Severe voice disorders are often observed in the hard-of-hearing and deaf populations.

SUMMARY

Diagnosis is probably the most important single aspect of a remedial program. (Moore, 1971, p. 108)

A systematic diagnostic voice evaluation may be utilized with all types of voice disorders, with minor modifications in the format made as needed. The major goals are to discover the causes of the voice disorder and to describe the present vocal components. Once discovered a management program may be planned in which the causes are modified or eliminated leading to an improved voice quality.

The goal of describing the vocal components has been greatly enhanced with the use of more objective procedures and techniques for describing voice function. Chapter 6 introduces you to the concept of instrumental measurement of voice through a thorough review of acoustic analysis of voice, aerodynamic measurement of voice function, and laryngeal imaging techniques. When combined with the more subjective voice evaluation, these techniques, along with the team care concept of voice treatment, have greatly enhanced the treatment of voice disorders. The diagnostic voice evaluation not only determines the causes of the voice disorder, it also teaches and educates the patient about the disorder. In this manner, the evaluation tool may be viewed, in its own right, as a primary **therapy** tool.

SAMPLE REPORT

Name:_____   Type of Case: Bilateral vocal fold nodules
Age: 44 years   Address:_____
Date of Birth: 2-14-50   Phone:_____
Date: 4-22-94   Examiner: JCS

SR#1   **Referral:** The patient was referred by_____, M.D.,
        otolaryngologist, Dayton, Ohio.

SR#2   **Reason for Referral:** The patient was referred for both evaluation
        and treatment, with a diagnosis of small, bilateral vocal fold nodules.

SR#3   **History of the Problem:** The patient reported first experiencing vocal
        difficulties in April of 1993. At that time, she contracted a cold that
        created an excessive amount of coughing and throat clearing. She
        also then experienced dysphonia, which persisted after the cold
        symptoms resolved. Another cold was experienced over the Labor
        Day weekend at which time the patient became aphonic for two
        days. This motivated her to seek the medical examination. The
        patient reported that her voice quality is currently better in the
        morning and worsens with use as the day progresses. An increased
        amount of hoarseness has been noted following church choir
        rehearsals. Motivation for modifying these vocal difficulties appeared
        to be high due to the patient's vocal needs in her work setting.

SR#4   **Medical History:** The patient was hospitalized in 1979 for a
        tonsillectomy and in 1981 for a complete hysterectomy. Chronic
        disorders reported by the patient included excessive sinus drainage,
        which creates coughing and throat clearing, and nightly heartburn
        which is exacerbated by stress and nervousness. The patient reported
        that she presently takes no medications and that she stopped smoking
        three weeks prior to this evaluation. Her liquid intake was poor and
        consisted of mostly caffeinated products. She had previously smoked
        one package of cigarettes per day for twenty-two years. On a day-to-
        day basis, the patient reported that she generally felt "good."

SR#5   **Social History:** Mrs._____ was divorced in 1984 and has four
        children, ages 20, 21, 22, and 25 years. Three children still live at
        home. She is a civilian employee at Wright Patterson Air Force
        Base where she works as an Equal Employment Opportunity
        program manager. This position involves managing a federal
        woman's job program; career counseling of female employees; and
        the conduction of management relations seminars. Much speaking
        is required on a daily basis, which the patient continued during the
        initial cold and the onset of dysphonia.
            Nonwork interests and activities include playing the piano,
        singing in the church choir, teaching Sunday School to pre-schoolers,
        and conducting church youth meetings, sewing, and reading. The
        patient reported that singing, teaching Sunday School, and the youth
        meetings all tax her voice, creating increased dysphonia. Mrs.
        _____ also admitted to some shouting in the home environment.
        Other than job tension, no emotional difficulties were reported.

SR#6   **Oral-Peripheral Examination:** The structure and function of the oral mechanism appeared to be well within normal limits for speech and voice production. Laryngeal sensations reported included dryness, burning, occasional pain, and a "lump-in-the-throat feeling." The patient reported having difficulty swallowing pills. Food and liquids were swallowed well. Laryngeal area muscle tension was not noted, subjectively.

VOICE EVALUATION

SR#7   *General Quality:* The patient demonstrated a mild dysphonia characterized by breathiness and intermittent glottal fry phonation. She further reported that the voice quality worsened with use and toward the end of every day.

SR#8   *Respiration:* A supportive, thoracic breathing pattern was demonstrated. The patient was able to sustain the /a/ for 14 seconds, the /s/ for 27 seconds, and the /z/ for 22 seconds.

SR#9   *Phonation:* Occasional glottal fry phonation and breathiness were noted. No hard glottal attacks were observed.

SR#10   *Resonation:* Normal.

SR#11   *Pitch:* The patient demonstrated almost a two octave pitch range with good inflection and variability noted conversationally. Habitual pitch level was within normal limits for the patient's sex and age.

SR#12   *Loudness:* Loudness was appropriate for the speaking situation. The patient was readily able to increase intensity to a shout.

SR#13   *Rate:* Normal

SR#14   *Impressions:* It is my impression that this patient presents with a voice disorder with a primary etiology of voice abuse. These include the abusive behaviors of:

1. coughing and throat clearing which have persisted since recovering from the April cold;
2. straining the voice while singing; and
3. raising the voice during youth meetings and in her home.

Secondary precipitating factors include:

1. the contribution of gastroesophageal reflux;
2. poor hydration
3. the necessity to speak excessively on a daily basis in the presence of the current dysphonia;
4. the use of breathy phonation; and
5. general weakness and imbalance of the laryngeal musculature.

SR#15   *Prognosis:* The prognosis for modifying these etiologic factors and resolving the laryngeal pathology is good. This is based on the small size of the nodules, the continued fluctuation of the voice quality, and the patient's apparent desire to return to normal voicing. Estimated time for completion of the vocal management program is 8 to 10 weeks.

SR#16   *Recommendations:* It is recommended that the patient be enrolled in a voice therapy program on a weekly basis with therapy focusing on:

1. vocal hygiene counseling;
2. elimination of the abusive behavior of habit throat clearing;
3. vocal function exercises designed to strengthen and balance the laryngeal musculature; and
4. formal hydration program.

In addition, the patient will return to her family physician to discuss the possibility of being placed on an anti-reflux regimen.

REFERENCES

Blood, G., Mahan, B., & Hyman, M. (1979). Judging personality and appearance from voice disorders. *Journal of Communication Disorders, 12*, 63–67.

Cooper, M. (1973) *Modern techniques of vocal rehabilitation.* Springfield, IL: Charles C. Thomas.

Eckel, F., & Boone, D. (1981). The s/z ratio as an indicator of laryngeal pathology. *Journal of Speech and Hearing Disorders, 6*, 147–149.

Gelfer, M. (1988). Perceptual attributes of voice: Development and use of rating scales. *Journal of Voice, 2*, 320–326.

Herrington-Hall, B., Lee, L., Stemple, J., Niemi, K., & McHone, M. (1988). Description of laryngeal pathologies by age, sex, and occupation in a treatment seeking sample. *Journal of Speech and Hearing Disorders, 53*, 57–65.

Hirano, M. (1981). *Clinical examination of voice.* New York: Springer Verlag.

Koufman, J., & Isaacson, G. (1991). The spectrum of vocal dysfunction. In J. Koufman & G. Isaacson (Eds.), *The Otolaryngologic Clinics of North America: Voice Disorders, 24*, 985-988.

Moore, P. (1971). *Organic voice disorders.* Englewood Cliffs, NJ: Prentice- Hall.

Sander, E. (1989). Arguments against the aggressive pursuit of voice treatment for children. *Language, Speech, and Hearing Services in the Schools, 20*, 94–101.

Stemple, J. (1993). *Voice therapy: Clinical studies.* St. Louis, MO: Mosby Year Book.

Wilson, D. (1979). *Voice problems of children,* (2nd ed.). Baltimore: Williams and Wilkins.

Wilson, F. (1970). The voice disordered child: A descriptive approach. *Language, Speech, and Hearing Services in the Schools, 1.*

Yanagasawa, E. & Yanagasawa, R. (1991). Laryngeal photography. In J. Koufman & G. Isaacson (Eds.), *The Otolaryngologic Clinics of North America: Voice Disorders, 24*, 999–1022.

6

INSTRUMENTAL MEASUREMENT OF VOICE

In the past decade, clinicians and researchers who examine vocal function and rehabilitation have witnessed a rapid explosion of new technology designed to assist in the measurement and documentation of voice production. Several factors account for this rapid buildup of voice and speech analysis tools, including increased accessibility to microprocessing equipment, development of clinically applicable packages for easier recording and analysis of speech and voice events, and the availability of enhanced imaging and video recording techniques (Sataloff et al., 1990).

Unfortunately, the existence of a large armamentarium of speech and voice analysis tools does not necessarily mean better reliability or validity of so-called "objective" measures. Indeed, the utility and application of any tool is only as appropriate as the knowledge of the user. Although product developers and vendors provide continual upgrades in the quality and accessibility of their devices, they necessarily maintain a marketing and business interest that may not always coincide with the best needs of the individual clinician or researcher.

Thus, this chapter examines a range of measurement instruments that are common in clinical voice laboratories and discusses the scientific principles that underlie their development, application, and interpretation. Because no publication can remain current with the continuing technological advances, this discussion addresses general principles, equipment, and measurement techniques, without making specific reference to products in the marketplace.

If instrumental voice measurements are to be useful clinically, the information provided must contribute to the diagnosis, etiology, severity, prognosis, or measurable change in the phonatory disorder (Hicks, 1991). The clinical utility of instrumental measures can be assessed on three levels: **(1) detection, (2) severity,** and **(3) diagnosis.** Can the voice measurement validly and reliably:

1. identify the existence of a voice problem? **(Detection)**
2. assess the severity or stage of progression of the voice problem? **(Severity)**
3. identify the differential source of the voice problem? **(Diagnosis)**

Technologic advances and continued product development seek to enhance the validity of instrumental measures. However, evaluation of instrument efficacy is a complex task, because clinical voice measurements represent a wide range of tools, analysis routines, and recording protocols (Table 6–1). Furthermore, many vocal function measures have limited normative data available to ensure reasonable interpretations or comparisons across laboratories (Bless, Glaze, Biever-Lowery, Campos, & Peppard, 1993) Finally, all equipment is subject to artifact and error, especially when calibration techniques have not been provided. A need for standardization of measurement techniques is recognized clearly among voice pathologists and scientists (Titze, 1991a, 1993).

Table 6–1. Instrumental Measures in the Voice Laboratory

TECHNIQUE	INFORMATION
Stroboscopic imaging of the larynx	Gross structure Gross movements Vibratory characteristics
Acoustic recording and analysis	Fundamental frequency Intensity Signal/harmonics to noise ratio Perturbation measures Spectral features
Aerodynamic measurement	Airflow rate and volume Subglottal (intraoral) pressure Laryngeal resistance Phonation threshold pressure
Electroglottography (EGG)	Measure of vocal fold contact area
Photoglottography (PGG)	Measure of glottal area
Electromyography (EMG)	Direct measures of muscle activity; used for localization of muscle

Today, the clinical voice pathologist is faced with myriad choices in vocal function measures and limited time and resources for testing, analysis, and interpretation. To help discriminate the most useful and expedient tools and measures among the large array of options, Bless (1991) offered considerations to assess the utility and interpretability of various voice measurements. First, are **restraints** posed on the speech mechanism during the measurement process? If so, is the speech product sufficiently **representative** of typical behavior? For example, equipment or speech task artifacts (e.g., tight-fitting face masks, rigid endoscopes in the mouth, sustained /i/ vowel) may limit or alter the voice product to the extent that the measured signal is no longer representative of the voice pathology.

Have the recording equipment, procedures, and analysis routines demonstrated **reliability** across time? Are there adequate **normative references** to allow useful comparison and interpretation of the resulting data? Does the measurement protocol and analysis routine prevent unnecessary and inefficient **redundancy** so that the series of test events is both **efficient** and **cost effective?** No measurement technique will satisfy all of these criteria. Yet, greater awareness of the limits of a particular measure minimizes the possibility of inappropriate or misleading interpretation of the resulting data.

Justifications of voice laboratory equipment and measurements are awash in flattering descriptors: "objective," "documentable," "high resolution," and "noninvasive." But, the user must always recognize that all noninvasive voice laboratory measurements are **indirect** estimates of vocal function from which one might make inferences about voice quality or laryngeal status. (Note that the only direct measure of vocal function is percutaneous electromyography, which is invasive and requires collaboration with an otolaryngologist or neurologist in the clinical setting.) Thus, the levels of observation that are represented by various measurement tools also dictate the limits to interpretation of data (Titze, 1991a). A purpose of this chapter is to clarify both **utility** and **limitations** of the clinical voice laboratory data.

PRINCIPLES OF INSTRUMENTAL MEASUREMENT

Baken (1987) provides thorough explanations of the general principles of electronics, physics, and mechanics that underlie the development and process of signal measurement using many of the voice laboratory tools. These principles have also been described in a laboratory manual format by Orlikoff and Baken (1993). Essentially, speech and voice measures rely on three events: **signal detection, signal manipulation or conditioning,** and **signal reconversion.** In these three processes, the physical phenomenon is:

1. **detected** and **input** by a device, such as a microphone, pressure transducer, flow meter, or electrode
2. **manipulated** in some form, such as **filtering, amplification,** or **editing,** for use with a specific type of equipment or analysis routine.
3. **reconverted** for **output** and display in some readable form, such as a numerical value, oscilloscope tracing, or speaker.

Because most voice measurement equipment relies on a series of inputs and outputs between electronic components (e.g., microphone to tape recorder to computer to loudspeaker or oscilloscope), it is important that users are familiar with some of the technical specifications of standard equipment. Knowledge of the sequence of connections and conditioning events that occur at each point also helps ensure that added error is not transmitted along the component pathways.

For acoustic measurement, signal detection generally begins with a **microphone.** Vibrating sound waves oscillate against an internal diaphragm or other sensing device that has electronic connections to an amplifier and, eventually, an output device, such as a monitor, oscilloscope, or speaker. The free field sound pressure level energy excites the internal diaphragm, changing into mechanical energy, then changing again into electronic energy for transmission through the system. The process of changing energy from one form to another is called **transduction,** and any device that converts the energy is called a **transducer** (Baken, 1987).

Amplification means increasing the magnitude of a signal for capture and processing by a piece of equipment. The exact magnitude of this amplification is **gain,** usually expressed as an input to output ratio (Baken, 1987). **Linearity** of an amplifier is the degree to which gain is constant across all input magnitudes. For example, the amplifier gain across a speech signal should be equal across all frequencies. If the amplifier characteristic is nonlinear, then distortions of the speech signal will be produced. When the linear range is too small for the amount of amplification (gain) applied, a distortion called **peak clipping** occurs. The amplitude peaks and troughs of the waveform are literally cut off or flattened (Baken, 1987).

Frequency response of a component refers to the range of frequencies that can be detected. If the frequency range is too small to apply equal manipulation of the entire speech signal, then the signal will be distorted. Frequency response is commonly expressed as a range (e.g., 20 to 20,000 Hz) and can apply to microphones, recording devices, and speakers (Baken, 1987).

Impedance refers to the electronic current available at the output and input ports of different components. To avoid distortion, the input and output impedances must match. Without this interface matching, errors in the resolution and accuracy of the signal will be passed to the second component, resulting in inaccuracies in the final signal presented for analysis. A typical impedance standard for electronic components is 200 Ohms (Baken, 1987).

Filtering is a process of eliminating energies above or below a certain range. **Low pass** filters allow energy in the lower frequencies to be passed through (high energy rejected). **High pass** filters allow the high frequency energy to pass through (rejecting low frequency energy). A **band pass** filter rejects energy above and below a certain range (band) (Baken, 1987; Kent & Read, 1992).

ELECTRICAL ERROR

These specifications described here are important to avoid electrical error, or artifact. Biomedical technology teams or electronics engineers can provide guidance and recommendations specific to the voice laboratory site and equipment. However, some general recommendations apply. **Cables** must be of sufficient strength and quality and devoid of any breaks or weakness to allow accurate transmission of the current (signal). It is recommended that the cables be coaxial or tri-axial and well-insulated to avoid functioning as an antenna by picking up extraneous electrical signals or 60 cycle (60 Hz) noise from other electrical equipment in the room (e.g., lights, lamps, heating units, etc.). The longer the cable, the greater the resistance along its path, and the greater the likelihood for increased error to be transmitted (Baken, 1987).

ELECTRICAL SAFETY

To ensure protection of the patient, examiner, and equipment in the voice laboratory, certain precautions are needed. Always use **grounded** (three-prong) plugs for all electrical equipment. If old, ungrounded (two-prong) plugs or outlets are still present in the laboratory, have them replaced. Never use a two-prong adapter to override a three-prong plug in a ungrounded outlet (Baken, 1987). **Fuses** should be replaced carefully, using the exact size and strength recommended by the manufacturer. If a piece of equipment blows fuses repeatedly, the source of electrical overload must be examined and repaired. Fuses should never be replaced with a larger size to avoid blowout; this tactic only masks the real problem and can create dangerous electrical safety conditions.

Patients must be protected from inappropriate grounding and low resistance current. Equipment should be stored on nonmetal racks, if possible. If water is used in the laboratory, it should not come in contact with electrical wiring. Never use any equipment that shows signs of distressed wiring (cracks, taped connections, breaks in insulation seal) (Baken, 1987; Orlikoff & Baken, 1993). The wiring and electrical connections between the many components in a voice laboratory should be appropriately labeled and stored off the ground. Wires that are repeatedly pulled, stretched, stepped on, or rolled over will be easily damaged, which creates unnecessary repair expense and a potential electrical hazard. Finally, most facilities have a **biomedical engineering** office that ensures compliance with electrical safety requirements for the particular institution. These personnel can recommend strategies to ensure safety standards in the voice laboratory.

HYGIENIC SAFETY

All laboratory equipment that comes in contact with patients must be sterilized as recommended by the manufacturer. Frequently, disposable items may be substituted for reusable (e.g., airflow tubes), however, this practice can increase expense and waste. Most nursing staff or medical hygiene standards committees can assist the voice laboratory in achieving compliance with the institutional requirements for equipment sterilization.

The examiner, too, must practice stringent and rigid adherence to hygiene. Currently, voice laboratories are recommended to utilize Universal Precautions guidelines, as established by Occupational Safety and Health Association (OSHA) (Hirano & Bless, 1993). This includes thorough handwashing *before* and *after* having contact with a patient and using gloves during any procedure that puts your hands or equipment (e.g., endoscope) in contact with their mouth, nose, throat, or ears (Orlikoff & Baken, 1993).

ACOUSTIC MEASUREMENTS

Acoustic measures of voice production provide objective and noninvasive measures of vocal function. Increasingly, these measures are available at affordable cost, and voice pathologists find them a convenient indirect measure to document voice status across time. Figure 6–1 shows an acoustic analysis system for recording, storing, and analyzing the speech signal.

Although normative information for acoustic measures is not complete, many acoustic measurement tools provide some guidelines for comparison so that a user can discriminate normal performance from abnormal ranges based on that equipment. The validity of acoustic measures can be assessed on three levels:

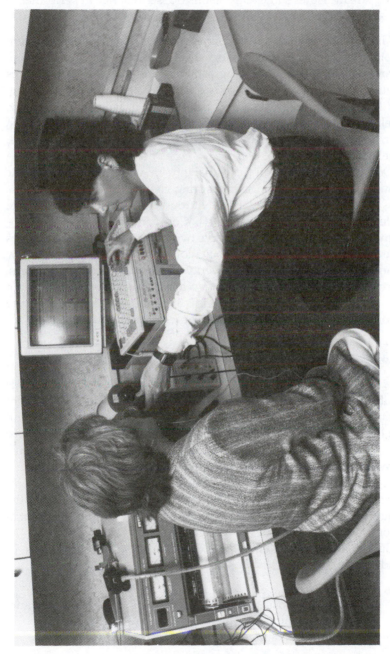

Figure 6–1. An acoustic analysis system for recording, storing, and analyzing the speech signal. (Photo by Rick Berkey, St. Elizabeth Medical Center, Dayton, Ohio)

1.   Can the measure(s) discriminate normal from pathologic voice?
2.   What association exists between acoustic measures and the clinical standard, audio-perceptual judgments of voice quality?
3.   Are measures sufficiently stable to assess change in performance across time?

The efficacy of acoustic measures in discriminating normal from pathologic voice to detect phonatory disorders has been demonstrated. However, there is inconsistent agreement between acoustic measures and audio-perceptual ratings of voice quality (Askenfelt & Hammarberg, 1986; Davis, 1981; Hill, Meyers, & Scherer, 1990; Hillman, Holmberg, Perkell, & Walsh, 1990; Kempster, Kistler, & Hillenbrand, 1991; Laver, Hiller, & Beck, 1992; Ludlow, Bassich, Connor, & Lee, 1987; Wolfe, Cornell, & Palmer, 1991).

Despite known intrasubject variability in vocal function, acoustic measures appear to succeed in measuring change in vocal productions across time (Garrett & Healey, 1987; Nittrouer, McGowan, Milenkovic, & Beehler, 1990; Stone & Rainey, 1991). Comparison of pre- and post-treatment acoustic measures may serve two purposes. First, the measures help evaluate the effects of the rehabilitation plan. Second, they may allow an indirect inference about the severity of the voice pathology. Thus, acoustic measures reflect the status of vocal function generally and do not relate specifically to various etiologies. To date, no acoustic measure purports to differentially diagnose the source of the voice pathology.

Equipment

A large, and ever increasing number of acoustic measurement tools is available for clinical, research, and teaching purposes. Two independent surveys of a representative range of technology (Read, Buder, & Kent, 1990; 1992) attempted to provide information about the available options, utility, capacity, ease of applications, and user friendliness of the most common tools. In the short time since those surveys were conducted, the published reports are virtually obsolete, due to the advent of new tools and the continual upgrade of current existing products. Nonetheless, the critique model proposed by these authors is worthwhile for any potential user or consumer of acoustic analysis equipment.

Buder, Read, and Kent (1992) outline the following points of consideration:

1.   **System Utility**
     Overall purpose and application of the system: clinic, research, teaching
     Number of users involved

Project expandability
Cost limits
Technology support limits at site or institution

2. **Analysis Capability**
    Specific analysis routines desired: vocal function, spectral processing, speech synthesis
    Integration with other speech measurement signals: airflow, pressure, EGG signal, kinematics

3. **Equipment Specifications**
    Hardware and software capabilities: signal capacity, number of channels, memory, speed
    Data management facility: save, edit, replication, manipulation of signal
    Configurability of analysis features: filtering characteristics, sampling rates, original analysis routines to address specific task or population

4. **Speed and Ease**
    Number of keystrokes, processing time needed to conduct analyses

The potential consumer of acoustic analysis programs may wish to add the following selection criteria:

1. **Technical support** and training tutorials available for the novice user and for troubleshooting over the long-term use of the device.
2. Adequacy and readability of the **user's manual,** including normative information and references, if possible.
3. Clinical **macros,** or test routines, that can serve as a convenient framework for developing a standard clinical analysis protocol.
4. **Comparability of data** measures across laboratories, which enhances the standardization and interpretability of findings (Karnell, Scherer, & Fisher, 1991).

Digital Signal Processing

The basis for current acoustic analysis capabilities is digital processing of the speech signal, which has been described by Kent and Read (1993). Speech and voice are **analog signals,** which means **continuous** and **time-varying.** For digital speech processing, this continuous analog signal must be divided up into small discrete bits of information that can be represented numerically. This process is called **digitization** and is achieved by a hardware device called an analog-to-digital (A/D) board or converter.

When a signal is divided up or "discretized" for numerical representation, the process must record faithfully the **change** in this continuous signal across **time.** Thus, two parameters are of interest: the **time-varying** component, as seen on the horizontal axis and the **amplitude** units, as displayed on the vertical axis. To convert this analog signal to digital form, two operations are conducted simultaneously: **sampling rate** and **quantization level.**

The **sampling rate** defines the spacing of the digital points across the original analog signal and is expressed in number of samples per second. For digital voice analysis, most sampling rates are 20,000 Hz or higher. In other words, the original analog signal is "sampled" at least 20,000 times per second. Thus, the sampling rate divides the signal based on time units. The **quantization level** converts the continuous changes in waveform amplitude height into discrete steps or levels. The greater number of quantization levels, the better representation of amplitude changes in the original analog signal. Together, sampling and quantization operations determine the adequacy of the conversion from a continuous analog signal to a digitized waveform.

An important source of error for digitization is in undersampling or "overwide" spacing between sampling points. This undersampling can lead to an artifact known as **aliasing,** where high frequency information is misrepresented due to too few sampling points (Kent & Read, 1993). A similar type of error can occur if the quantization levels are too few, and amplitude changes are insufficiently replicated in the digital signal. Although higher sampling rates and greater quantization levels improve the representation of the analog signal, they also require greater computer speed and memory. For this reason, the minimal standards for sampling rate and quantization level have increased as microprocessing capabilities have expanded.

Kent and Read (1993) described five overall steps in the analog to digital process. These steps incorporate both signal conditioning (filtering) and conversion (sampling and quantization).

Signal Conditioning
1. **Pre-emphasis:** Because low frequency energy tends to be greater than high frequency energy in the speech signal, pre-emphasis is a normalizing procedure designed to equalize the strength of acoustic energy across all frequencies so that low frequency energy does not disproportionally dominate the analysis.
2. **Pre-sampling filter:** a low pass filtering procedure designed to reject high frequency energy above a specified level and limit the threat of undersampling the acoustic signal and the resulting aliasing artifacts.

Digital Conversion
1. **Sampling:** division of time units of the continuous signal into finite units for numerical assignment.

2. **Quantization:** division of amplitude height into discrete steps or levels for numerical representation
3. **Encoding:** the process of assigning numerical values to discrete points along the analog waveform.

Pitch Detection Algorithm

The first acoustic determination for acoustic signal analysis is the fundamental frequency, known commonly as "pitch detection." Examination of the digitized waveform reveals a complex, but quasi-periodic repetition of pitch periods across time. Various schemes have been used to extract the pitch of an acoustic signal. Historically, two approaches were used: **peak-picking** and **zero-crossing.** The peak-picking method identifies the highest point of amplitude excursion in successive periods and calculates the period distance between "peaks" to reveal the pitch period. Zero-crossing uses a similar technique by identifying the point of waveform crossing on the horizontal axis. When the waveform resolution is deteriorated, as in a severely aberrant or dysphonic voice, the amplitude peaks and axis crossing points can be highly irregular or difficult to detect. No pitch detection algorithm can account for extreme acoustic distortion, but zero-crossing and peak-picking algorithms are particularly susceptible to error if multiple peaks or axis crossings occur within a pitch period, thus masking the true distance between waveform periods (Davis, 1981; Titze & Liang, 1993).

A more recent technique (Milenkovic, 1987) utilizes more than one point along a waveform to identify the endpoints of a pitch period. This method has been termed **waveform matching,** because it tracks the entire shape of successive waveforms and uses a mathematical cross-comparison (autocorrelation) of the shape and length of successive waveforms across cycles, with interpolation between waveform deviations. A composite waveform shape emerges, which may be more resistant to error from fluctuations in peak amplitude or axis crossing (Titze & Liang, 1993).

Fundamental Frequency

Once the pitch period (T) is detected, then fundamental frequency (F_0) can be calculated from the reciprocal ($F_0 = 1/T$). Fundamental frequency is the rate of vibration of the vocal folds, and is expressed in Hertz (Hz), or cycles per second. Fundamental frequency is the acoustic measure of an audio-perceptual correlate, pitch. Several frequency measures are useful in assessing vocal function. The **mean fundamental frequency** can be measured during sustained vowels or extracted from connected speech. **Variation** in fundamental frequency during connected speech can be used to reflect changes in intonation. Fundamental frequency range, also called **phonational range,** measures the highest and lowest pitch a patient can produce. The numeric values of fundamental frequency are nonlinear; the pitch difference between 200 and 400 Hz is far greater than the perceptual difference between 600 and 800 Hz. Therefore, the top and bottom frequencies measured in phonational range can be "normalized" on the musical scale and expressed as a number of notes, or **semitones** (Hirano, 1981).

Perturbation Measures

There are many fine waveform analysis routines, but most acoustic analysis programs offer measures of **voice perturbation.** Perturbation is defined as the cycle-to-cycle variability in a signal, and two common expressions of this term are **jitter** (frequency perturbation) and **shimmer** (amplitude perturbation). There is a range of mathematical calculations for these terms, which may vary based on three general parameters (Baken 1987; Orlikoff & Baken, 1993):

1. Length of the analysis window: short versus long-term averages
2. Absolute or relative measurement units: ratio or percentage
3. Statistical expression: central tendency (e.g., mean jitter) or variability (e.g., coefficient of variation of frequency)

There is poor agreement among voice laboratory users, including speech scientists, clinicians, and vendors who develop these tools as to the preference of one measure over another. This lack of comparable measures has limited the development of a coherent normative base of acoustic measures and has impeded cross-comparison of studies conducted in different sites with different measurement tools (Karnell, Scherer, & Fisher, 1991). Another point of confusion in assessing the validity of derived values of perturbation measures is the independent variable of technology advancement. Titze (1991a) observed that so-called "normal" measures of jitter values have dropped across four decades of analysis, as the increased fidelity of microphones and increased speech and memory of signal processing provided better waveform resolution in the acoustic analysis. Technical capabilities continue to improve, and optimal recording standards and equipment specifications may lead to increased stability and validity of acoustic measures (Titze, 1993; Titze, Horii, & Scherer, 1987; Titze & Winholtz, 1993).

Harmonics to Noise Ratio

Acoustic analysis programs often produce a ratio measure of the energy in the voice signal over the noise energy in the voice signal. Like perturbation measures, signal to noise ratios are often derived from different algorithms and expressed in various units, limiting comparison across laboratories. However, the general principle is retained; greater signal or harmonic energy in the voice is thought to reflect better voice quality. Large noise energy (random aperiodicity in the voice signal) represents more abnormal vocal function (Colton & Casper, 1990; Milenkovic, 1987).

Intensity

Vocal intensity (I_0) is the acoustic correlate of another perceptual attribute, loudness. It is referenced to sound pressure level (SPL) and measured on the logarithmic decibel (dB) scale. Both mean intensity and intensity range (maximum and minimum) are useful measures of vocal function. Intensity measurements can be made with a number of different instruments, including sound level meters, acoustic analysis programs, and some aerodynamic measurement devices. However, intensity measures are subject to several artifacts, including influence of ambient or background noise, inconsistencies in mouth to microphone distance, and variations with changes in speech task, vowel production, or fundamental frequency. A standard, well-monitored elicitation protocol will help minimize the potential sources of error in intensity measures.

Phonetogram

The phonetogram, also known as the **physiological frequency range of phonation (PFRP)** has been used by voice pedagogues and phoniatricians in Europe for many years and has gained recent attention for its wide application to functional changes in voice production. In a systematic progression from lowest to highest pitch, the patient produces his frequency range at lowest and highest intensity levels. The resulting plot is an ellipse-shaped frequency/intensity profile, and its dimensions are expressed in semitones. This comprehensive assessment is a useful measure for before and after treatment and for long-term monitor of vocal range development in professional voice users (Bless, 1991; Titze, 1992).

Spectral Analysis

The sound **spectrogram** displays the glottal sound source and filtering characteristics of the speech signal across time. Both formant frequency energy (vocal tract resonation) and noise components (aperiodicity, transient or turbulent noise) of the speech production are presented in a three-dimensional scale. The horizontal axis is time. The vertical axis is frequency, with the lowest energy band representing the fundamental, and formant trajectories above. A third scale is the darkness or "gray" scale (or color difference) that represents intensity change. Spectrogram analysis can provide an estimate of the harmonic to noise ratio of a speech production.

Another form of spectral analysis is the **line spectrum,** which plots all harmonic energies at a single time point. Frequencies are plotted on the horizontal axis; amplitude on the vertical axis. Advanced mathematical routines, such as Fast Fourier Transform (FFT) and Linear Predictive Coding (LPC), have been applied to spectral analysis to identify formant characteristics (Baken, 1987; Kent & Read, 1992). These microprocessing capabilities have increased the speed and accessibility of spectral processing greatly. However, as with other forms of acoustic analysis, FFT and LPC routines are highly sensitive to noise and other signal artifacts. To avoid error, care must be taken to ensure that a clean, undistorted signal is presented to the system for analysis. For voice pathologists, spectral analysis is useful to assess the interaction between the sound source and vocal tract (supraglottic) influences.

Acoustic Recording Considerations

Acoustic analysis routines are written based on assumptions of a quasi-periodic, stable sound source, and recording protocols must accommodate this underlying principle. A sustained or extracted vowel portion must be of sufficient **length** to preserve the validity of acoustic measurement (Karnell, 1991). If the pathologic sound source is so aphonic or dysfluent (e.g., spasmodic dysphonia) that the patient cannot produce a sustained vowel, then acoustic analysis cannot be used with confidence for that speaker.

Variations in **fundamental frequency, intensity,** and **vowel selection** will all affect the resulting acoustic measures (Glaze, Bless, & Susser, 1990; Horii, 1982; Orlikoff & Kahane, 1991). The **number of trials** must be adequate to represent the speech behavior. Occasionally, patients will offer a very unrepresentative first trial production (e.g., too loud, too high pitched) due to some form of uncertainty with the task, or test anxiety. It is crucial that the voice pathologist observe the patient's production carefully to elicit the most representative production. The **test-retest reliability** has also been a concern for users of acoustic analysis data. There is an inherent amount of intrasubject variability in all speech and voice productions. To use acoustic measures for pre- and post-treatment comparison, it is critical to exact a stable baseline measure. A sample recording protocol for acoustic measures is contained in this chapter appendix.

AERODYNAMIC MEASUREMENT

Aerodynamic measurements are interpreted as a reflection of the valving activity of the larynx, representing both vocal fold configuration and movement, structure and function (Schutte, 1992). Air flow and pressure can be measured under stable and transient speech productions. Average airflow rate or flow volume during sustained productions would reflect long-term or average aerodynamic measures. Momentary changes in oral pressure measured during production of plosive or fricative consonants are examples of transient, or short-term aerodynamic measures (Miller & Daniloff, 1993; Scherer, 1991). Combination terms, such as laryngeal resistance or glottal power, integrate pressure and flow in a single measure (Hirano, 1981; Hoit & Hixon, 1992; Melcon, Hoit, & Hixon, 1989). Figure 6–2 displays an aerodynamic recording system for measurement of airflow and pressure during speech production.

The utility of aerodynamic measures is limited by similar constraints as other instrumental measures, including technological error (Miller & Daniloff, 1993), type of speech sample (Holmberg, Hillman, & Perkell, 1989), and intrasubject variability (Higgins, Netsell, & Schulte, 1994). Measures of intraoral pressure, transglottal flow, and combination quotients (e.g., laryngeal resistance) have been used to discriminate normal and pathologic vocal function, assess severity, and in some cases, suggest implications for the diagnostic source of the voice pathology (e.g., hyper- or hypo-functional valving of the vocal folds) (Hillman, Holmberg, Perkell, Walsh, & Vaughn, 1990; Iwata, 1988). An emerging normative data base for aerodynamics expands the clinical utility of these measures and allows some comparison across clinical sites (Higgins, Netsell, & Schulte, 1994; Higgins & Saxman, 1991; Kitajima & Fujita, 1992; Sawashima, Niimi, Horiguchi, & Yamaguchi, 1988).

Pressure, Flow, and Resistance

The instrumentation used for aerodynamic measurement exploits the integral relationship between pressure, flow, and resistance. These physical events behave in predictable ways. Molecules in fluid (air or water) will always flow from a region of higher density (tight, compressed) to lower density (more space). Imagine a hundred people crowded together in a small room. Suddenly a small door opens to the outside. Feeling crowded, the people start pushing toward the door, trying to get outside. The flow of people spreading out into a wider space mimics the activity of compressed molecules or electrons. The molecular movement from regions of higher to lower density is **flow;** when electrons do the same, it is called **current.** Current (electrons) and flow (molecules) are analogous. **Resistance** is simply the impediment to flow, whether molecular or electronic. In the crowded room, the flow of people out the door is limited by the physical constraints of the walls and small door, which pose a restriction or constriction on the natural tendency of people who wish to spread out.

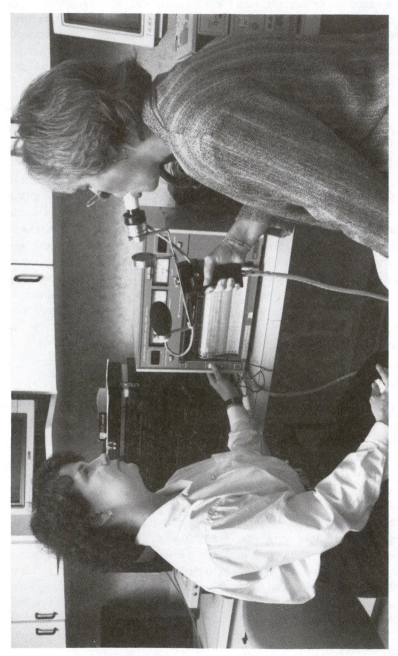

Figure 6–2. An aerodynamic recording system for measurement of airflow and pressure during speech production. (Photo by Rick Berkey, St. Elizabeth Medical Center, Dayton, Ohio)

Asymmetries in the concentration of molecules (or electrons) result in flow. The differences in concentration between two points creates a **driving pressure** and a **potential** for molecular flow. In aerodynamic terms, this asymmetry is represented as **differential pressure**, which is defined as the difference in pressure between two points, and thus the potential to do work. In the electronic form, this potential is called **voltage.** Recall the pressure of crowded people pushing up against the door jam, trying to ease through the small opening. The pressure just inside the doorway is far greater than the pressure just outside of it, where newly unconstrained people are wandering about freely. The relative pressure inside (p1) versus outside (p2) are different. This differential pressure represents the flow asymmetry on either side of the constriction.

Ohm's Law

The relationship between differential pressure, flow, and resistance have been clarified in the electrical principle known as **Ohm's Law,** which states that **voltage** (E) is equal to **current** (I) times the **resistance** (R): E = IR. In the analogy with aerodynamic processes, **differential pressure** (p1 vs. p2) is equal to **flow** (V) times the **impediment to flow** (R): [p1 - p2] = VR. This means that two separate pressure points, measured on either side of a known resistance, can be used to calculate the magnitude of flow (Figure 6–3).

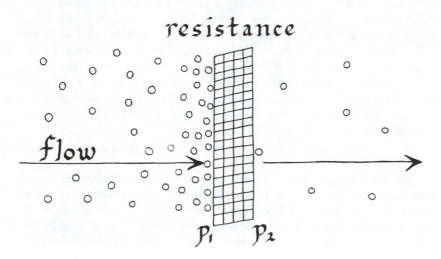

Figure 6–3.   Flow, resistance and differential pressure.

Equipment

Two simple instruments can be used to measure static pressure and static flow directly. The pressure meter is called a **U tube manometer** and consists of a glass tube shaped into a long U standing upright with a calibrated index along the tube. The tube is filled with water or mercury, depending upon the type of pressure measurement needed. Pressure is applied to one side of the U, and the displaced amount of liquid is read directly off the contralateral side in appropriate units (cm H_2O or mm Hg). Airflow rate can be similarly measured, using a **rotameter**, which is a tall glass tube with a small float inside and a calibrated index along the side. When airflow is blown into a port at the base of the tube, the float rises to level that corresponds with the rate of flow. Again, the measure is read directly (ml or cc per second). The significant limit to these two measurement devices is that they can only measure static, or long-term, sustained pressure and flow. Because many pressure and flow measurements in speech production are short-term and rapidly varying, the manometer and rotameter cannot be used conveniently. However, when combined with a compressed air source, they are useful as external measures for calibrating other devices used to measure pressure and flow (Baken, 1987; Orlikoff & Baken, 1993).

Flow Measurement

There are two basic measurements of airflow used in speech production: flow volume and flow rate. **Volume** is the total amount of flow that is used during a certain production, such as a maximum phonation time. Volume is generally measured in liter or milliliter units. The **spirometer** is a respiratory measurement device that records volume measures. Two forms of this instrument are available: wet and dry spirometers. The wet spirometer has two chambers with known volumes of air and water contained within. As the patient blows air into the upper chamber, the volume of water displaced by the flow is measured directly. The dry spirometer utilizes a turbine mechanism. As air passes across the turbine, the number of rotations is calibrated with specific volume amount (Baken, 1987; Colton & Casper, 1990).

The measurement of airflow rate is somewhat less direct, and a range of devices and techniques is available. The most common airflow device is the **pneumotachograph,** which uses the principle of differential pressure across a known resistance to estimate flow rate. A pneumotachograph is essentially a metal tube, with a mechanical resistance (usually a wire mesh screen or a series of small tubes) inside. As airflow is blown through the tube and its resistance, differential pressures are measured at sites directly upstream and downstream to the resistance. Recalling Ohm's Law, flow is calculated using the differential pressure divided by the resistance. The amount of flow divided over the amount of time equals flow rate. A second device used to measure airflow is the **warm wire anemometer.** When flow passes over a warm wire within this instrument, the wire is cooled, changing the electrical resistance of the wire with the change in temperature. The change in resistance in the wire is proportional to the flow, and flow rate can be calculated from that change (Baken, 1987; Miller & Daniloff, 1993).

When airflow is measured, the transducer must be coupled to the face through some form of airflow mask or valve. Flow masks must be airtight to avoid measurement error, but this creates some artifact due to a sensation of "backpressure," which may cause the patient to perform differently. Occasionally, coaching will be needed to ensure that performance is representative of free speech conditions. Rothenberg (1977) developed a mask with screen vents, which gives acoustic feedback to the speaker and alleviates the problem of excess backpressure. The Rothenberg technique measures airflow indirectly from the radiated acoustic power in the glottal source.

Subglottal Air Pressure Measurement

Pressure is defined as the force per unit area, acting perpendicular to the area. In voice production, respiratory (subglottal) pressure acts as a force building up below the adducted vocal folds, rising until the folds open and are set into oscillation. Subglottal air pressure is essentially the power supply, and variables such as vocal fold stiffness, hyperfunctional compression, and incomplete glottic closure will influence the amount of subglottal effort needed to initiate phonation. Thus, voice pathologists use measures of subglottal pressure as an indicator of the valving characteristics of the vocal folds. Subglottal pressure can only be measured directly through an invasive procedure that requires a needle puncture into the tracheal space directly below the vocal folds. This technique is not used clinically.

Estimating Subglottal Pressure

A noninvasive, indirect estimate of subglottal pressure has been used clinically by measuring the intraoral pressure during production of an unvoiced plosive consonant. This pressure is an accurate estimate of the subglottal pressure only under the following assumptions:

1. The oral plosive constriction creates a momentary airtight seal, which provides a continuous opening from the lungs to the lips. Note that velopharyngeal incompetence would violate this assumption.
2. The vocal folds are open so that the oral pressure produced in the plosive production is analogous with the respiratory effort that

would be available as driving pressure to set the vocal folds in oscillation (Netsell, 1969).

Subglottic pressure is estimated from repeated production of an unvoiced plosive + vowel syllable (e.g., /pi/). An oral tube is placed between the closed lips and connected to a pressure transducer. The oral catheter must be placed carefully in the mouth, sealed by the lips, and not occluded by the tongue. The length, diameter, and angle of the tube can influence the pressure measurement (Baken, 1987). The peak intraoral pressure recorded during the plosive production is considered to equal the tracheal pressure.

Phonation Threshold Pressure

Titze (1991b, 1994) defines **phonation threshold pressure** as the minimal pressure required to set the vocal folds into oscillation. The measure has been estimated indirectly using intraoral pressures described above, measured at the exact moment of voice onset for barely audible phonation (Verdolini-Marston, Titze, & Drucker, 1990). Titze (1994) defines the theoretical relationship between phonation threshold pressure and the tissue properties of the vocal folds. Phonation threshold pressure decreases when:

1. the pre-phonatory glottal width is smaller;
2. vocal fold edge is thicker, more rounded;
3. tissue damping (gradual loss of oscillation amplitude) is less; and
4. mucosal wave velocity is less.

These favorable conditions for lower phonation threshold pressure are met when the fundamental frequency drops. In general terms, phonation threshold pressure can be interpreted as a measure of the effort needed to begin phonation. Because speakers with vocal pathologies frequently report greater effort in "turning the voice on," this new measure may prove highly useful for assessing effects of treatment or phonosurgical results.

Laryngeal Resistance

Combination measures that utilize measures of pressure and flow in a ratio or product have also been examined (Hirano, 1981; Smitheran & Hixon, 1981). Laryngeal resistance is the quotient of peak intraoral pressure (estimated from production of an unvoiced plosive) divided by the peak flow rate (measured from production of a vowel) as produced in a repeated train of a consonant + vowel syllable. This measurement is intended to reflect the overall resistance of the glottis, and by extension, serve as an estimate of the valving characteristic, whether too tight (hyperfunctional), too loose (hypofunctional) or normal (Hoit & Hixon,

1992; Melcon, Hoit, & Hixon, 1989). Unfortunately, combination measures pose some limits to interpretability. The magnitude of the derived value (e.g., high laryngeal resistance) is not meaningful without examining the separate contributions of pressure and flow. For example, a measure of increased laryngeal resistance values might be attributable to excessive subglottal pressure, insufficient transglottal flow, or both.

Aerodynamic Recording Considerations

Like all instrumental measures, aerodynamic assessment must be observed carefully to avoid equipment or task artifact. Airflow masks, oral pressure sensing tubes, and oral coupling tubes for spirometry all require an airtight seal with the face or lips. The examiner must attempt to ensure patient compliance and comfort to elicit as natural a speech production as possible. Multiple trials are always useful to secure a stable baseline. Finally, the validity of aerodynamic measures should be verified by conducting a standard calibration routine prior to each examination session. A sample recording protocol for aerodynamic measures is contained in the chapter appendix.

STROBOSCOPY

Laryngeal imaging offers the greatest potential for detection, severity assessment, and diagnosis of the voice problem in patients with voice disorders. Historically, the voice pathologist relied on the otolaryngologist's verbal description of gross laryngeal structure and function, and on audio-perceptual judgments of voice quality to assess, diagnose, and plan remediation for a voice disorder. The advent of endoscopy with stroboscopy not only adds a bigger, brighter, and longer look at the larynx, it provides inspection of the vibratory pattern of the vocal folds during phonation. Figure 6–4 shows the stroboscopic unit used for laryngeal imaging.

Increasingly, the technique of endoscopy with a stroboscopic light source has been used to augment the indirect examination. The diagnostic utility of stroboscopy, which is usually combined with video recording capabilities for documentation and review, has been reported (Woo, Colton, Casper, & Brewer, 1991; Hirano & Bless, 1993). Clearly, the endoscopic examination is **never** a substitute for the otolaryngologist's indirect examination, but the two procedures offer complementary information.

Talbot's Law

The science of stroboscopy is founded on the principle of Talbot's Law, which defines an optical phenomenon called "persistence of vision"

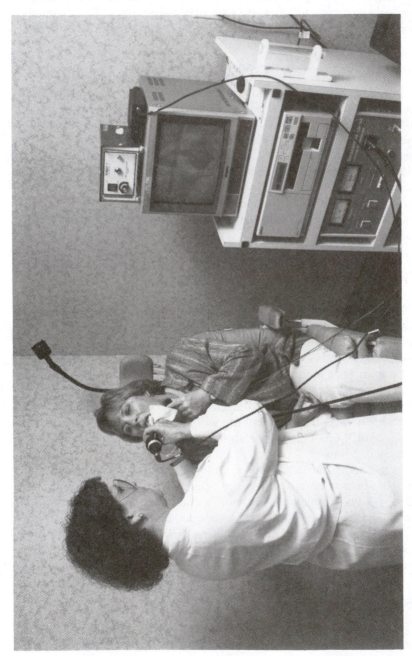

Figure 6–4. The stroboscopic unit used for laryngeal imaging. (Photo by Rick Berkey, St. Elizabeth Medical Center, Dayton, Ohio)

of the human retina. The retina can only perceive a maximum of five separate images per second, at a rate not faster than 0.2 second per image. If separate images are presented at this speed, then the eye will perceive each image independently. However, if images are presented to the eye at faster rates, they will be perceived visually as "fused" or connected images. When a strobe light illuminates the larynx at a pulse rate faster than five images per second, the result is a visual-perceptual composite of the images, perceived as continuous motion (Hirano & Bless, 1993).

The vocal folds vibrate at rates from approximately 60 (low bass) to greater than 1200 (high soprano) Hz. Therefore, these rapidly oscillating vocal fold vibratory cycles are repeated at rates far faster than could be perceived by the naked eye. Stroboscopy light pulses achieve a systematic sampling of these quasi-periodic waveforms, to allow a composite vibratory cycle, sampled from many single points along multiple waveforms, and fused together based on Talbot's Law of optics. Thus, the stroboscopy image, though representative of the general pattern of vocal fold vibration, is actually a composite of separate points sampled across many repetitions.

Mechanics of the Stroboscope

The lighting of the strobe unit is usually achieved by two separate sources: a steady **halogen** light, and a flashing **xenon** light. (Note that one strobe manufacturer offers a unit with only a xenon light source.) The halogen light presents a static view of the anatomical structures similar to the view obtained on an indirect examination. A halogen light is a filament bulb that will burn out after a finite number of hours of use. The strobe pulse light is achieved by the xenon light, which is composed of a xenon gas, and the brightness of the light source dissipates over time instead of burning out at one moment (Hirano & Bless, 1993).

The timing of the xenon strobe flash is triggered by the fundamental frequency of the voice, as detected by a contact microphone placed tightly over the neck (usually near the thyroid lamina). The strobe flash pulses are very short (<40 microseconds) and are triggered under two operating modes to create either a **still** or **travelling** image of the vocal folds.

1. In the **still** mode, the strobe flashes occur at exactly the same point within the vibratory cycle, and the resulting image appears stable or "locked" (Figure 6–5).
2. In the **travelling** mode, the strobe flashes occur at different points within the vibratory cycle, and the resulting image appears as a moving or "walking" wave of vibration (Figure 6–6). Most strobe units achieve this slow motion effect by strobing at a rate that is slightly slower than the fundamental frequency (-1 to -2 Hz).

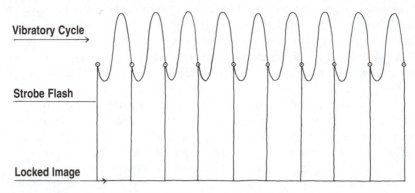

Figure 6–5.   Strobe flash at the same point in the vibratory cycle: still image.

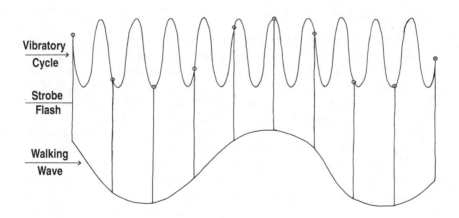

Figure 6–6.   Strobe flashing at different points in the vibratory cycle: travelling image.

The fundamental frequency for most speakers is between 90 to 300 Hz. However, current video technology only allows 50 to 60 separate images (video fields) per second. Therefore, strobing at or near the fundamental frequency results in multiple exposures per video field. For example, if the fundamental frequency is 120 Hz, then approximately two strobe flashes will occur in each video field. These multiple exposures per frame create a "blinky" and sometimes blurred image.

Note that one strobe manufacturer provides the ability to strobe at the fundamental frequency rate or, alternatively, at the video field rate. The resulting strobe image is clearer than under traditional flashing rates because only one strobe flash is generated in each video field. The contact microphone is still used to trigger where within the glottic cycle phase to flash the strobe pulse (J. Crump, Kay Elemetrics, personal communication, 1993).

Endoscopes

Both flexible and rigid endoscopes may be coupled to a strobe generator for the examination (Figures 6–7, 6–8, and 6–9). In general, the flexible endoscope offers a more natural production, allowing the patient to perform multiple speech tasks and the examiner to observe the supraglottic region. However, the flexible endoscope is slightly more invasive than the rigid endoscope and is subject to intermittent changes in elevation as the patient alters position of the velum, base of tongue, and swallows. Consequently, it is more difficult to achieve a stable image, especially during connected speech. Because of the smaller diameter of the fiberoptic light bundle, the image may be darker, although camera peripherals also influence lighting (Casper, Brewer, & Colton, 1988; Hibi, Bless, Hirano, & Yoshida, 1988). The fiberoptic scope is ideal when minimal distortion of the speech pattern is sought, as for patients with a motor speech disorder or for professional voice users.

The rigid endoscopes offer larger, more stable, and often brighter images of the vocal folds, but require a sustained vowel for visualization of the larynx. Rigid endoscopy also avoids some of the optical artifacts due to a stable lens to object distance (Yanigasawa, 1987). Ninety and 70° scopes offer similar views, but require different positioning in the oral cavity (see Figures 6–7 and 6–8).

If the patient has a hypersensitive gag reflex, then the rigid endoscope may be more difficult to tolerate. Usually, patients can be relaxed through coaching, with instructions to keep the eyes open, breathe gently, and watch an image or picture during the examination. Approximately 5 to 10% of all patients may not be able to tolerate the rigid examination without use of topical anesthesia to suppress the gag reflex. Peppard and Bless (1991) have demonstrated that the use of topical does not alter the resulting visual image of the larynx. Topical anesthesia should not be administered without a standing order from a physician and only in a medical setting that is prepared to handle the remote, but possible complications (Hirano & Bless, 1993).

Levels of Error

At this point, it is useful to consider four levels of error that underlie the stroboscopic images.

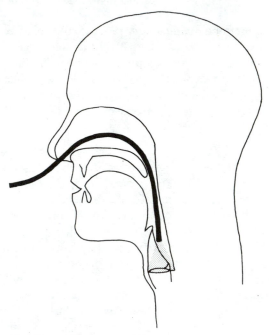

Figure 6–7. Flexible endoscope position.

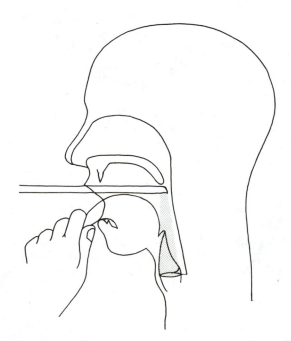

Figure 6–8. Ninety degree endoscope position.

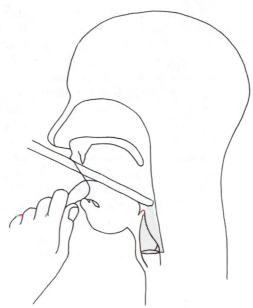

Figure 6–9.   Seventy degree endoscope position.

1. **Stroboscopy is not real-time.** The vibratory image achieved is a result of pulsed flashes timed at various phases across many waveforms, and does not represent a true continuous waveform "slowed down," but rather a composite group of single flashes across time.

2. **Image is seen through optic devices.** The resulting image seen on the monitor screen has been projected through optic devices, including an endoscope, a camera lens (sometimes magnified), and pixels on a monitor screen. Consequently, variables such as lighting, lens focus, lens-to-object distance, uneven angle of lens, color, and video system resolution all contribute to the adequacy and accuracy of the resulting image. The possibility for visual artifacts and distortions from these optic devices must be considered critically as possible limits to the interpretation.

3. **Speech sample may not be representative.** If stroboscopy is conducted using rigid endoscopy, then the speech sample is limited to sustained vowels (usually /i/), sometimes at pitches higher than conversational connected speech, and certainly in a posture unnatural for speech (e.g., mouth open, tongue and neck extended). Certain voice pathologies are masked under these speech conditions, and the resulting vibratory image may not be

fully representative of vocal fold patterns during uninhibited speech. Even use of a flexible fiberscope can alter the patient's voice performance sufficiently to pose a level of error in the recording and interpretation process. Thus, task-based artifacts do exist and must be explored with caution.

4. **Individual subject variability is large.** Many patient factors can influence the success and interpretability of the image, including anatomical limits to full visualization, the levels of comfort and compliance with the tasks, and the severity of the voice disorder. Because the accuracy of the strobe flashing rate is dependent upon stable pitch tracking from the contact microphone, a very aperiodic or aphonic voice may not trigger the strobe light accurately. When this occurs, the image will flicker in a rapid, irregular fashion and is not representative of the vocal fold vibratory pattern. Consequently, individual variability may influence the interpretability of the resulting image.

Criteria for Videostroboscopic Examination

Is a videostroboscopic examination warranted for every patient with a voice disorder? The answer to this question will depend upon the medical delivery model and can be decided ultimately by the professionals who use and interpret this technique. Certainly, permanent documentation of the vocal pathology or status of vocal fold function is worthwhile. However, more critical rationales for using this diagnostic tool are essential if stroboscopy is to be justified to both patients and insurers. The central questions to be addressed include:

1. What information does stroboscopy provide that is not available in the otolaryngologist's indirect examination? Voice pathologists have recognized the unique importance of assessing the vibratory pattern of phonation, an event which cannot be seen without this special lighting technique.

2. How might the stroboscopic imaging influence (in fact, change) either the diagnosis or the treatment plan (whether medical or rehabilitative)? If the diagnosis or treatment plan is not affected by findings on stroboscopy, then the utility of the procedure is limited to documentation and may not be seen as essential to case reviewers.

One set of conservative indications criteria includes the following profiles:

1. Patients with persistent dysphonia (greater than 3 weeks' duration) unexplained by findings on indirect exam (normal or inconclusive).

2. Patients who are professional voice users and have noted changes or decrements in voice performance (e.g., range, quality, stability, or endurance).

3. Whenever phonosurgery is planned, to allow adequate pre-operative examination of the vocal fold status, and post-operatively, to assess recovery from the procedure.

4. To clarify the etiology of the voice disorder, when organic and/or functional contributors are unclear.

5. To determine an optimal management plan, whether medical, surgical, or rehabilitative.

These criteria are far from all-inclusive, and do not purposefully exclude any particular patient group, but are designed to address the questions posed above and provide justifiable utilization criteria for using stroboscopic imaging to make decisions in the assessment and treatment process.

Recording Protocol

The recording protocol will also vary across sites, but generally includes:

1. Full face recording with a connected speech sample (e.g., counting, standard passage, sustained vowels). This allows the examiner to assess overall perceptual quality and free field speech and voice behaviors.

2. The endoscopic recording must utilize a sustained /i/ vowel to bring the epiglottis forward and allow observation of the vocal folds during vibration. The sustained vowels will include habitual and range tasks of pitch and loudness capabilities.

3. Laryngeal diadochokinesis, using both repeated /i i i i/ and /hi hi hi hi/ allows inspection of the medialization and rapid ab- and adduction of the vocal folds.

4. Vegetative maneuvers, including inhalation, rest breathing, coughing, laughing, and throat clearing also allow observation of the function of the laryngeal valve and can assist in detection of any movement aberrancies or left/right imbalance.

5. It is important to use multiple trials of all speech tasks, if possible, to assess individual variability. Often, patient compliance with the exam will improve with time and accommodation to the scoping.

Finally, it important during all recordings to adjust for a stable vertical level (lens-to-object distance) on the left versus right side, working toward achieving a full image (anterior commissure to posterior rim of the glottis), a clear, well-lit and well-focused image, and no mucus, which can obscure the anatomy and mask the presence of lesions.

Observations

Both steady (halogen) light and strobe (xenon) light observations will be made from the recorded image. Although a variety of rating scales and schemes exist, some consensus has been achieved about the salient features for visual perceptual judgments (see Table 6–2). Steady light observations include shape and configuration of the **glottic closure,** whether complete, irregular, hourglass, posterior, anterior, or central (bowing) gap(s). **Supraglottic hyperfunction** refers to the level of medial compression of the lateral ventricular folds, and the anterior-to-posterior "squeeze" of the epiglottis and arytenoids. Often, evidence of supraglottic hyperfunction is also accompanied by a general lowering of the larynx during phonation. Because excessive mucus on the vocal folds may signal dehydration or irritation of the mucosa, its presence is also notable and may be described by location and appearance (e.g., tacky, pooling, etc.). Structural appearance of the entire larynx, including vocal folds, epiglottis, posterior glottic rim, ventricular folds, and pyriform sinuses should be explored, along with movement (ab- and adduction) of the vocal folds, to reveal gross asymmetry or abnormality.

Table 6–2.   Visual Perceptual Judgments of Stroboscopic Image

Steady Light
>   Glottic closure
>   Supraglottic hyperfunction
>   Mucus
>   General appearance
>   General movement

Strobe Light
>   Periodicity
>   Symmetry
>   Amplitude
>   Mucosal wave
>   Stiffness/nonvibrating portion/adynamic segment
>   Phase closure

Other Observations
>   Patient tolerance
>   Endoscope type
>   Topical anesthesia
>   Perceptual quality
>   Fundamental frequency and Intensity: range and habitual

Drawing/Sketch Ad- and Abduction Pattern
>   Midline closure pattern (adduction)
>   Lateral excursion of the vocal folds (abduction)
>   Sites of notable features (e.g., hemorrhage, lesions, mucus, etc.)

Vibratory features for visual perceptual judgments include ratings of timing factors and shape-changing factors. The regularity of timing, called vibratory **periodicity,** refers to the cycle-to-cycle stability of the vocal fold oscillation. **Phase closure** is the relative ratio of glottis open to glottis closed within a single vibratory cycle. Shape-changing factors include **mucosal wave** and **amplitude,** which assess the movement or excursion of the vocal folds in several dimensions during one vibratory cycle. Absence of mucosal wave, called **nonvibrating portion,** stiffness, or adynamic segment, can be described in terms of its location and extent of the vocal fold. **Symmetry** refers to the shape-changing relationship between left and right vocal folds: Do they move in the same manner at the same time? A sample rating form for stroboscopy judgments is contained in the chapter appendix.

Finally, general comments related to the adequacy, compliance, and tolerance of the examination are useful and help ensure test-retest reliability for re-examinations. If the pre-test fundamental frequency, intensity, and audio-perceptual judgments of voice quality are noted at the initial endoscopy, then these factors may be controlled for, or help account for, changes in subsequent exams. Peppard and Bless (1990) described a technique for increasing reliability of repeated stroboscopic examinations. A plastic transparency is placed over the still video image on the monitor, and anatomical landmark boundaries are traced to form a "template." This transparency record is affixed to the monitor in follow-up exams to line up the retest image for comparable size and angle of view.

NORMATIVE INFORMATION FOR ACOUSTIC, AERODYNAMIC, AND STROBOSCOPIC MEASURE OF VOICE

Normative information is crucial to establishing the clinical utility of instrumental measures of voice. Following collection of reliable normative standards, comparisons with pathologic groups may be made. Normative information also gives information about the range and variability of performance in speakers without voice complaints. Ideally, the collection of a normal data base for clinical comparisons should account for many factors that might influence the instrumental results. For example, the **demographic groups** of speakers, including different sex, age, health history, and local dialect should be reported. **Elicitation techniques** and **sample tasks** may vary across studies, as well as **equipment standards** and **analysis routines.** These factors limit the ability to compare findings across studies or sites. Finally, the technologic advances in instrumental performance and fidelity have rendered older data somewhat obsolete. Perturbation measures obtained prior to high speed digital sampling may not be comparable to data collected under different (enhanced) signal processing techniques (Titze, 1991a).

A practical resolution to the problem of limited or incomparable normative data is available to any voice pathologist. Collection of "local norms" can be generated readily by soliciting volunteers from the local community or institution where the voice laboratory is located. Many normal speakers are willing to volunteer as subjects in the clinical test protocol of acoustic recording, aerodynamic measures, and video-stroboscopic imaging. By having the opportunity to run a large group of normal speakers through the voice laboratory equipment, the user can develop a normative data base that is easily referenced for demographics (age, sex, vocal behaviors, health history). More importantly, the findings can be interpreted with confidence because data are collected on the same equipment, using the exact elicitation methods and recording techniques applied to pathologic speakers in that clinical laboratory.

A synopsis of some of the published normative information available for fundamental frequency, intensity, aerodynamics, and stroboscopy is presented below. The purpose is to offer some of the normative levels that have reached consensus among various reports across time. Unfortunately, perturbation measures and signal/harmonic-to-noise ratios employ such disparity in recording techniques, analyses, units of measurement, and equipment variables that no coherent standards have been achieved. Recently, acoustic analysis programs have begun to include normal and disordered speaker data banks specific to their technology and equipment as part of the system package. However, the emerging normal data base for instrumental measures of voice must continue to be expanded with cooperative contributions across laboratories.

Fundamental Frequency

Many studies have examined the speaking fundamental frequency sampled from spontaneous speech or reading passages. Because variables in speech utterance, loudness, and intonational patterns may influence the resulting fundamental frequency, other researchers have used a stable, sustained vowel at comfortable pitch and loudness to minimize variability in findings. The data in Table 6–3 were collected during production of a sustained neutral /ɑ/ vowel, and are commensurate with other reported fundamental frequency data.

Intensity Range

Recording considerations for intensity measurements are both task- and equipment-based. Measures are known to vary based on the vowel or speech utterance, mouth to microphone distance, and filtering characteristics of the sound level meter. The data in Table 6–4 were collected on vowel /ɑ/, using a sound level meter with C scale weighting held a constant 12 inches from the mouth.

Table 6–3.   Normative Fundamental Frequency

	Mean	Minimum	Maximum
Children 6–10 years[1]			
Boys (N = 59)	226 Hz	179 Hz	272 Hz
Girls (N = 62)	238 Hz	193 Hz	294 Hz
Adults [2]			
Males (N = 58)	106 Hz	77 Hz	482 Hz
Females (N = 61)	193 Hz	137 Hz	634 Hz

[1]*Source:* Adapted from Glaze, L. E., Bless, D. M., Milenkovic,P. H., & Susser, R. D. (1988). Acoustic characteristics of children's voice. *Journal of Voice, 2*(4), 312–319.

[2]*Source:* Adapted from Bless, D. M., Glaze, L. E., Biever-Lowery, D. M., Campos, G., & Peppard, R. C. (1993). Stroboscopic, acoustic, aerodynamic, and perceptual attributes of voice production in normal speaking adults. In I. R. Titze (Ed.), *Progress report 4* (pp. 121–134), Iowa City, IA: National Center for Voice and Speech.

Airflow Rate

Airflow rate is will be affected based on the speech sample measured. Sentence productions yielded greater intrasubject variability in airflow than sustained vowels in 11 male and 10 female speakers measured within and across sessions (Higgins, Netsell, & Schulte, 1994). The data in Table 6–5 were collected using a Nagashima Phonatory Function Analyser and sampled during production of a sustained /ɑ/ vowel at comfortable pitch and loudness.

Intraoral Pressure Estimates

Holmberg, Hillman, and Perkell (1988) reported intraoral estimates of subglottal air pressure for normal adult speakers under three conditions: normal, soft, and loud productions, and findings confirmed the covarying proportional relationship between subglottic pressure and loudness. In a follow-up study using low, normal, and high pitch conditions, the authors found increased pressure in both low and high pitch (Holmberg, Hillman, & Perkell, 1989) (see Table 6–6).

Stroboscopic Judgments

Bless, Glaze, Biever-Lowery, Campos, and Peppard (1993) examined visual-perceptual ratings of stroboscopic vibratory features in a study of 121 normal speakers ranging in age from 16 to 92 years. The vibratory features that regressed significantly with increased age were **supraglottic activity, amplitude, and mucosal wave.** Older female speakers also displayed significantly less **regularity** in vocal fold vibration with increased age.

Table 6-4.   Normative Intensity

	Mean	Range
Children[1] 6–10 years (N = 97)	70 dB	60–99 dB
Adults[2]		
Males (N = 58)	70 dB	<60–110 dB
Females (N = 61)	68 dB	<60–106 dB

[1]*Source:* Adapted from Glaze, L. E., Bless, D. M., & Susser, R. D. (1990). Acoustic analysis of vowel and loudness differences in children's voice. *Journal of Voice, 4*(1), 37–44.

[2]*Source:* Adapted from Bless, D. M., Glaze, L. E., Biever-Lowery, D. M., Campos, G., & Peppard, R. C. (1993). Stroboscopic, acoustic, aerodynamic, and perceptual attributes of voice production in normal speaking adults. In I. R. Titze (Ed.), *Progress report 4* (pp. 121–134), Iowa City, IA: National Center for Voice and Speech.

Table 6–5. Normative airflow rate

	Mean	Range
Adults		
Males (N = 67)	119 cc/sec	40–320
Females (N = 78)	115 cc/sec	50–220

Source: Adapted from Bless, D. M., Glaze, L. E., Biever-Lowery, D. M., Campos, G., & Peppard, R. C. (1993). Stroboscopic, acoustic, aerodynamic, and perceptual attributes of voice production in normal speaking adults. In I. R. Titze (Ed.), *Progress report 4* (pp. 121–134), Iowa City, IA: National Center for Voice and Speech.

Table 6–6.   Normative Intraoral Pressure Estimates

	Normal	Soft	Loud
Adults[1]			
Males (N = 25)	5.91 cm H_2O	4.79 cm H_2O	8.39 cm H_2O
Females (N = 25)	6.09 cm H_2O	4.79 cm H_2O	8.46 cm H_2O
	Normal	**Low Pitch**	**High Pitch**
Adults[2]			
Males (N = 25)	6.3 cm H_2O	7.0 cm H_2O	7.5 cm H_2O
Females (N = 20)	5.8 cm H_2O	6.7 cm H_2O	6.1 cm H_2O

[1]*Source:* Adapted from Holmberg, E. B., Hillman, R. E., & Perkell, J. S. (1988). Glottal airflow and transglottal air pressure measurements for male and female speakers in soft, normal, and loud voice. *The Journal of the Acoustical Society of America, 84,* 511–529.

[2]*Source:* Adapted from Holmberg, E. B., Hillman, R. E., & Perkell, J. S. (1989). Glottal airflow and transglottal air pressure measurements for male and female speakers in low, normal and high pitch. *Journal of Voice, 3*(4), 294–305.

OTHER PHYSIOLOGIC MEASURES OF VOCAL FUNCTION

Inverse Filter

Any signal measured at the mouth is a product of two components, the glottal sound source and the resonance characteristic from the vocal tract. Inverse filtering is a technique that theoretically isolates these two components; the supraglottic or vocal tract influence is removed, leaving intact the glottal waveform only. Inverse filtering has been applied to both acoustic waveforms and airflow measurements. The pattern of the inverse filtered waveform can be described in terms of opening and closing slopes, speed and open quotients, and waveform minima and peaks (Colton & Casper, 1990; Fritzell, 1992). One limit to the inverse filter process is the imprecise estimation of vowel formant frequencies and vocal tract area functions for the individual speaker (Titze, 1994).

Electroglottography (EGG)

Electroglottography is a noninvasive technique that uses electrical current passing through the neck to measure vocal fold contact across time. Two electrodes are placed on either side of the thyroid alae, with a small electrical current passing through as the vocal folds vibrate. Tissue conducts the current better than air, so the resistance will increase when the vocal folds are opening and decrease during the closing phase. The EGG waveform displays this variable resistance and serves as an analog of vocal fold opening and closing gestures during vibration, with peaks and troughs representing maximum points of ab- and adduction (Childers, Alsaka, Hicks, & Moore, 1987). The technique is not without artifact, however, because variations in tissue thickness, electrode placement, mucous interference, and laryngeal movements can produce error in this measure (Colton & Contour, 1990). Nonetheless, EGG has been used in combination with other physiologic measures of vocal function, for cross-validation through simultaneous measurement. A most useful application was suggested by Karnell (1989), who synchronized an EGG signal with stroboscopy flash pulses to offer a real-time monitor of the vibratory phase points across the stroboscopic image. A recent improvement in the recording technique was reported by Rothenberg (1992), who has developed a dual channel EGG. This device positions two electrodes vertically on each side of the thyroid to achieve better representation of the upper and lower dimensions of vocal fold contact during the vibratory cycle.

Photoglottography (PGG)

While electroglottography plots vocal fold contact across time, photoglottography plots glottal area across time. The technique uses a light source in the supraglottis (usually a flexible fiberoptic scope) and a light sensing device (photodiode) held against the neck, below the level of the vocal folds. As the patient phonates, the variable light pattern emitted by the opening and closing gestures of the glottis is detected by the sensor and recorded as a glottal area waveform. The validity of this measure is based on the consistency of light transmission through neck tissues. Unfortunately, many speech and voicing gestures can interfere with the light pattern (e.g., epiglottis drift, tongue movements, laryngeal height) and create error. Often, PGG is used in combination with EGG and other physiologic measures. Measures of clinical interest include opening and closing slopes, duty cycle, and speed and open quotients. (Baken, 1987; Colton & Casper, 1990; Gerratt, Hanson, Berke, & Precoda, 1991).

Electromyography (EMG)

Electromyography is a direct measure of laryngeal function and, as an invasive procedure, it must be performed clinically by a neurologist or otolaryngologist. Electrodes are inserted percutaneously into the laryngeal muscles, and the pattern of electrical activity is studied. Because the insertions are essentially "blind," a series of vocal tasks have been described to validate placement of electrodes in the correct muscles. The electrical signals recorded from the muscles are interpreted as normal or pathologic based on four basic features: timing (onset and offset) of muscle activity, and the pattern, number, and amplitude of muscle action potentials. The interpretation of muscle activity patterns is not always straightforward (Hirose, 1986). The widest application of laryngeal EMG is for diagnosis and prognosis in vocal fold neuropathy, including paralysis, dystonia, and other neuromuscular disorders, and for discriminating vocal fold paralysis from mechanical fixation of the cricoarytenoid joint. A more recent clinical application of percutaneous EMG is to identify the correct site of BOTOX injection for treatment of spasmodic dysphonia (Bless, 1991; Harris, 1981; Hirose, 1986; Ludlow, 1991).

THE CLINICAL VOICE LABORATORY

The data generated by instrumental measures of voice constitute the first step toward objective description of voice quality. Increasingly, knowledge of anatomy and physiology of the larynx can be interfaced with vocal function measures. This complementary information improves understanding of the capabilities in normal and professional speakers and the voice production limits of disordered patients. The clinical utility of the laboratory has been defined as a function of pathology **detection,** assessment of **severity,** or differential **diagnosis** of a voice problem. Instrumental measures offer varying success at each of these levels. However, in the rehabilitation process, instrumental measures constitute a fourth level of clinical application as a **primary treatment** tool. Objective measures of vocal function and observation of the laryngeal image can both be used by the voice pathologist to display, instruct, motivate, and justify treatment needs. Instrumental feedback may assist with achieving target behaviors. Repeated pre- and post-test measurements may reinforce the patient's progress. Finally, information about the vocal pathology offers an illustration or documentation of the pathology that may be more convincing than perceptual judgments of voice quality alone.

SUMMARY

Instrumental measures of voice have expanded greatly over the past decades. Acoustic, aerodynamic, imaging, and physiologic measures of vocal function have been enhanced by better recording devices, signal processing techniques, and analysis routines. Voice pathologists have recognized the clinical applications of these measurement tools to integrate instrumental measurements in the diagnosis and treatment of voice disordered patients. Yet, interpretation must be done with care, and users must be knowledgeable about the risks of artifact and error to ensure valid application of these measures. Normative information is still insufficient in most areas, but improving.

GLOSSARY

Acoustics

Acoustic Waveform

Frequency: The rate of vibration, represented by a number of waveform periods per unit time, for example, hertz (Hz) as the number of cycles per second.

Fundamental frequency: The lowest periodic waveform of vocal fold vibration. Fundamental frequency is the reciprocal of the pitch period ($F_0 = 1/T$).

Harmonics (Signal) to noise ratio: The mathematical ratio of periodic energy (signal) to random or aperiodic energy (noise) in a given signal.

Intensity: Sound energy present in a signal, represented by waveform amplitude.

Perturbation: Measures of variability or instability in a quasi-periodic waveform.

Jitter: Also known as pitch perturbation; a measure of cycle-to-cycle variability in fundamental frequency. Can be expressed in absolute measures or as a percentage referenced to the fundamental frequency.

Shimmer: Also known as amplitude perturbation; a measure of the cycle-to-cycle variability in waveform amplitude.

Pitch: The perceptual correlate of the fundamental frequency, based on a judgmental rating from low to high.

Pitch Detection Algorithm (PDA): A mathematical equation designed to detect the fundamental frequency of a speech waveform. Several methods are used commonly: zero-crossing, peak-picking, and waveform matching with autocorrelation.

Pitch period: The length of time for one waveform of vocal fold vibration. The pitch period is the reciprocal of fundamental frequency ($T = 1/F_0$).

Semitone: A unit devised for comparison of frequencies (e.g., 200 Hz to 400 Hz represents a 12 semitone range). The semitone scale includes all of the notes (sharps and flats included) on the musical scale, and is logarithmic. The semitone scale reflects perceptual attributes of the human ear, as the difference in hertz between semitones lower on the musical scale is smaller than semitones that reflect higher frequencies.

Spectrogram: A visual display of a speech signal across time (horizontal axis), giving information about frequency (vertical axis) and intensity (gray or color variation) in the display.

Spectrum: A plot of signal energy (intensity) by frequency.

Signal Processing

Amplification: Increasing the amplitude of a signal to increase the "gain" (measurable or detectable changes) in time-variation for purposes of recording, playback, data measurement, or signal processing.

Analog-to-digital (A/D) processing: Conversion of an analog signal to digital form, using a computer hardware device (A/D board or converter). An analog signal is time- and amplitude-varying and continuous. Digital processing, or digitization, divides the signal into discrete bits of information which are encoded numerically.

Filters: A method of including (passing) and excluding (filtering) specified levels of energy in the signal, usually in the course of signal processing. A "low pass" filter excludes energy at high frequencies; a "high pass" filter excludes energy at low frequencies; and a "bandpass" filter excludes energies higher or lower than a specified band of frequencies.

Sampling rate: The number of samples per second of a digital signal. The greater the sampling rate, the more information obtained for signal processing.

Transducer: A device that converts energy from one form to another, for example, flow or pressure into an electrical signal.

Quantization: The division of amplitude in an analog signal into discrete numeric values. The greater the quantization levels, the more adequately the amplitude waveform is represented.

Aerodynamics

Pressure

Pressure: Force per unit area acting perpendicular to the area.

Differential pressure: Referenced to some other pressure (e.g., between two measured sites, such as left and right nares).

Driving pressure: Flow of a gas from higher to lower regions of molecular concentration.

Intraoral pressure: Obtained from the closed oral cavity when the vocal folds are abducted, as in an unvoiced plosive consonant; an indirect estimate of subglottal pressure (Smitheran & Hixon, 1981).

Phonation threshold pressure: The minimal pressure needed to set the vocal folds into oscillation, considering variables of tissue damping, mucosal wave, vocal fold thickness, pre-phonatory glottal width, and transglottal pressure (Titze, 1994).

Subglottal pressure: Measured directly from the lung pressures below the glottis, when the vocal folds are adducted. Subglottic pressure: estimated clinically using intraoral pressure peaks produced during an unvoiced plosive consonant; a measure of the tracheal (respiratory) driving pressure used during phonation.

Airflow and Volume

Flow: The movement of a quantity of gas through an area.
Flow rate (volume velocity): Speed (and direction) of flow per unit time.

Flow volume: Quantity of flow.

Pneumotachograph: A differential pressure sensing device that measures the drop in pressure when airflow passes across a known mechanical resistance (e.g., wire-mesh screen or narrow tubes).

Rotameter (flow meter): Airflow measurement device; a cylindrical tube with a ball "float" within and an external measurement index. As flow passes through the bottom of the tube, the float rises to a level corresponding to the flow rate.

Spirometer: Flow volume measurement device (wet and dry varieties); records the total amount of air blown across a sensing device (dry) or volume of water displaced (wet) during exhalation.

U-tube Manometer: Pressure measurement device; a bent glass tube with external measurement index, filled with liquid (usually water or mercury). As pressure is applied to one side of the U, the direct reading can be taken from the liquid displacement on the other side.

Warm-wire Anemometer: Flow measurement device; as airflow passes over (and cools) the warm metal wire, its electrical resistance changes, and flow magnitude can be predicted from the change in resistance of the wire.

Stroboscopy

Talbot's Law: Persistence of vision on the retina; the human retina cannot perceive more than five separate images per second (each image "rests" 0.2 second on the retina) and, when presented in succession, are fused into one apparent continuous image. Thus, a series of still images presented at this rate (or faster) will be perceived visually as a connected, moving image.

Vibratory Features

Amplitude: The lateral excursion of the vocal folds.

Mucosal wave: The movement of the vocal fold cover in lateral, longitudinal, and vertical waveform motion.

Periodicity: Regularity of the TIMING of successive cycles.

Phase closure: Ratio of open to close phase of the glottis during one full vibratory cycle.

Stiffness / Nonvibrating portion / Adynamic segment: Commonly expressed as a percentage of the full length of the membranous portion of the vocal fold.

Symmetry: The extent to which the left and right vocal folds appear to move as mirror images; changes in phase are identical.

REFERENCES

Askenfelt, A., & Hammarberg, B. (1986). Speech waveform perturbation analysis: A perceptual-acoustic comparison of seven measures. *Journal of Speech and Hearing Research, 29*(1), 50–64.

Baken, R. J. (1987). *Clinical measurement of speech and voice.* Boston: College-Hill Press.

Bless, D. M. (1991). Assessment of laryngeal function. In C. N. Ford & D. M. Bless (Eds.), *Phonosurgery* (pp. 91–122). New York: Raven Press.

Bless, D. M., Glaze, L. E., Biever-Lowery, D., Campos, G., & Peppard, R. C. (1993). Stroboscopic, acoustic, aerodynamic, and perceptual attributes of voice production in normal speaking adults. In I. R. Titze (Ed.), *Progress report 4* (pp. 121–134). Iowa City, IA: National Center for Voice and Speech.

Casper, J. K. , Brewer, D. W., & Colton, R. H. (1988). Pitfalls and problems in flexible fiberoptic videolaryngoscopy. *Journal of Voice, 1*(4), 347–352.

Childers, D. G., Alsaka, Y. A., Hicks, D. M., Moore, G. P. (1987). Vocal fold vibrations: An EGG model. In T. Baer, C. Sasaki, K. Harris (Eds.), *Laryngeal function in phonation and respiration* (pp. 11–202). Boston: College-Hill Press.

Colton, R. H., & Casper, J. K. (1990). *Understanding voice problems.* Baltimore: Williams and Wilkins.

Colton, R. H., & Contour, E. G. (1990). Problems and pitfalls of electro-glottography. *Journal of Voice, 4*(1), 10–24.

Davis, S. (1981). Acoustic characteristics of normal and pathologic voices. *ASHA Reports, 11,* 97–115.

Fritzell, B. (1992). Inverse filtering. *Journal of Voice, 6*(2), 111–114.

Garrett, K. L., & Healey, E. C. (1987). An acoustic analysis of the fluctuations in the voices of normal adult speakers across three times of day. *Journal of the Acoustical Society of America, 82,* 58–62.

Gerratt, B. R., Hanson, D. G., Berke, G. S., & Precoda, K. (1991). Photoglottography: A clinical synopsis. *Journal of Voice, 5*(2), 98–105.

Glaze, L. E., Bless, D. M., Milenkovic, P., & Susser, R. D. (1988). Acoustic characteristics of children's voice. *Journal of Voice, 2*(4), 312–319.

Glaze, L. E., Bless, D. M., & Susser, R. D. (1990). Acoustic analysis of vowel and loudness differences in children's voice. *Journal of Voice, 4*(1), 37–44.

Harris, K. (1981). Electromyography as a technique for laryngeal investigation. *ASHA Reports, 11,* 70–87.

Hibi, S. R., Bless, D. M., Hirano, M., & Yoshida, T. (1988). Distortions of videofiberoscopy imaging: Reconsideration and correction. *Journal of Voice, 2*(2), 168–175.

Hicks, D. M. (1991). Functional voice assessment: What to measure and why. In *Assessment of speech and voice production: Research and clinical applications* (pp. 204–209). Bethesda, MD: National Institute on Deafness and Other Communicative Disorders.

Higgins, M. B., Netsell, R., & Schulte, L. (1994). Aerodynamic and electroglottographic measures of normal voice production: intrasubject variability within and across sessions. *Journal of Speech and Hearing Research, 37*(1), 38–45.

Higgins, M. B., & Saxman, J. H. (1991). A comparison of selected phonatory behaviors of healthy aged and young adults. *Journal of Speech and Hearing Research, 34*(5), 1000–1010.

Hill, D. P., Meyers, A. D., & Scherer, R. C. (1990). A comparison of four clinical techniques in the analysis of phonation. *Journal of Voice, 4*(3), 198–204.

Hillman, R. E., Holmberg, E. B., Perkell, J. S. Walsh, M., & Vaughn, C. (1990). Phonatory function associated with hyperfunctionally related vocal fold lesions. *Journal of Voice, 4*(1), 52–63.

Hirano, M. (1981). *Clinical examination of voice.* New York: Springer-Verlag.

Hirano, M., & Bless, D. M. (1993). *Videostroboscopic examination of the larynx*. San Diego: Singular Publishing Group.

Hirose, H. (1986). Electromyography of the laryngeal and pharyngeal muscles. In C. W. Cummings, J. M. Frederickson, L. A. Harker, C. J. Krause, & D. E. Schuller (Eds.), *Otolaryngology-Head and Neck Surgery* (pp. 1823–1828). St. Louis: The C. V. Mosby Co.

Hoit, J. D., & Hixon, T. J. (1992). Age and laryngeal airway resistance during vowel production in women. *Journal of Speech and Hearing Research, 35*(2), 309–313.

Holmberg, E. B., Hillman, R. E., & Perkell, J. S. (1988). Glottal airflow and transglottal air pressure measurements for male and female speakers in soft, normal and loud voice. *Journal of the Acoustical Society of America, 84,* 511–529.

Holmberg, E. B., Hillman, R. E., & Perkell, J. S. (1989). Glottal airflow and transglottal air pressure measurements for male and female speakers in low, normal and high pitch. *Journal of Voice, 3*(4), 294–305.

Horii, Y. (1982). Jitter and shimmer differences among sustained vowel phonations. *Journal of Speech and Hearing Research, 25*(1), 12–14.

Iwata, S. (1988). Aerodynamic aspects for phonation in normal and pathologic larynges. In O. Fujimura (Ed.), *Vocal physiology* (pp. 423–432). New York: Raven Press.

Karnell, M. P. (1989). Synchronized videostroboscopy and electroglottography. *Journal of Voice, 3*(1), 68–75.

Karnell, M. P. (1991). Laryngeal perturbation analysis: Minimum length of analysis window. *Journal of Speech and Hearing Research, 34*(3), 544–548.

Karnell, M., Scherer, R. S., & Fischer, L. B. (1991). Comparison of acoustic voice perturbation measures among three independent voice laboratories. *Journal of Speech and Hearing Research, 34*(4), 781–790.

Kempster, G., Kistler, D. J., & Hillenbrand, J. (1991). Multidimensional scaling analysis of dysphonia in two speaker groups. *Journal of Speech and Hearing Research, 34*(3), 534–543.

Kent, R. D., & Read, C. (1992). *The acoustic analysis of speech*. San Diego: Singular Publishing Group.

Kitajima, K., & Fujita, F. (1992). Clinical report on preliminary data on intraoral pressure in the evaluation of laryngeal pathology. *Journal of Voice, 6*(1), 79–85.

Laver, J., Hiller, S., & Beck, J. M. (1992). Acoustic waveform perturbations and voice disorders. *Journal of Voice, 6*(2), 115–126.

Ludlow, C. L. (1991). Neurophysiological assessment of patients with vocal motor control disorders. In *Assessment of speech and voice production: Research and clinical applications* (pp. 161–171). Bethesda, MD: National Institute on Deafness and Other Communicative Disorders.

Ludlow, C. L., Bassich, C. J., Connor, N. P., Coulter, D. C., & Lee, Y. J. (1987). The validity of using phonatory jitter and shimmer to detect laryngeal pathology. In T. Baer, C. Sasaki, & K. Harris (Eds.), *Laryngeal function in phonation and respiration* (pp. 492–508). Boston: College-Hill Press.

Melcon, M., Hoit, J. D., & Hixon, T. J. (1989). Age and laryngeal airway resistance during vowel production. *Journal of Speech and Hearing Disorders 54*(2), 282–286.

Milenkovic, P. H. (1987). Least mean squares of waveform perturbation. *Journal of Speech and Hearing Research, 29*(4), 529–538.

Miller, C.J., & Daniloff, R. (1993). Airflow measurements: Theory and utility of findings. *Journal of Voice, 7*(1), 38–46.

Netsell, R. (1969). Subglottal and intraoral air pressures during intervocalic contrast of /t/ and /d/. *Phonetica, 20*(1), 68–73.

Nittrouer, S., McGowan, R. S., Milenkovic, P. H., & Beehler, D. (1990). Acoustic measurements of men's and women's voice: A study of context effects and covariation. *Journal of Speech and Hearing Research, 33*(3), 761–775.

Orlikoff, R. F., & Baken, R. J. (1993). *Clinical voice and speech measurement.* San Diego: Singular Publishing Group.

Orlikoff, R. F., & Kahane, J. C. (1991). Influence of mean sound pressure level on jitter and shimmer measures. *Journal of Voice, 5*(2), 113–119.

Peppard, R. C., & Bless, D. M. (1990). A method for improving measurement reliability in laryngeal videostroboscopy. *Journal of Voice, 4*(3), 280–285.

Peppard, R. C., & Bless, D. M. (1991). The use of topical anesthesia in videostroboscopic examination of the larynx. *Journal of Voice, 5*(1), 57–63.

Read, C., Buder, E. H., & Kent, R. D. (1990). Speech analysis systems: a survey. *Journal of Speech and Hearing Research, 33*(2), 363–374.

Read, C., Buder, E. H., & Kent, R. D. (1992). Speech analysis systems: an evaluation. *Journal of Speech and Hearing Research, 35*(2), 314–332.

Rothenberg, M. (1977). Measurement of air flow during speech. *Journal of Speech and Hearing Research, 2*(1), 155–176.

Rothenberg, M. (1992). A multichannel electroglottograph. *Journal of Voice, 6*(1), 36–43.

Sataloff, R. T., Spiegel, J. R., Carroll, L. M., Darby, K. S., Hawkshaw, M. J., & Rulnick, R. K. (1990). The clinical voice laboratory: practical design and clinical application. *Journal of Voice, 4*(3), 264–279.

Sawashima, M., Niimi, S., Horiguchi, S., & Yamaguchi, H. (1988). Expiratory lung pressure, airflow rate, and vocal intensity: Data on normal subjects. In O. Fujimura (Ed.), *Vocal physiology* (pp. 415–422). New York: Raven Press.

Scherer, R. C. (1991). Aerodynamic assessment in voice production. In *Assessment of speech and voice production: Research and clinical applications* (pp. 42–49). Bethesda, MD: National Institute on Deafness and Other Communicative Disorders.

Schutte, H. K. (1992). Integrated aerodynamic measurements. *Journal of Voice, 6*(2), 127–134.

Smitheran, J., & Hixon, Y. J. (1981). A clinical method for estimating laryngeal airway resistance during vowel production. *Journal of Speech and Hearing Disorders, 46*(1), 138–146.

Stone, R. E., & Rainey, C. L. (1991). Intra- and intersubject variability in acoustic measures of normal voice. *Journal of Voice, 5*(3), 189–196.

Titze, I. R. (1991a). Measurements for assessment of voice disorders. In *Assessment of speech and voice production: Research and clinical applications* (pp. 42–49). Bethesda, MD: National Institute on Deafness and Other Communicative Disorders.

Titze, I. R. (1991b). Phonation threshold pressure: A missing link for glottal aerodynamics. In I. R. Titze (Ed.), *Progress report 1* (pp. 1–14). Iowa City, IA: National Center for Voice and Speech.

Titze, I. R. (1992). Acoustic interpretation of the voice-range profile (phonetogram). *Journal of Speech and Hearing Research, 34*(5), 21–35.

Titze, I. R. (1993). Towards standards in acoustic analysis of voice. In I. R. Titze (Ed.), *Progress report 4* (pp. 271–280). Iowa City, IA: National Center for Voice and Speech.

Titze, I. R. (1994). *Principles of voice production.* Englewood Cliffs, N.J.: Prentice Hall.

Titze, I. R., Horii, Y., & Scherer, R. C. (1987). Some technical considerations in voice perturbation measurements. *Journal of Speech and Hearing Research, 30*(2), 252–260.

Titze, I. R., & Liang, H. (1993). Comparison of F_0 extraction methods for high-precision voice perturbation measurements. *Journal of Speech and Hearing Research, 36*(6), 1120–1133.

Titze, I. R., & Winholtz, W. S. (1993). Effect of microphone type and placement on voice perturbation measurements. *Journal of Speech and Hearing Research, 36*(6), 1177–1190.

Verdolini-Marston, K., Titze, I. R., & Drucker, D. G. (1990). Changes in phonation threshold pressure with induced conditions of hydration. *Journal of Voice, 4*(2), 141–151.

Wolfe, V., Cornell, R., & Palmer, C. (1991). Acoustic correlates of pathologic voice types. *Journal of Speech and Hearing Research, 34*(3), 509–516.

Woo, P., Colton, R., Casper, J., & Brewer, D. (1991). Diagnostic value of stroboscopic examination in hoarse patients. *Journal of Voice, 5*(3), 231–238.

Yanagisawa, E. (1987). Fiberoptic and telescopic videolaryngoscopy—A comparative study. In T. Baer, C. Sasaki, K. Harris (Eds.), *Laryngeal function in phonation and respiration* (pp. 475–484). Boston: College-Hill Press.

APPENDIX

IVAR Recording Forms

Phonatory Function Test (Acoustic and Aerodynamic Analysis)

**Institute for Voice Analysis
and Rehabilitation**
369 West First Street
Suite 408
Dayton Ohio 45402-3065
(513) 496-2622 FAX (513) 496-2610

Joseph C. Stemple, Ph.D.
Bernice K. Gerdeman, Ph.D.

Name: _____   Date: _____   Age: _____

Occupation: _____   Physician: _____

Type: _____

PHONATORY FUNCTION TEST

ACOUSTIC ANALYSIS

SUSTAINED VOWEL /a/	f$_0$ (Hz)	jitter (%)	shimmer (dB)	H/N (dB)
Comfort	_____	_____	_____	_____
	_____	_____	_____	_____
Ave	_____	_____	_____	_____
High	_____	_____	_____	_____
	_____	_____	_____	_____
Ave	_____	_____	_____	_____
Low	_____	_____	_____	_____
	_____	_____	_____	_____
Ave	_____	_____	_____	_____

PHONATION DYNAMIC RANGE	Glide from mid-voice to as **low** as possible	Glide from the mid-voice to as **high** as possible
	_____ (Hz)	_____ (Hz)

SPEAKING FUNDAMENTAL FREQ	Reading	Conversation
	_____ (Hz)	_____ (Hz)

INTENSITY	Habitual level	Loudest tone level	Softest tone level
	_____ (dBSPL)	_____ (dBSPL)	_____ (dBSPL)

Comments:

_____

_____

_____

AERODYNAMIC ANALYSIS

SUSTAINED VOWEL /a/	Phonation Flow Volume (mL)	Phonatory Flow Rate (mL/s)	Peak Air Flow Rate (mL/s)	Intensity (dB)	Maximum Phonation Time (sec)
Comfort	————	————	————	————	————
Ave	————	————	————	————	————
High	————	————	————	————	————
Ave	————	————	————	————	————
Low	————	————	————	————	————
Ave	————	————	————	————	————

SUBGLOTTIC PRESSURE   Repeat Ipipi
(cm H_2O)

GLOTTAL RESISTANCE

Comfort

———————— (Ns/m5)

Ave

GLOTTAL EFFICIENCY

High

———————— (ppm)

Ave

GLOTTAL POWER

Low

———————— (watt)

Ave

Perceptual Quality:

_____

_____

Comments & Recommendations:

_____

_____

_____

_____

Stroboscopic Evaluation

Institute for Voice Analysis and Rehabilitation
369 West First Street
Suite 408
Dayton Ohio 45402-3065
(513) 496-2622 FAX (513) 496-2610

Joseph C. Stemple, Ph.D.
Bernice K. Gerdeman, Ph.D.

Name: _____   Date: _____   Age: _____

Occupation: _____   Physician: _____

Type: _____

STROBOSCOPIC EVALUATION

VOICE QUALITY	Normal	Mildly Dysphonic	Mild-Mod Dysphonic	Moderately Dysphonic	Mod-Severely Dysphonic	Severely Dysphonic	Aphonic

GLOTTIC CLOSURE	Cannot Rate	Complete	Anterior	Irregular	Spindle	Posterior	Hourglass	Incomplete

SUPRAGLOTTIC ACTIVITY Latero-Medial Compression	(0) None	(1) Mild compression of vent. folds	(2) Mild-Mod	(3) Moderate	(4) Mod-severe	(5) Severe	(6) Dysphonia Plica Ventricularis TVF not visible

Antero-Post Compression	(0) None	(1) Mild	(2) Mild-Mod	(3) Moderate	(4) Mod-Severe	(5) Severe

VERTICAL LEVEL APPROX.	(0) Cannot Rate	(1) Equal	(2) Right Lower	(3) Left Lower	(4) Questionable

VOCAL FOLD EDGE	LEFT	(0) Cannot Rate	(1) Smooth Straight	(2)	(3)	(4)	(5)	(6) Rough Irregular
	RIGHT	(0)	(1)	(2)	(3)	(4)	(5)	(6)

VOCAL FOLD MOBILITY	LEFT	(0) Cannot Rate	(1) Normal	(2) Limited Adduction (mild) (mod) (sev)	(3) Limited Abduction (mild) (mod) (sev)	(4) Fixed (mild) (mod) (sev)
	RIGHT	(0)	(1)	(2)	(3)	(4)

AMPLITUDE	LEFT	(0) Cannot Rate	(1) Normal	(2) Mildly Decreased	(3) Mild-Mod Decreased	(4) Mod Decreased	(5) Mod-Sev Decreased	(6) Severely Decreased	(7) No Visible Movement
	RIGHT	(0)	(1)	(2)	(3)	(4)	(5)	(6)	(7)

MUCOSAL WAVE	LEFT	(0) Cannot Rate	(1) Normal	(2) Mildly Decreased	(3) Mild-Mod Decreased	(4) Mod Decreased	(5) Mod-Sev Decreased	(6) Severely Decreased	(7) Absent
	RIGHT	(0)	(1)	(2)	(3)	(4)	(5)	(6)	(7)

NON-VIBRATING PORTION	LEFT	(0)	(1)	(2)	(3)	(4)	(5)
		None	20%	40%	60%	80%	100%
	RIGHT	(0)	(1)	(2)	(3)	(4)	(5)

PHASE CLOSURE	Cannot Rate	(-5) Open Phase Predominates (Whisper dysphonia)	(-4)	(-3)	(-2)	(-1)	(0) Normal	(1)	(2)	(3)	(4)	(5) Closed Phase Predominates (Glottal fry-extreme hyperadduction)

PHASE SYMMETRY	Cannot Rate	(0) Regular always symmetrical	(1) Irregular during end or begin tasks	(2) Irregular during extremes pitch or loud	(3) 50% asymmetrical	(4) 75% asymmetrical	(5) always asymmetrical

OVERALL LARYNGEAL FUNCTION	(0) Normal	(1) Hypofunction	(2) Hyperfunction	(3) Laryngeal tremors (sust. v) (speech) (mild) (mod) (severe)	(4) Phonatory spasms (add) (abd) (mild) (mod) (severe)

Strobe Comments and Interpretations:

7

SURVEY OF VOICE MANAGEMENT

The extensive diagnostic voice evaluation has provided the voice pathologist with answers to what has caused the voice disorder and a description of the current vocal symptoms. The answers to the etiologic questions include primary causes as well as other secondary etiologic factors. A systematic management approach must now be initiated with the purpose of modifying or eliminating the etiologic factors and improving the quality of the voice production. This chapter is designed to survey the basic philosophies of voice therapy and to introduce the reader to some specific voice therapy techniques. Although the information contained in this chapter is by no means an exhaustive presentation of all voice therapy techniques, it is hoped that the reader will find this a useful point of departure for the study of vocal management.

VOICE THERAPY ORIENTATIONS

As stated in Chapter 1, the management of voice disorders by "speech correctionists" began in the 1930s. Since that early beginning, a rich and interesting history of voice therapy approaches has evolved leading to several philosophical orientations of therapy. These orientations include *symptomatic, psychogenic, etiologic, physiologic,* and *eclectic* voice therapies.

167

Symptomatic Voice Therapy

The focus of *symptomatic voice therapy* is on the modification of the deviant vocal symptoms or components which were identified by the voice pathologist during the diagnostic voice evaluation. These symptoms may be breathiness, low pitch, glottal fry phonation, the use of hard glottal attacks, and so on. Daniel Boone (1971) was the first voice pathologist to organize previous literature and introduce to the profession the symptomatic therapy orientation. Symptomatic voice therapy is based on the premise that most voice disorders are caused by the functional misuse or abuse of the voice components including pitch, loudness, respiration, and so on. When identified through the diagnostic process, the misuses are eliminated or reduced through various voice therapy **facilitating techniques.** Boone (1971) stated:

> In the voice clinician's attempt to aid the patient in finding and using his best voice production, it is necessary to probe continually within the patient's repertoire to find that one voice that sounds "good" and which he is able to produce with relatively little effort. A **voice therapy facilitating technique** is that technique which, when used by a particular patient, enables him easily to produce a good voice. Once discovered, the facilitating technique and resulting phonation become the symptomatic focus of therapy.... This use of a facilitating technique to produce a good phonation is the core of what we do in symptomatic voice therapy for the reduction of hyperfunctional voice disorders. (p. 11)

Boone's (1971) original facilitating techniques included:

1. altering tongue position
2. change of loudness
3. chewing exercises
4. digital manipulation
5. ear training
6. elimination of abuses
7. elimination of hard glottal attack
8. establish new pitch
9. explanation of the problem
10. feedback
11. hierarchy analysis
12. negative practice
13. open mouth exercises
14. pitch inflections
15. pushing approach
16. relaxation
17. respiration training
18. target voice models
19. voice rest
20. yawn-sigh approach.

As you read through this chapter, many of these approaches are described in greater detail as they continue to be well utilized in the treatment of voice disorders. (A complete description of each facilitating technique as well as kinds of problems for which the techniques are useful and procedural aspects may be found in Boone and McFarlane, 1988.) From this list, it may be observed that the main focus of symptomatic voice therapy is direct modification of the vocal symptoms. The voice pathologist constantly probes for the "best" voice in the presence of the disorder. When the best voice is found, attempts to stabilize that voice with the various facilitating techniques are made. Symptomatic voice therapy assumes voice improvement through direct symptom modification (Stemple, 1993).

Psychogenic Voice Therapy

Psychogenic voice therapy is based on the assumption of underlying emotional causes for the voice disturbance. The relationship of emotions to voice production has been well documented in the literature starting as early as the middle 1800's (Goss, 1878; Russell, 1864; Ward, 1877). West et al. (1937) and Van Riper (1939) discussed the need for emotional retraining in voice therapy, while Murphy (1964) and Brodnitz (1971) presented excellent information related to the psychodynamics of voice production.

Aronson (1980) first articulated the most complete description of a psychogenic voice disorder when he stated that:

> A psychogenic voice disorder is broadly synonymous with a functional one but has the advantage of stating positively, based on an explanation of its causes, that the voice disorder is a manifestation of one or more types of psychological disequilibrium—such as anxiety, depression, conversion reaction, or personality disorder—which interfere with normal volitional control over phonation. (p. 131)

Aronson (1990), Case (1984), and Colton and Casper (1990) further discussed the need for determining the emotional dynamics of the voice disturbance from the perspectives of emotions as a cause for voice disorders and voice disorders being the cause of emotional disequilibrium.

Psychogenic voice therapy focuses on identification and modification of the emotional and psychosocial disturbances associated with the onset and maintenance of the voice problem. When the psychogenic causes are resolved, so too will there be a resolution of the voice disorder. Voice pathologists must develop and possess superior interview skills, counseling skills, and the skill to know when the emotional or psychosocial problem is in need of more intensive evaluation and therapy by other professionals (Stemple, 1993).

Etiologic Voice Therapy

Etiologic voice therapy is based on the reasonable assumption that there is always a cause for the presence of the voice disorder. If that cause (or causes) can be identified, then appropriate treatments can be devised for modifying or eliminating those causes. Once modified, the voice production has the opportunity to improve or return to normal (Stemple, 1984). During the diagnostic evaluation, much effort is focused on identifying the direct and indirect causes of the voice disorder. To be successful, the voice pathologist must understand the many etiologic factors that may possibly contribute to the voice disorder (see Chapter 3). Once the etiologic factors are treated, the vocal symptoms often improve without direct manipulation of the voice components. A common example may be the reduction of the abusive behavior of shouting in children who have vocal nodules. By modifying the shouting behavior, the nodules are given the opportunity to resolve and the voice improves without modification of the voice components which may have **resulted** from the presence of the nodules (such as lower pitch, breathiness and so on).

Direct symptom modification (i.e., raising the pitch, reducing breathiness, and so on) is reserved for situations where the inappropriate use of a voice component is found to be the primary etiologic factor. For example, we recently evaluated a patient who attempted to sound more authoritative by using a pitch that was too low with intermittent glottal fry phonation. The use of the inappropriate pitch was found to be the primary cause of the patient's dysphonia and laryngeal fatigue and was therefore modified leading to improved voice production.

Etiologic voice therapy presumes that every voice disorder has a cause. Once identified, the cause can be modified or eliminated leading to improved voice production. If the primary etiologic factor is found to be the inappropriate use of a voice component, then direct symptom modification is used to resolve the problem.

Physiologic Voice Therapy

Physiologic voice therapy is the term used to describe direct voice therapies which have been devised to alter or modify the physiology of the vocal mechanism. Normal voice production is dependent upon a balance among airflow, supplied by the respiratory system; laryngeal muscular strength, balance, coordination, and stamina; and coordination among these and the supraglottic resonatory structures. In addition, physiologic voice therapy concentrates on developing and maintaining the health of the vocal fold cover. Any disturbance in the physiologic balance of these vocal subsystems may lead to a voice disturbance. As stated by Stemple (1993):

These disturbances may be in laryngeal muscle strength, tone, mass, stiffness, flexibility, and approximation. Disturbances may also manifest in respiratory volume, power, pressure, and flow. The overall causes may be mechanical, neurologic or psychological. Whatever the cause, the management approach is direct modification of the inappropriate physiologic activity through direct exercise and manipulation. (p. 4)

Physiologic voice therapy strives to balance the physiology of voice production through direct physical exercise and manipulations of the laryngeal, respiratory, and resonatory systems. In addition special care is taken to account for the health of the vocal fold cover. This care may be related to proper mucosal hydration, attention to voice abuse reduction, or anti-reflux regimens as examples.

Eclectic Voice Therapy

Eclectic voice therapy is the combination of any and all of the other orientations of voice therapy. Successful voice therapy is dependent upon the voice pathologist using all of the therapy techniques that seem appropriate for individual patients. Many patients may share the same diagnosis, however, the etiologies and personalities, vocal needs and emotional reactions to their voice problems may be very different. Because of these differences, the same pathologies may require very different management approaches. Therefore, the voice pathologist is advised not to adhere to any one philosophical orientation of voice therapy, but rather to learn a broad range of management approaches. Utilizing a case study format, let us examine a typical patient with a voice disorder from the perspective of each voice therapy orientation.

Case Study 1

The patient was a 48-year-old woman who was diagnosed by the laryngologist as having moderate bilateral Reinke's edema with the left fold suggesting a more severe draping, polypoid degeneration. The patient was referred for a voice evaluation and a trial voice therapy program. Should short-term therapy not prove successful in improving her vocal fold condition and voice quality, then the patient would be scheduled for surgical intervention.

History of the Problem

The patient was referred to the otolaryngologist by her internist when, during a regular physical examination, she noticed that the patient's voice quality "sounded as deep as a man's." The patient stated that her voice had always been deep and that she really didn't think there was much of a problem. However, when the otolaryngologist told her that she had vocal fold polyps, she became concerned enough to throw her cigarettes in the exam room trash can and, by the time of the voice evaluation, had not smoked for two weeks. She reported that her voice quality was essentially the same throughout the day, though it tended to become "huskier" toward the end of a work day.

Medical History

The patient reported undergoing thyroid surgery five years ago during which her left thyroid lobe was excised. In addition, she underwent a tonsillectomy and appendectomy as a teenager. In addition to the surgeries, she was hospitalized for chronic depression on two different occasions. The last hospitalization lasted for three weeks and occurred 18 months ago. The patient continues to be treated for depression with medication and remains in bimonthly counseling.

Chronic medical conditions included asthma and frequent bronchitis; high blood pressure; elevated blood sugar; and rheumatoid arthritis. Daily medications were taken for depression, "nerves" (a sleep aid), thyroid, high blood pressure, and pain associated with the arthritis. Until 2 weeks prior, she had smoked $1^1/_2$ to 2 packages of cigarettes per day for approximately 30 years. Her liquid intake was poor, consisting of approximately three cups of caffeinated coffee and four cans of caffeinated soda per day. Chronic throat clearing was noted throughout the evaluation. The patient indicated that on a day to day basis she felt "fair-to-poor" due to stress, fatigue, and arthritis pain.

Social History

The patient was married for 29 years, but had presently been separated from her husband for 3 months, causing much stress and tension. She had three grown children. The middle child, a 26-year-old son, had recently divorced and temporarily moved back into the house. Again, the patient pointed to the stress of this situation. The patient was not reticent to talk about her depression and indicated that an unhappy marriage and the feeling of an unfulfilled life were the causes.

The patient had been employed for 6 years by a factory that made latex gloves for medical use. She indicated that her specific job was in the "powder room" where the gloves were filled with powder and packaged. Apparently the powder dust caused much coughing during the day. In addition, the packaging machines were noisy requiring the workers to talk loudly to be heard. Most talking on the job was social among eight people who worked in a large, well-ventilated room.

Nonwork activities included walking her two dogs nightly, talking on the telephone with her daughter, and actively shopping at yard sales and flea markets with a close friend. However, all of these activities were curtailed when she didn't feel well physically or emotionally.

Oral-Peripheral Examination

The structure and function of the oral mechanism appeared to be well within normal limits for speech and voice production. The laryngeal sensations of dryness and occasional thickness were reported by the patient. Laryngeal area muscle tension and neck tension were demonstrated by the patient.

Voice Evaluation

The patient's voice quality was described as mild-to-moderately dysphonic, characterized by low pitch, inappropriate loudness, and husky hoarseness.

Respiration: s/z = 25 sec/10 sec; Patient demonstrated a thoracic, supportive breathing pattern. She tended to speak on residual air especially toward the end of phrases.

Phonation: A slight breathiness was noted during conversational voice. Occasional glottal fry was noted toward the end of phrases.

Resonation: Normal

Pitch: Patient demonstrated an unusually low pitch conversationally.

Loudness: Patient spoke unusually loud for the speaking situation.

Rate: Normal

Acoustic measures and aerodynamic analyses revealed the following:

- fundamental frequency = 136 Hz
- frequency range = 106 to 320 Hz
- jitter percent: sustained vowels = .56
- shimmer dB: sustained vowels = .67
- intensity (habitual) = 76 dB
- airflow volume = 2,300 ml
- airflow rate = 180 ml/sec, all pitch levels
- phonation time = 12.7 sec
- subglottic air pressure = 8.6 cm/H_2O

Laryngeal videostroboscopic observation revealed a moderate bilateral vocal fold edema, worse left than right. Prominent blood vessels were noted bilaterally. Glottic closure was complete with a mild ventricular fold compression. The amplitude of vibration was moderate-to-severely decreased left and moderately decreased right. The mucosal waves were severely decreased bilaterally. The open phase of the vibratory cycle was slightly dominant, while the symmetry of vibration was irregular by 50%. In short, the patient demonstrated an edematous, stiff, out of phase vocal fold system.

Impressions

The patient presented with a voice disorder secondary to these possible etiologic factors:

- long-term cigarette smoking
- harsh employment environment in terms of dust and talking over noise
- poor hydration and large caffeine intake
- asthma and frequent bronchitis
- prescription medications causing mucosal drying
- frequent coughing and throat clearing
- emotional instability
- talking too loudly in general conversation
- using a low pitch
- laryngeal area muscle tension

Recommendations

Symptomatic Voice Therapy   General focus would use facilitating techniques to:

1. raise pitch
2. reduce loudness
3. reduce laryngeal area tension and effort

This direct symptom modification would follow an explanation of the problem and would run concurrently with modification of the vocally abusive behaviors including:

1. smoking
2. caffeine intake
3. coughing and throat clearing

Psychogenic Voice Therapy   General focus would explore the psychodynamics of the voice disorder. This exploration would include:

1. detailed patient interview to determine the cause and effects of stress, tension, and depression
2. determination of the exact relationship of emotional problems and voice problem
3. counsel the patient regarding the effects of emotions on voice problems
4. reduction of musculoskeletal tension caused by emotional upheaval
5. support of ongoing psychological counseling.

Secondary focus would deal with modification/elimination of the abusive behaviors including:

1. smoking
2. caffeine
3. coughing and throat clearing

Inappropriate use of pitch and loudness would most likely be viewed as obvious symptoms of the voice problem. As the psychodynamics improve, the voice symptoms would be expected to improve.

Etiologic Voice Therapy   General focus would be to identify the primary and secondary causes of the voice disorder and then to modify or eliminate these causes. The primary causes would include:

1. smoking
2. laryngeal dehydration from poor hydration, caffeine intake, and drugs
3. voice abuse such as talking loudly over noise at work, coughing, and throat clearing
4. inhalation of large quantities of powder

Secondary causes that may be more the result of the problem as opposed to a cause would be:

1. laryngeal area muscle tension due to increased mass and stiffness
2. low pitch due to increased mass
3. increased loudness due to effort to force stiff, heavy folds to vibrate

Therapy would focus on modification or elimination of the primary etiologic factors. The patient would be supported in her effort to stop smoking, encouraged to begin a hydration program and to reduce caffeine intake, given vocal hygiene counseling in an effort to reduce the vocally abusive habits, and encouraged to wear a mask to filter her breathing at work. The secondary causes of tension, low pitch and increased loudness would be expected to spontaneously improve as the primary causes were modified and the vocal fold condition improved.

Physiologic Voice Therapy   General focus would be to evaluate the present physiologic condition of the patient's voice production and develop direct physical exercises or manipulations to improve that condition. This patient demonstrated increased mass and stiffness of the vocal folds changing the physical dynamics of vocal fold vibration. Indeed, she was required to build greater subglottic air pressure to initiate and maintain vibration which required a borderline high airflow rate. This increased pressure caused her to speak too loudly in conversation. She also attempted to overcome these problems by making physical adjustments such as increasing supraglottic tension in an effort to maintain her voice. When added to the mucosal and muscular stiffness, vocal hyperfunction was the result. The management program would therefore include:

1. Vocal Function Exercises designed to restrengthen and balance the laryngeal musculature and to balance airflow to muscular activity and improve supraglottic placement of the tone (vocal function exercises are discussed later in this chapter)
2. hydration program and decrease in caffeinated products to improve the mucous membrane of the vocal folds
3. discussion of medications with the patient's physician
4. elimination of habit coughing and throat clearing
5. vocal hygiene counseling for elimination of direct voice abuse

Eclectic Voice Therapy   It is obvious in the review of these orientations, that each management approach has certain strengths as well as inherent weaknesses. You will be able to best treat your patients with the understanding and use of all of these orientations. Therefore, eclectic voice therapy is obviously the treatment of choice with any voice disordered patient. This patient would best be served when the management plan included

1. symptom modification
2. elimination/modification of the causes
3. attention to the psychodynamics of the problem
4. direct physiologic exercise and attention to the mucosal covering of the vocal folds.

The remainder of this chapter presents specific treatment strategies for voice disorders caused by voice abuse and misuse, personality-related etiologies, and some special cases of voice disorders. Chapter 8 describes treatments for the medically related voice disorders.

TREATMENT STRATEGIES FOR VOCAL ABUSE

Hyperadduction of the vocal folds is vocally abusive, especially when the abuse occurs frequently. Some common vocally abusive behaviors that may be modified through voice therapy include shouting, loud talking, screaming, the production of vocal noises, and habitual throat clearing. There are many reasons for the occurrence of vocal abuse among both adults and children. For example, homemakers may shout at their children for discipline; factory workers talk loudly over noise for extended periods of time; and teachers and lecturers may talk too loudly with inappropriate tone focus on a routine basis. Most children shout and make vocal noises. They shout during unsupervised play; they are encouraged to shout while participating in team sports; and they shout when they are angry. Both children and adults are also susceptible to the development of throat clearing either primarily as the result of frequent colds or allergies or secondary to the development of laryngeal pathologies. Let us examine some of the techniques utilized for modifying vocally abusive behaviors.

Therapy Approaches

The most effective way of dealing with vocal abuse is through **vocal hygiene counseling.** Once the abuses have been identified, the first step of this approach is patient education. Patient education involves making the patient aware of the effects that abuse has on the laryngeal mechanism by utilizing graphic pictures and descriptions of the anatomy and physiology. Indeed, the most effective educational tool is the patient's own video of the stroboscopic evaluation. It is much easier for patients to resolve their vocal problems when they truly understand the cause and effect relationships that may be displayed visually.

After the general abuses have been identified and explained in detail, it is important to determine exactly why the patient presents with the specific abuses. For example, if the abuse is shouting, the voice pathologist will want to know when and why it occurs and whether the patient feels it is required. Once these factors are determined, the treatment plan will involve, (a) eliminating those abusive behaviors that may be eliminated; (b) modifying those abusive behaviors which cannot be totally eliminated to reduce the abusive impact on the vocal mechanism; and (c) environmental manipulation to secure more favorable voicing conditions.

We may synthesize the vocal hygiene approach to a four-step outline.

1. identify the abuse
2. describe the effects

3. define the specific occurrences
4. modify the behavior

Let us examine several cases in the context of the vocal hygiene therapy approach.

Case Study 2: The Homemaker

A 35-year-old patient was referred with the diagnosis of bilateral vocal fold nodules. She had a several year history of intermittent dysphonia that became persistent approximately three months before the voice evaluation. She reported that her voice was better in the morning than in the evening and that she had never experienced aphonia.

The patient's medical history was unremarkable except for a large intake of caffeine and little other liquid. She had never smoked and had always lived in a non-smoking environment. Socially, she was a homemaker with three sons, ages 3, 8, and 12 years. She enjoyed crafts, decorating her newly purchased Victorian home, and, until recently, sang soprano in the church choir. Her voice problem precluded singing. Her 8- and 12-year-old sons played soccer, and her oldest son also played baseball and basketball. The patient's husband was a manufacturer's representative and was on the road three out of five working days. The patient admitted to frequent shouting when disciplining her children and cheering loudly during their many sporting events.

The patient's voice quality during the evaluation was moderately dysphonic, characterized by low pitch and a breathy hoarseness. Respiration was thoracic and supportive for conversational voice. She was able to sustain the /z/ for 7 seconds and the /s/ for 21 seconds. Phonation was characterized by voice breaks and the production of occasional glottal fry. A limited pitch range was demonstrated with the habitual pitch located near the bottom of the range. Limited inflection was noted conversationally. Resonation was normal and the loudness level was appropriate for the speaking situation. She was able to readily increase the loudness level to a shout. Rate was normal. The abusive behavior of throat clearing was noted throughout the evaluation. The patient complained that her voice quality worsened with use suggesting laryngeal muscle fatigue. Instrumental measures yielded the following:

fundamental frequency	168 Hz
frequency range	156 Hz–460 Hz
jitter percent	.57%
mean intensity	68 dB SPL
shimmer dB	.47 dB

airflow volume	3200 ml
airflow rate	235 ml/sec
maximum phonation time	13.6 sec
subglottic air pressure	5.2 cm/H_2O

Vocal abuse is common in many homemakers as was demonstrated by Herrington-Hall et al. (1988). Homemakers often shout for disciplinary purposes and call their children home from long distances. Abusive behaviors in the home that may not be easily recognized include calling or reprimanding a pet; shouting from one room to another; calling someone to the telephone; talking to a spouse or relative who is hard of hearing; and talking loudly over the television or stereo. By discussing the specific situations that relate to the patient, the voice pathologist and the patient may devise alternatives to the abusive behaviors. The alternatives may be as simple as turning the stereo volume down when speaking, or as creative as blowing a whistle to call the children home for dinner. Some patients are advised not to answer when someone calls from another room but rather to make the caller seek them or to go to the caller before replying. Again, once the specific abusive behaviors are identified, most motivated patients are well able either to eliminate the abuse or devise creative nonabusive alternatives to aid in their own treatment processes.

The homemaker in Case Study 2 developed vocal nodules as a result of shouting and maintained inappropriate vocal health through habitual throat clearing, laryngeal dehydration, and laryngeal muscle strain and weakness. Following the four-step vocal hygiene plan, this problem was managed as follows:

1. Identify the abuse:
   shouting; throat clearing; caffeine intake; laryngeal muscle strain
2. Describe the effect:
   accomplished with illustration as well as the patient's own video of the stroboscopic evaluation
3. Define specific occurrences:
   shouting to discipline children and at sporting events; chronic habit throat clearing; and heavy coffee drinker
4. Modify the behavior:
   attempt to discipline through discussion and deprivation; substitute a mechanical noisemaker for vocal enthusiasm at sporting events; eliminate habitual throat clearing through behavior modification program (discussed later in this chapter); introduce formal hydration program (6–8 eight ounce glasses of water or juices per day); and direct Vocal Function Exercise to strengthen and balance the physiologic vocal system.

Case Study 3: The Noisy Job Environment

Communication is often very difficult and potentially vocally abusive for people who work in noisy job environments. In these situations, the vocal abuse usually takes the form of talking loudly or shouting over noise for extended periods of time. In defining specific occurrences, it is necessary to determine how much talking is job-related, that is, is necessary for the worker to carry out the duties of the job, and how much is simply social discourse. Unnecessary communication may certainly be reduced, but this is not the total answer. You also want to know the type of noise, constant or intermittent, to determine if there are more appropriate times than others to talk.

Strategies for modifying this behavior may include moving as far away from the noise sources as possible, shielding the voice with the body by turning away from the noise source, and wearing ear protectors so background noise is masked and the speaker is better able to hear his or her own voice. Another beneficial principle to teach patients who must talk in noisy environments is to make the listener strain to hear them; not for them to strain their voices to be heard by the listeners. An explanation of the Lombard effect, where the speaker will always talk slightly louder than the noise source, is often helpful for patients. Many patients do not realize how loudly they are talking in the noisy background because of the Lombard. Direct voice therapy may also be used to teach the patient how to raise the voice in this environment without causing abuse. Finally, the most drastic step in working with the voice-disordered patient in a noisy environment is to explore the possibility of removing the patient, through job transfer, to a less noisy environment.

For example, a 50-year-old male with a diagnosis of a post-surgical left unilateral vocal fold polyp was referred for voice evaluation and treatment. He worked as a foreman at a local automobile assembly plant. Being a nonsmoker, the development of the polyp was thought to be associated with the need to raise his voice in the work environment. The following vocal hygiene management plan was developed during the diagnostic evaluation:

1. Identify the abuse:
   talking loudly over noise on a daily basis.
2. Describe the effect:
   accomplished with illustrations and discussion of physiology.
3. Define specific occurrences:
   discussing daily work duties with 22 workers;
   reporting daily activities to supervisor; and
   social discussions.

4. Modify the behavior:
    meet with workers, two to four at a time, in office away from
    noise source;
    make inspections on the line, then ask workers to come into
    office as needed;
    decrease social conversations;
    make workers strain to hear; and
    direct voice therapy concentrating on increasing loudness with
    improved breath support, appropriate pitch, and proper
    breath support.

Case Study 4: The Public Speaker

Excessive loud talking with inappropriate tone focus and breath
support by teachers, lecturers, politicians, preachers, actors, and other
professional voice users may often be the cause of vocal difficulties.
These inappropriate vocal behaviors or misuses may lead to laryngeal
muscle strain and fatigue and in some cases to vocal fold mucosal
changes, including mass lesions. In the early stages of the problem, the
public speaker will quite often describe to the voice pathologist, in a
perfectly normal voice, extreme vocal difficulties that occur during
presentations or lectures. The history of the problem normally includes strong voice in the morning that weakens as the day progresses.
Some of these patients report that by the end of the day they are "lucky
to have any voice at all."

Often, as the voice is tested during the diagnostic, there is a good
chance that it will test out rather normal and the misuse behaviors will
not be evident. It is important to secure a sample of the public speaking voice to determine the presence of vocal misuse during the presentation. This is easily accomplished by having the patient ask a
lecture participant to tape-record 10-minute samples at both the beginning and the end of the presentation.

If it is determined, after reviewing the tape, that excessive loudness, inappropriate pitch, and poor tone focus are causing strain of the
vocal mechanism, then the need to define the specific situation is present. For example, how large is the room? Are the acoustics adequate?
How many people are being addressed? Is amplification available?
What is the seating arrangement in relation to the podium? How many
hours of public speaking are done each day? When do breaks occur?
What is the subject matter?

After defining the situations, the occurrences, and the specific
environment of the speaker, the modifications are made. These may
include moving the lecture site closer to the audience, using amplification, building vocal time-outs into daily lesson plans, or simply talk-

ing softer while monitoring the back row of the audience to see if the speaker can still be heard.

If the patient continues to speak with the inappropriate voice components following these environmental controls, then direct modification of loudness, pitch, and focus may prove necessary. In the latter stages of therapy, large room presentations should actually be practiced using the improved voice components. (Modification of specific components is described later in this chapter.) Finally, direct Vocal Function Exercises for rebalancing airflow, muscle activity, and tone focus may be utilized.

For example, a 32-year-old female was referred for voice evaluation and treatment with a diagnosis of bilateral vocal fold nodules The patient was a new college professor who taught courses in special education and remedial reading. The following vocal hygiene management plan was developed during the diagnostic evaluation.

1. Identify the abuse:
    excessive loudness during lectures, use of a high pitch, and back tone focus.
2. Describe the effect:
    accomplished with illustrations and discussion of physiology.
3. Define specific occurrences:
    during 9 hours of lecture per week to an average class size of 25 students; and
    during occasional (average once per month) guest lectures that involved 1/2-day workshops.
4. Modify the behavior:
    ask the students to sit in the front of the room;
    build in more classroom discussion and less straight lecture;
    have more audience participation during workshops;
    use amplification when possible;
    direct modification of the voice components of loudness, pitch, and tone focus; and
    Vocal Function Exercises.

Case Study 5: Vocal Abuse in Children

By far the most common cause of voice disorders in children is vocal abuse including the abusive behaviors of shouting, loud talking, vocal noises, and throat clearing. Most children shout, and some shout more than others. Part of the natural childhood expression is through shouting. The problem, of course, arises when some children who abuse their voices develop laryngeal pathologies such as vocal fold nodules or chronic vocal fold edema.

When laryngeal pathologies occur, the traditional management approaches have focused on ways of reducing or eliminating the abusive behaviors through behavior modification programs (Wilson, 1987). These programs involve identifying the specific vocal abuses and then **charting** their occurrences on daily graphs prepared by the voice pathologist. Reduction in the occurrences of the abuses is rewarded in some manner. While this approach has proved to be successful with many children, its limited scope proves less than adequate for many others. We would suggest that several questions must be considered when planning management strategies for vocally abusive children. These questions include:

1. How does the child shout?
2. Does the child make vocal noises?
3. Does nonplay shouting occur?
4. Has the laryngeal pathology created a physiologic imbalance of the vocal mechanism?
5. Does habitual throat clearing occur?

Let us examine each question individually.

1. How and why does the child shout? A question that is often asked involves why, if most children shout, do some children develop laryngeal pathology while others do not? We might speculate that some children simply shout more than others; children are differentially susceptible to the development of laryngeal pathology; or maybe some vocal mechanisms are not as resilient as others. Another reason that appears clinically significant is that different children shout in different ways perhaps with some of the shouting behaviors being more physiologically balanced and supported than others, and therefore not as abusive to the vocal mechanism.

These speculations have led us to attempt a treatment strategy that we find to yield successful results. That strategy is to teach the child how to shout. It is our belief that it is not practical or totally fair to ask a child to stop all shouting behaviors. Rather than trying to extinguish all shouting (especially during play), it is possible and effective to teach children to shout using a low-pitched voice with improved breath support. We believe that use of the lower pitch reduces the natural stiffness and tension of the vocal folds which is inherent when a higher pitch is used. This may be accomplished by teaching the child to use a "grown-up voice," "daddy's voice," or a "papa bear voice," depending on the child's age. With older children, we simply explore their lower pitch range and choose a pitch level toward the bottom of the range. The patient practices speaking at that level in a comfortable conversational loudness level. They are then instructed in gradual steps to increase the loudness level until an appropriate "shout" is attained. At the same time, respiratory support, using proper breathing patterns, is established. This is the method that we successfully use with cheerleaders who develop voice disorders.

Why does the child shout ? This question explores the psychodynamics of the shouting behaviors. Andrews (1991, 1993) explains the importance of modifying the psychosocial aspects of the child's shouting behavior in order for the more direct therapy interventions to be successful. The exploration and modification of these behaviors must involve cooperation of the parents and, at times, major changes in family interactions and reactions to the vocally abusive child and change in interpersonal strategies. In extreme cases, family counseling may be helpful in developing more appropriate family psychodynamics.

2. Does the child make vocal noises? An abusive vocal behavior that is often neglected by many voice pathologists is the production of vocal noises. Most children have abusive noises, which they make often during play, but, unless they are specifically asked about vocal noises during the evaluation, the noises will go undetected. Some favorite noises include machine guns, cars, trucks, motorcycles, sirens, and various animal noises. Each year there appears to be a popular new noise which is most often influenced by popular toys, movies, television shows or video games. Modification or elimination of these abusive noises is often desirable as a part of the treatment plan. Various mouth sounds and whistles that do not involve phonation may serve as substitutions. Extinguishing these abusive behaviors rarely proves to be difficult as the noises change or self-extinguish as play behavior and maturity levels change.

3. Does nonplay shouting occur? Another factor that needs to be identified and modified is nonplay shouting. Again, it is extremely helpful to have a parent involved in the entire management process. If such cooperation is available, then education of that parent may help to modify occurrences of shouting in the home, such as shouting from room to room, calling people to the phone, and arguing with brothers and sisters. Suggestions for the parent may include (a) not responding when the child calls from another room, forcing the child to physically seek the person being called, (b) not shouting for the child and expecting a response, and (c) attempting to control vocal sibling arguments. Without the parent's cooperation, nonplay shouting will probably continue, ideally with the modified low-pitched shout.

4. Has the laryngeal pathology created a physiologic imbalance? Both children and adults with laryngeal pathologies are likely to develop an imbalance in the respiratory, muscular, and resonatory aspects of voice production. A general weakness of the laryngeal muscles may also result as the vocal mechanism adjusts itself to accommodate the presence of the pathology. When a physiologic imbalance or a muscle weakness is suspected, direct Vocal Function Exercises and the Accent Method (Koschkee, 1993; Smith & Thyme, 1976) are voice therapy techniques that are recommended. Both of these management approaches, described later in this chapter, provide a holistic method of dealing with improvement of the entire physiologic vocal mechanism.

5. Does habitual throat clearing occur? In a study by Stemple and Lehmann (1980), more than two-thirds of the patients studied with vocal hyperfunction demonstrated a habitual throat clearing behavior. As a primary etiology, throat clearing most commonly develops as a result of mucous drainage due to colds, flu, and allergies or as a secondary symptom of esophageal reflux. While drainage itself is not abusive to the laryngeal mechanism, the throat clearing habit that results is extremely abusive because of the mechanical impact of the vocal folds and the grinding of the posterior laryngeal structures. In addition, acid burning caused by reflux in the posterior larynx creates a globus, or "lump in the throat" feeling leading to habitual throat clearing. The behavior often continues even after the medical condition has resolved due to the inherent edema and irritation that leads to more throat clearing or simply as a result of habit. At times, this cycle continues until a laryngeal pathology results.

Throat clearing may also develop secondary to laryngeal pathologies. This behavior occurs especially in the presence of mass lesions and vocal fold edema. Many patients report that they "feel" something in their throats that they try to clear. Some patients clear their throats to prepare the voice for phonation before they talk; others have no awareness of their throat clearing habit.

The importance of eliminating this behavior cannot be denied. We have seen cases in which all etiologic factors except throat clearing were resolved, and the abusive nature of this behavior maintained the pathology. Although we are discussing vocal abuse in children, the techniques for significantly reducing throat clearing apply to adults as well. The following example first reported by Stemple (1984) and repeated in Stemple (1993) is a management approach that is appropriate for all ages; the language used will vary, of course, with the age of the patient.

> Throat clearing is one of the most abusive things you can do to your vocal folds. When you clear your throat like this (demonstrate), you create an extreme amount of movement of your vocal folds, causing them to slam and rub together (demonstrate using your hands). You should understand that it is not unusual for you to have developed this habit. The vast majority of patients we see with your type of voice problem also have this habit. Sometimes people do not even know that they are doing it. But often they say that they feel something in their throat, like a lump or mucus. The majority of the time, however,

when you clear your throat, there is simply nothing there. The only thing you have accomplished is to create more vocal fold abuse.

We have demonstrated to you with the tape recording of this evaluation that most of the time when you clear your throat, it occurs right before you begin to speak. Also, you are clearing many more times than you realized. This is a sign that throat clearing is very much a habit. Like all habits, it is difficult to break. We are, therefore, going to try to make it easier by giving you a substitute habit that will (a) take the place of throat clearing, (b) accomplish the same thing as throat clearing, and (c) is not abusive. This substitute, nonabusive habit is a hard, forceful swallow. If you do, in fact, occasionally have an increased amount of mucus on your vocal folds, a hard swallow will accomplish the same thing as throat clearing—minus the abuse. The only difference is that throat clearing feels good. It psychologically gives you more relief than the hard swallow, even though it physically accomplishes no more. It is your goal to overcome this psychological dependence. Understand that this habit is harmful and that it must be broken.

In order to break this habit, you need to tell everyone in your family and any friends who are around you often (and whom you feel comfortable in telling) that you are not permitted to clear your throat anymore. When these "helpers" hear you clear your throat, and they will, they are to immediately point it out to you. Your task then is to "swallow hard". Obviously, it will not be necessary to swallow, since you just cleared your throat. However, this is your first step in substituting the hard swallow for the throat clearing.

After your family and friends have pointed out your throat clearing to you several times, you will begin to catch yourself. You will clear your throat and almost immediately thinks "OOPS! I am not supposed to do that". Your response again should be to swallow hard. When you have caught yourself clearing your throat several times, you will begin to halt yourself just prior to clearing. Once again, you will substitute the hard swallow, but this time the throat clearing was stopped. By the time you have reached this point, you will be very close to breaking the habit totally. The final goal will be met when you realize that you are swallowing many fewer times than the number of times you used to clear your throat.

I want you to work very hard on this problem. I think you will be very surprised just how quickly you are able to break this habit. As a matter of fact, the majority of our patients have significantly reduced the habit within 1 to 2 weeks. Most patients, though, cannot do it alone. So please, find other people to help you by having them point out when this occurs. Any questions? (pp. 22–23)

Following this explanation, the patient will typically clear his or her throat more times than usual. Each event is immediately pointed out by the voice pathologist, and the hard swallow substitution is initiated. Often, great gains in habit modification are made during this initial session.

Another suggestion for modification of throat clearing was made by Zwitman and Calcaterra (1973). These authors suggested a "silent cough" substitution for this behavior. The silent cough is accomplished by breathing deeply and then forcing air strongly through abducted vocal folds. This technique also reduces the abuse of coughing.

As stated previously, several factors must be considered when planning therapy strategies for vocally abusive children. Charting and graphing may certainly serve as a positive behavior modification approach in modifying or eliminating abuses, however, many more factors may be considered and other approaches utilized. A summary of a vocal hygiene plan for vocally abusive children would include

1. Identify the abuses:
    shouting;
    loud talking;
    vocal noises; and
    throat clearing.
2. Describe the effect:
    utilize pictures, diagrams, drawings, and video.
    Do not hesitate to give simple explanations of anatomy and
        physiology to children.
3. Define specific occurrences:
    These will be distinctly different for every individual child.
    Therefore, no two children will follow the same management plan.
    Psychodynamics of the behavior must also be described.
4. Modify the behavior:
    teach the child *how* to shout;
    modify or eliminate vocal noises;
    eliminate nonplay shouting;
    eliminate throat clearing; and
    balance the physiology of the voice production through direct
        therapy.

Case Study 6: Can We Always Expect Success?

Vocal abuse may occur in many settings under many different circumstances. These settings might include nightclubs, bars, bowling alleys, swimming pools, auction houses, sporting events, work environments, homes, schools and churches. Wherever we communicate, the possibility of vocal abuse is present. Often, the life-styles of patients dictate the ease or difficulty they will have in attempting to make vocal modifications. Some patients are not willing to modify their life-styles even for the health of the laryngeal mechanism. Voice pathologists must realize that their own concern for a patient's voice disorder does not always match that of the patient. For example, the patient who enjoys getting rowdy in bars may not respond well to the voice pathologist's greatest efforts for vocal reeducation. Or the patient who enjoys bowling in two winter leagues may continue to bowl and abuse the voice by laughing, talking, and shouting above the noise level as well as drinking dehydrating liquids. These are the patients who provide us with interesting challenges, but, we must remember that ultimate responsibility for change rests with the patient. The following is an interesting example of a patient who failed to respond to a four-step vocal hygiene counseling program.

The patient was a 30-year-old female who was referred with a diagnosis of chronic vocal fold edema for evaluation and treatment. The patient reported experiencing intermittent dysphonia for several years, but the dysphonia became persistent about six months prior to the evaluation. The diagnostic evaluation yielded the following management plan.

1. Identify the abuses:
   shouting; and
   straining the singing voice.
2. Describe the effect:
   accomplished with illustrations and discussion of physiology.
3. Define specific occurrences:
   shouting to discipline her children; and
   straining the voice during church singing on Sunday mornings and Wednesday evenings.
4. Modify the behavior:
   discussed various other strategies for disciplining children; and
   patient agreed to discontinue singing until her voice improved. Singing without strain would then be discussed.

The patient's voice quality during the evaluation was moderately dysphonic, characterized by a low pitch, glottal fry phonation, pitch breaks, and breathiness. No significant change or improvement in voice quality was observed during a 3-week period of therapy sessions which were held twice weekly. The patient denied shouting at her children and singing in church during this time.

Also during this period an interesting pattern of dysphonia was noted. The patient reported experiencing severe dysphonia and almost total aphonia every Sunday night and Thursday morning. When the patient was seen in therapy on Tuesdays and Fridays, the original moderate dysphonia was noted. Further questioning yielded the true cause of the patient's disorder.

As you may have guessed, she attended church services on Sunday mornings and Wednesday evenings. Although she refrained from singing, she joined the many people in the congregation who responded with vigorous vocal enthusiasm to the preacher's message. The need to add this behavior to those requiring modification was explained to the patient.

Although she made concentrated efforts to reduce her vocal enthusiasm during the church service, she had little success in doing so. Final attempts were made to counteract these periods of extreme vocal abuse through direct symptom modification. Because of the frequency of the abuse however, this, too, proved unsuccessful. The patient eventually was terminated from therapy with no improvement noted in her vocal condition. This patient made the informed decision that her vocal behaviors during the church service were more important to her than improving the quality of her voice.

Can we always expect success? Yes! Otherwise we may be guilty of a self-fulfilling prophecy. Will we succeed with all patients? The answer, unfortunately, is no. But only a concerted effort for a reasonable period of time will give us that answer.

TREATMENT STRATEGIES FOR INAPPROPRIATE VOCAL COMPONENTS

Chapter 3 describes the components of voice that include respiration, phonation, resonation, pitch, loudness, and rate. The inappropriate use of any one vocal component or combination of components may lead directly to the development of a voice disorder. Voice disorders my occur in patients who simply have faulty vocal habits and use, for example, a functionally breathy voice, soft voice, or a voice that is too high or too low in pitch. Other patients may use the resonatory system inefficiently or may focus the laryngeal tone inappropriately while others talk either too fast or slow. When inappropriate vocal components are used, direct symptom modification may be in order.

Inappropriate vocal components may also be the result of the laryngeal pathologies. For example, the voice of the patient with Reinke's edema may be breathy and low in pitch. Although the vocal components of pitch and respiration are inappropriate, they are not the primary cause of the pathology but merely two of the symptoms. Modification of the primary etiology (such as smoking in the case of Reinke's edema) is the first line of treatment, with symptom modification following only when necessary.

THERAPY APPROACHES

Respiration

Very few voice patients have breathing patterns so faulty that they interfere with normal phonation. Boone (1971), Brodnitz (1971), and

Murphy (1964) all suggested that little need exists for the formal training of breathing for speech. In fact, little, if any, benefit is seen in changing breath support from thoracic to diaphragmatic. It has been our experience that attempts to bring conscious control over this subconscious action of breathing often confuses rather than helps patients. Having said this, however, the reader should understand that some patients do have the need to modify certain functional respiratory habits. Respiration is one of three major physiologic components of voice production which may be modified by a voice disorder or may primarily contribute to the development of a voice disorder. As a primary cause, breathing modifications that are most common in contributing to voice problems occur in individuals who talk on residual air and in public speakers who may require greater breath support during presentations than during normal conversational speech.

Patients who continue to talk following the normal expiration of air are talking on residual air. Because this type of phonation requires increased laryngeal muscle tension, this behavior may strain the vocal mechanism and lead to the development of a voice problem. Suggestions for reducing this behavior include the following:

1. **Identification.** Identify the problem for the patient and describe its effect in detail, utilizing illustrations and descriptions of vocal fold anatomy and physiology.
2. **Ear training.** Monitor the patient's respiration strategy utilizing tape-recorded samples of the voice.
3. **Component modification.** (a) Practice breathing for voice by saying as many numbers as possible on one normal expiration. Stop before any force or strain is evident. (b) Mark a paragraph with phrase markers. Read the paragraph aloud with normal inhalations occurring at each phrase marker. (c) Tape-record an open discussion between the voice pathologist and the patient during the structured therapy period. Monitor the tape for inappropriate breathing patterns.
4. **Stabilization.** Structure nontherapy conversational times in which the patient is to monitor the voice on a daily basis. Often, a good time to do this is during dinner with the family.

Some patients, especially those who use their voices for some type of public speaking, request strategies for learning diaphragmatic breathing. Although thoracic, or chest breathing, is normally adequate for voice support, the most efficient means of breathing for speech is the diaphragmatic method. A suggested approach for training this method follows.

1. By utilizing a box diagram (Figure 7–1), describe the various means of air exchange, including clavicular, thoracic, and diaphragmatic.

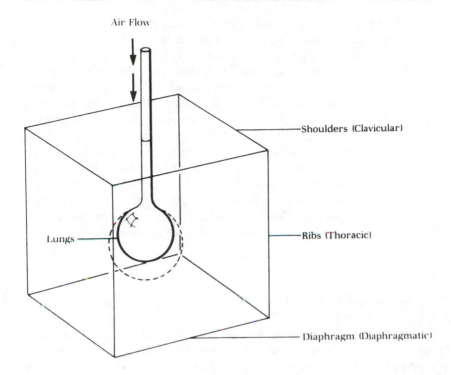

Air Flow

Shoulders (Clavicular)

Lungs

Ribs (Thoracic)

Diaphragm (Diaphragmatic)

Figure 7–1.   Box diagram representing breathing patterns.

The voice pathologist may say, "There are three ways in which air may be made to flow into the lungs. All three ways require some expansion of the thoracic cavity, where the lungs are located. The least efficient way to expand the cavity is to raise the top of the box or the shoulders. This allows for poor cavity expansion and would require much vocal effort given the small amount of air that enters the lungs. I'm not even sure that anyone even uses this type of breathing pattern. The most common way of expanding the cavity is to raise the sides, or the rib cage. This larger expansion normally allows enough air to be inhaled to support voice during normal conversational speech. If you watch people breathe as they talk, you'll notice that most are using this inhalation method."

"The most efficient method of air intake for the support of voice is through the downward contraction of the bottom, or the diaphragm. The diaphragm is a dome-shaped elastic muscle that forms the bottom of the thoracic cavity. When it contracts downward, the muscles of the abdomen are forced outward, and the cavity expands to its maximum extent. This permits a greater flow of air into the lungs. This air may then be used to better support your voice."

2. Following this explanation, the patient is requested to place one hand on the chest and the other hand on the upper abdominal wall. When inhaling diaphragmatically, the abdominal wall will expand outward while the chest remains in a nearly fixed position with only minimal movement. Contraction of the diaphragm cannot be seen. The patient is asked to breathe in this manner without phonation while observing the proper hand movement on both inhalation and exhalation. Practice is then gradually expanded, utilizing vowels, words, phrases, paragraph reading, and conversational speech. The public speaking voice may also be practiced in the therapy session utilizing the new breathing method.

Phonation

Inappropriate phonation is demonstrated by the use of hard glottal attacks, glottal fry phonation, and breathy phonation. As usual, the first step in modifying these behaviors involves identifying their presence to the patient. This may be accomplished through evaluation of tape-recorded samples of the voice. The impact of the vocal misuse should also be identified through illustrations and the discussion of vocal fold anatomy and physiology. Finally, the specific misuse should be described in detail as follows.

1. Hard glottal attack.

"A hard glottal attack is made when subglottic air pressure, or air that you build up below your vocal folds, is increased to a very high pressure level just before you say a word that begins with a vowel sound. Then, when you say that word, the vocal folds literally blow apart (demonstrate the hard glottal attack) like this. This action is very harsh on the vocal folds. It causes them to squeeze together very hard to maintain the high air pressure. Then when the vowel sound is produced, they rub and bang together as the pressure is released."

Another way of describing this behavior is to use the example of a garden hose.

"A typical garden hose is attached to a faucet at one end and has a spray nozzle at the other end. When the nozzle is closed and the water is turned on at the faucet, a tremendous amount of pressure builds up through the whole system, with the greatest amount of pressure at the nozzle. If the nozzle is suddenly opened and then closed, the water gushes out and then slams against the nozzle valve. However, if the nozzle were slightly open and the water was con-

trolled at the faucet, the entire system would remain relaxed and little pressure would be exerted on the valve. We can relate the pressure
in the hose to your subglottic air pressure and the nozzle to your
vocal folds. What you need to do is to learn how to produce words
that begin with vowel sounds without building up that pressure."

The patient is then taught to produce a soft glottal attack or an
easy onset by initiating phonation with the sound /h/, utilizing vowels, vowel-consonant combinations, and progressing through words,
phrases, paragraph reading, and conversation. The /h/ is extinguished as soon as possible in the process. Negative practice is effective as a stabilization strategy.

2. Glottal fry phonation. The glottal fry is an unusual lower register voice produced at the very bottom the normal pitch range. It may be
recognized as an aperiodic staccato sound and is produce on tightly
approximated vocal folds with flaccid free edges (Zemlin, 1988). We
often observe glottal fry phonation at the end of phrases, as patients
drop their breath support, and in the voices of patients who complain
of voice fatigue. Extended use of glottal fry phonation appears to be
abusive to the vocal folds and should be modified. Because it normally
occurs in conjunction with the use of an inappropriately low pitch,
modification is made by training a slight increase in pitch and loudness.

3. Breathy phonation. Some patients have the habit of speaking
with an incomplete adduction of the vocal folds, yielding a weak,
breathy voice. Although some actors cultivate this type of voice to project an image of sultriness or sexiness, it is a vocal misuse, and its prolonged use could lead to laryngeal pathology.

Again, therapy would begin with identification of the problem
and education of the effects that breathy phonation may have on the
vocal mechanism. When phonation is breathy, causing a wastage of air
during phonation, the vocal folds are forced to vibrate inefficiently.
The inherent poor breath support impairs vocal quality by causing secondary abusive glottal or supraglottal tension.

The major therapy approaches for modifying the breathy voice
involve training the patient to produce a more firm or engaged vocal
fold approximation. The specific approach used will depend on the
severity of the breathiness.

1. Mild breathiness may be modified through patient education and
    often through the use of a more precise articulation, especially on
    the plosive sounds /p/, /t/, and /k/ (Canfield, 1964).

2. A moderate amount of breathiness may often be modified by
    training the speaker to increase vocal intensity. A slightly
    louder voice will force the vocal folds to approximate more
    firmly, thus decreasing the wastage of air. Ear training, by com-

paring the breathy voice to the louder voice on a tape recorder, and negative practice are excellent modification approaches.

3. A more than moderate amount of breathiness may require these approaches as well as a more rigorous therapy approach. This may include actually teaching the patient to approximate the vocal folds utilizing the previously described "misuse" of hard glottal attacks. Hard glottal attacks will give the patient an awareness of the vocal fold approximation and muscle engagement. The vowel produced in this manner will have clearer tones that can be compared to the patient's breathy tones. An even more rigorous approach would be the use of Froeschel, Kastein, and Weiss's (1955) pushing exercises. These exercises combine the isometric pushing of the arms at the same moment of phonation. These simultaneous activities create firmer adduction of the vocal folds through overflow muscular tension, thus decreasing breathiness. (See Vocal Fold Paralysis in Chapter 8 for a complete description of pushing exercises.)

Resonation

The inappropriate use of resonation may be one of the more difficult properties of voice to modify. Thus far in our discussion we have been concerned with functional voice behaviors. When considering therapy for resonance disturbances, it is important for the voice pathologist to be certain that the disorder is, in fact, functional, and not organic in origin. There are many organic causes for resonance disturbances including various palatal clefts, insufficient function of the velopharyngeal port, surgical trauma, and neurological disease and disorders. Organic causation may be determined through medical examination, cineflouroscopy, and manometric measures. The major characteristic of functional resonance disorders is the lack of consistency in the resonatory quality and the positive stimulability of a more normal resonation.

Resonance characteristics of speech vary greatly from one geographic location to another. For example, resonation judged appropriate in the East may not be acceptable in the Midwest. These qualities often change naturally as speech and voice patterns are assimilated into the local patterns, or they may need to be modified through therapy. Other common causes of functional resonance disturbances are structural oral-pharyngeal changes following tonsillectomy and adenoidectomy, and imitation of other speakers with inappropriate resonance patterns.

Treatment of organic resonance problems is usually limited to surgical and orthodontic/prosthodontic procedures. These may include the closing of clefts, the creation of pharyngeal flaps for inadequate velar closure, or the molding and fitting of prosthetic obturators to provide posterior velar competence. Evaluation and treatment of organic resonance disturbances is most often provided by a formal team of professionals that comprise a Craniofacial Anomaly Team. Team members may include a speech pathologist, audiologist, orthodontist, prosthodontist, otolaryngologist, and general and plastic surgeons. Voice therapy often follows medical treatment to guarantee that maximum gain is received from the combined treatments.

The voice pathologist is most concerned with modifying both functional hypernasality and hyponasality as well as dealing with the more common use of an inappropriate tone focus. Treatment of resonance and focus problems often proves difficult and requires all the creative skills available. According to Aronson (1980), no management approach can be generalized to any population with nasal resonance. Techniques that work for one individual in improving voice quality may not work for others with the same problem.

For functional hypernasality and denasality problems, the direction of voice therapy is to manipulate articulation, resonation, and phonation boldly in as many combinations as proves necessary to locate the most efficient resonant quality.

Hypernasality

As usual, the first step in the modification of any vocal property is to identify the problem and to describe it in detail to the patient. Illustrations demonstrating the relationships between the resonance cavities are helpful. Tape-recorded samples of the patient's voice compared to the voices of other individuals of similar age are helpful for ear training. Other suggested modification approaches include:

1. Articulation therapy. Often, maximizing the precision of articulatory movements and decreasing any articulation errors will increase the intelligibility of the speech and decrease the perception of hypernasality (Arnold, 1965; McWilliams, 1954). Increasing articulatory precision will involve activating all the articulators in a somewhat exaggerated manner, with special emphasis placed on a wider mouth opening, thus decreasing the contribution of the nasal cavity in treating the glottal sound (Wilson, 1979).

2. Pitch and loudness modification. Boone (1977) discussed a positive decrease in the amount of nasal resonance in some patients who were taught to speak with an increased intensity at a lower pitch level.

3. Nonspeech phonation. The patient plays with the voice, making various nonspeech vocal sounds, such as animal and engine noises. If any of the nonspeech sounds demonstrates reduced nasality, then work from this sound by (a) comparing it to hypernasal sounds, (b) training similar sounds, and (c) expanding into speech sounds.

4. Utilize articulation deep test. A deep test of articulation is used to determine if any sounds in any phonetic contexts are made with normal or near normal amounts of nasal resonance. If so, these productions are expanded into similar sound clusters, first, then words, phrases, and conversational speech.

5. Do the obvious. The patient's ability to produce a voice "...like you have a cold" is explored. Some patients with functional hypernasality can easily produce a denasal voice quality when speaking in this manner. They simply were not aware that a slight modification of the "cold" voice would yield the normal nasal quality. It pays to explore this ability early in the therapy program.

6. Negative practice. Negative practice may also be an effective therapy tool used with resonance disorders. When the new normal resonance is first being produced, purposeful productions of the same sounds utilizing the "old" hypernasal voice may reinforce and strengthen the use of normal resonance. The patient's ability to use both voices upon dismissal from therapy shows a true mastery of the therapeutic goals.

Denasality

Functional denasality may occasionally occur, especially following the removal of nasal obstructions. Wilson (1979) suggested that the patient's auditory feedback system does not quickly adjust as it continues to attempt to maintain the status quo even though the nasal cavity is no longer obstructed. Once the disorder has been identified and described in detail, approaches used to modify the behavior include:

1. Utilizing the normal nasal sounds. In this approach the voice pathologist should determine the patient's ability to produce /m/, /n/, and /ng/ with normal resonance. If this is possible, /m/ and /n/ may be combined with vowel sounds and expanded through words, phrases, and so on.

If the nasal sounds are also produced with a denasal quality, attempts may be made to train the nasalization of /m/ using the singing voice. Humming, with the lips closed in the /m/ position, forces the production of more nasal resonance. These productions may be slowly modified by (a) opening the mouth while humming and saying /ma/, (b) expanding to other vowel sounds, (c) eliminating the hum, and (d) then expanding into other sounds, words, phrases, and so on.

2. Utilizing hypernasal resonance. Some patients who demonstrate a functional denasal voice are readily able to produce an exaggerated hypernasal voice quality. If this is so, then different gradients of velar closure may be demonstrated and stabilized, leading to normal velopharyngeal functioning.

3. Nonspeech phonation. (Explained under Hypernasality) This approach may also be an effective means of initiating normal voice resonance.

4. Negative practice. (Explained under Hypernasality.)

Tone Focus

Focus refers to the resonation of the voice in the supraglottic airways. Constriction of the airway at any point will alter the focus of the voice production. The ideal placement of the tone is forward as this placement allows the voice to resonate fully throughout the pharyngeal, nasal, and oral cavities without effort or tension. Tension at any point in the vocal tract will alter the free resonation of the tone and alter voice quality. In addition to changing the quality, less than ideal tone placement may result in a voice that fatigues easily and lacks flexibility and vibrancy.

Poor tone focus may be observed in patients who *functionally* constrict the pharynx, retract the tongue, and elevate the larynx as the habitual manner in which voice is produced. Poor tone focus may also be the *result* of laryngeal pathologies which, when present, force the patient to constrict the upper airway to accommodate the presence of the pathology. This constriction often leads to what is commonly termed a back-focused tone. The voice qualities associated with several laryngeal pathologies commonly present with a backward tone focus. These pathologies include edema and mass lesions of the vocal folds which require the patient to constrict the glottic and supraglottic structures due to the presence of the increased mass; bowed vocal folds and other incomplete closures caused by laryngeal myasthenia and laryngeal fatigue, paresis or paralysis; and adductor spasmodic dysphonia which forces the patient to tense the vocal mechanism as a means of pushing the voice through the spasms. As the inappropriate focus becomes habituated, it is common that direct voice therapy approaches must be utilized to reintroduced a more ideal and less tense placement of the tone.

A therapy approach that we have found useful for improving tone focus uses nasal sounds and sensory feedback to tune the patient into the nebulous concept of focus:

1. Patient education. We begin by teaching the patient about the concept of resonation by demonstrating how one sentence may be said with various resonance characteristics. Patients are made aware of how celebrity impersonators change the resonation of the voice to sound like other people. The concepts of frontal, back, and mid-focus are introduced by first demonstrating a tight, constricted, back-focused phrase which the patient is asked to imitate. Since this type of tone placement is most often implicated as the problem, most patients, though somewhat embarrassed, are able to produce this voice. Second, a breathy, poorly focused tone is imitated followed by an exaggerated, almost nasal forward focus. It is explained to the patient that, while the ultimate goal was not to talk in a nasal quality, this placement was closest to the desired focus. Practice of this exaggerated forward placement would be one step toward learning the desired placement.

2. Nasalized phrase production. The patient is instructed to slowly and softly chant the following phrases on a comfortable pitch level slightly above the fundamental frequency:

Oh my

Oh me

Oh no

Oh my no

Oh me oh my

The forward resonation of each phrase is exaggerated to the extreme and the patient is instructed to feel and sense the energy of the tone in the nose, on the lips, in the front of the face, and so on. Tape recordings of the phrases are made for both the clinician and the patient and ear training is accomplished as needed.

Once the phrases are produced to the satisfaction of the voice pathologist, negative practice is used. The patient is asked to alternate between forward and back-focuses to demonstrate the mastery of the focus technique on these simple phrases.

3. Introduce intensity and rate variations. Using the same phrases, patients are asked to repeat each phrase multiple times using the following routine:

very slow and very soft

faster-louder

fast-loud

slower-softer

very slow and very soft

Changing the rate and loudness of the chanted phrases adds a new dimension to the exercise that forces the patient to concentrate on maintaining the forward placement even as the intensity and rate are increased.

4. Introduce inflected phrase and normal speech. When the patient has succeeded in mastering the first three steps, the phrases may be modified from the single pitch chant to a more "sing-song" or inflected vocal presentation and then directly into a normally spoken phrase:

soft and slow

louder-faster

exaggerated inflection

normal speech

The proper focus of the tone is closely monitored during each one of these steps utilizing the phrases. Negative practice is judicially used throughout each session. Some patients move quickly through each of these steps and master a forward focus with ease. Others require many therapy sessions to master the appropriate focus. The final step is to expand the ability to produce a forward focus from these phrases into expanded phrases and sentences, paragraph reading, and conversational speech.

Other clues suggested by Lee (1993) to help make patients aware of forward focus include playing a comb wrapped with waxed paper with the lips (The lips are made to vibrate by phonation and the comb resonates this vibration making patients more aware of the forward placement of the tone); make a motorcycle noise by vibrating the lips together (This technique works well with children); and trilling the tongue on the top of the alveolar ridge while moving the lips to shape different sounds.

Pitch

Pitch levels that are either too high or too low are present in many laryngeal pathologies. The decision to modify pitch should be based on whether it is a primary etiologic factor or whether it is secondary to the pathology. If an inappropriate pitch is present due to laryngeal pathology, it is likely to reach a normal level without direct component modification once the pathology is resolved. Direct pitch modification is somewhat difficult and has the potential of causing laryngeal harm if the new pitch level is trained artificially high or low. Let us examine some of the more common reasons for the use of inappropriate pitch levels and identify those that may benefit from direct modification.

Increased vocal fold mass as a result of edema and mass lesions of the larynx may cause a lowering of the voice fundamental frequency. The primary etiology is whatever caused the pathology. If the cause proved to be the inappropriate use of pitch, then therapy would focus on direct pitch modification.

An example of inappropriate pitch as a primary cause of laryngeal pathology would be the use of the pseudoauthoritative voice. Conscious efforts by men and women to sound more authoritative or self-assured by using a forceful deep voice, especially in work settings, may lead to the development of a voice disorder. In this case, the therapy of choice would be a direct symptom modification approach as well as a discussion of why the need to use this voice is perceived by the patient.

Another example of an intentional pitch modification occasionally seen in therapy is the patient who is trying to "save" the voice. These are patients who are experiencing some vocal difficulties. In an attempt to counteract these difficulties, they try to "save" the voice by habitually lowering the pitch and volume. The patients have the misconception that by talking in this manner, they are reducing the impact of whatever is causing the vocal difficulty. In reality, just the opposite is true. Habitual use of an inappropriately low-pitched voice is a vocal misuse and can lead to the development of pathology. Direct pitch modification is then in order.

Patients who develop a hormonal imbalance due to surgery, malfunction of the endocrine system, or as a side effect to medications present an interesting problem. The interesting point about this etiologic factor is that laryngeal pathology is not likely to occur unless the patient's auditory feedback system attempts to modify the pitch level back to the original level. Counseling *against* direct pitch modification is often the treatment of choice.

Emotional and physical disturbances will often lead to a voice of depression. The way a person feels physically and emotionally is directly reflected in the vocal quality. People who are depressed, agitated, upset, physically ill, mourning, or going through other emotional conflicts often have a low-pitched, poorly supported voice. The primary etiology is the emotional stress, but secondary use of the inappropriate vocal components may lead to a voice disorder.

Two other factors that lead to the inappropriate use of pitch are whole body and laryngeal fatigue. The person who is constantly fatigued is likely to use poor breath support and permit the pitch level to lower due to a lack of effort behind the speaking voice. Fatigue may also affect the components of respiration and loudness. Laryngeal fatigue often leads to an *effort to talk*. As a result, patients often drop the pitch and respiratory support which actually exacerbates the problem of fatigue.

Upward pitch changes may also cause voice problems. As discussed under the abusive behavior of shouting, as vocal intensity increases so too does the frequency level. This problem may be remediated through direct pitch modification. Finally, pitch change may actually be desirable as requested by a male to female transsexual. Let us now look at some therapy approaches for pitch modification.

Case Study 7: The Pseudoauthoritative Voice

A 25-year-old male with a diagnosis of bilateral contact ulcers without evidence of reflux was referred for evaluation and treatment. Voice quality during the evaluation was moderately dysphonic, characterized by low pitch, glottal fry phonation, inappropriate loudness, and breathiness. The patient reported experiencing vocal difficulties soon after beginning a new job as a bank manager trainee five months prior to the evaluation. Other than occasional shouting at sporting events, no other vocal abuses were identified. Results of the evaluation revealed that the patient's contact ulcers were the result of using a loud, low-pitched pseudoauthoritative voice in his work setting. Being in his first position of authority, the patient attempted to project a "strong" image. Inappropriate use of the low, loud voice involved rubbing and grinding of the arytenoid cartilages that led to the development of the contact ulcers. The treatment plan involved three major steps.

The first step was to identify the causes and to explain to the patient in detail what contact ulcers are and what led to their development. When dealing with a male, it is not wise to explain that the pitch must be raised. The mental impression he gains would be that of a major pitch modification when, in fact, a very minor modification is needed. It is better to explain that he is talking at the very bottom of is voice and that therapy will be designed to return it to its normal level. Tape-recorded samples were then used to demonstrate the vocal symptoms in question. Examples of the voice components were also imitated by the voice pathologist.

The second step was an attempt to identify a more appropriate pitch level. As previously stated, this is somewhat risky with the pathological voice. However, a higher pitch that is comfortable for the patient, and produced with little effort, will normally prove adequate. Cooper (1973) suggested having the patient say, in a natural conversational voice, "um-hum," as if answering "yes" to a question. The "hum" part of the production is usually produced in a very relaxed tone near the patient's present, most comfortable pitch level.

The third step was to match the appropriate pitch level to a musical note on a pitch pipe which served as a reference note. The patient was then asked to match that level while repeating single-syllable words and short phrases. The phrases were gradually lengthened and inflectional patterns were introduced. Sentences, paragraph reading, and conversational speech marked his progress, which was monitored with audio replays (language master) and by tape-recorded samples. Negative practice was also used. It is positive for a patient to have total control of the voice, and negative practice helps the patient meet this goal.

Case Study 8: The Voice Saver

The patient was a 31-year-old male who was referred for evaluation and treatment with the diagnosis of mild, bilateral vocal fold edema. The patient had only recently begun experiencing vocal difficulties. As a young assistant pastor of a large Christian parish, he was required to hold meetings, counsel youth, visit the sick and elderly, teach a Bible studies class, and deliver a sermon one Sunday per month. He had noticed four weeks prior to the evaluation that his voice routinely tired and became hoarse every day in the early afternoon. The patient denied any vocal abuse and did not feel that he gave enough group presentations to cause the vocal problem. His medical history was unremarkable and the social history did not yield evidence of the typical forms of voice abuse except for throat clearing which was noted throughout the evaluation.

The patient's voice quality during the evaluation was described as moderately dysphonic, characterized by low pitch, low intensity, glottal fry phonation, and an unusual amount of breathiness. The use of these inappropriate voice components could account for this patient's voice difficulties, but the severity of the voice quality did not fit the observations made through laryngeal videostrobosopy or the diagnosis of mild edema.

The patient was therefore asked if this voice was typical of his voice when it would fatigue. "Oh, no!" he replied, and to the voice pathologist's surprise, his reply was in a normal voice. "I'm talking down like that to save my voice."

Further questioning revealed that the patient had a chest cold for two weeks prior to the onset of his daily voice fatigue. Much coughing and throat clearing during the cold was reported. When the cold subsided, the throat clearing persisted, continuing the mild edema and weakness of the vocal musculature. Introduction of the "saving" voice only caused more vocal misuse. Successful therapy focused on vocal hygiene counseling, elimination of throat clearing, and strengthening of the laryngeal muscles. Attempts to save the voice were extinguished.

It is said that experience is the best teacher. After that experience, we have found several patients who were trying to "save" the voice in much the same manner. This especially seems to occur in people who do a great deal of talking or singing on a daily basis. They report that they begin to experience laryngeal fatigue and therefore let the voice drop lower in pitch, decreasing the phonatory effort and respiratory support. This, of course, is a misuse of the vocal components that tax the muscular system, thus accelerating the laryngeal fatigue.

The most positive short-term approach to counteract fatigue is to train the patient to place more breath support under the voice, slightly increase loudness, and to maintain the higher, more appropriate pitch level. Even though this requires more perceived physical effort the improved balance of the vocal components will often reduce the fatigue and, indeed, refresh the voice production.

Case Study 9: Emotional Voice Changes

The patient was a 23-year-old woman who was referred for evaluation and treatment, with a diagnosis of mild to moderate vocal fold edema. The patient's voice quality during the evaluation was a mild dysphonia, characterized by a low pitch, low intensity, and breathiness. She reported that she experienced vocal difficulties just one month prior to the evaluation. The usual diagnostic questions were posed, probing for the etiologic factors associated with the development of the disorder. No form of vocal abuse could be identified, and the medical history was unremarkable.

However, questions regarding her social history, specifically "How long have you been married?" elicited an emotional and tearful response. This line of questioning was followed. The patient volunteered that just prior to the onset of her vocal difficulties she discovered that her husband of 11 months had been unfaithful. Rather than confront him with this information, she remained silent and was contemplating divorce.

The effect of emotional tension and depression on the vocal components and the resultant quality of voice were explained. Often the patient's understanding of why the voice lowers, weakens, becomes breathy, and tires easily is enough to relieve the additional anxiety of the vocal problem. In all cases, the need for further counseling is determined and the appropriate referrals made. This particular patient was referred for family counseling to attempt to resolve the primary cause of her laryngeal pathology. Direct vocal component modification was not appropriate or necessary in this situation.

Transsexual Voice Change

The voice pathologist may be called upon to aid in the feminization of the male to female transsexual voice and speech patterns. Individuals who desire gender reassignment therapy and surgery are often referred to Gender Dysphoria clinics. The programs offered by these clinics include step by step procedures leading to the final surgical modifications necessary to accomplish the permanent gender reassignment. The procedures also include psychological counseling, electrolysis for the removal of body hair, and hormone treatments to enhance female characteristics. In addition, patients are required to live the part of the desired sex for one year prior to surgery.

The effects of hormones administered for the purpose of feminization are minimal as related to voice change. Therefore, the individual is required to affect not only an elevation of the fundamental frequency, but also modification of the resonant characteristics, an alteration in inflection and intonation patterns, precision of articulation, and even type of vocalized pauses (Coleman, 1976; Nittrouer et al., 1990; Spencer, 1988;). It is desirable to modify these speech and voice characteristics even prior to the reassignment surgery.

Pitch modification is actually the first and easiest part of the feminization of the voice. We choose to test the entire frequency range of the patient and then attempt to place the new fundamental frequency as close to the comfortable mid-range as is possible. Modification of pitch in the normal laryngeal mechanism is potentially harmful if muscle tension is the result of the modification. Tension is monitored throughout therapy to assure that voice abuse does not result. The new pitch range is defined on a monitoring instrument (in our case a Visi-Pitch) and the patient practices producing words, phrases, sentences, paragraph readings, and conversations until the pitch level is habituated. At the same time, a slightly breathy phonation is taught and, when necessary the patient is taught to retract the tongue slightly which also tends to elevate the larynx in the neck. These slightly altered tongue and larynx positions tend to shorten the vocal tract and reduce the available area for supraglottic resonation which tends to feminize the voice (Spencer, 1988).

Along with the direct modification of the voice and vocal tract, patients must also learn to increase their rate of speech and lengthen their pauses, while at the same time increasing the precision of articulation (Terango, 1966; Wolfe, et al. 1990). Since female speakers use increased intonation, inflection patterns must be increased as well through practice with the voice pathologist. Finally, vocalized pauses, coughing, and throat clearing must also be modified. A harsh, low-pitched "uh" or throat clearing sound would certainly destroy the effect of the new voice and speech production. Patients must be trained to produce these sounds within a new acceptable range.

Loudness

Functional misuse of the intensities of voice may lead to the development of laryngeal pathologies. The vocally abusive behaviors of shouting and loud talking have already been discussed. However, habitual misuse of conversational voice levels that are either too loud or too soft may also lead to voice disorders. The first step in dealing with patients with either of these behaviors is to refer them for a complete audiological evaluation. The voices of patients with sensorineural hearing loss are often produced with too much intensity, caused by the inability to monitor the voice adequately. Those with conductive hearing losses may talk too softly, caused by their ability to hear through the bones in their heads and their inability to monitor competing background noise. When an auditory disorder has been ruled out or treated, several intensity modification approaches may be followed.

1. Make the patient aware of the problem by utilizing the diagnostic evaluation tape. Compare the patient's vocal intensity to that of the voice pathologist on the tape. Use illustrations and discussion to explain what effect the inappropriate use of loudness has had on the laryngeal mechanism.

2. Raise the patient's awareness level regarding how people react to the voice. For example, if the patient talks too loudly, do people back away, look away, or cut the patient short? Does the patient perhaps project an overbearing image? People who talk too softly may always be asked to repeat themselves, may be ignored, or may project a bashful or backward image.

3. Practice direct manipulation of many different intensities. Record these as short phrases for ear training purposes.

4. Utilize VU meter or a commercial intensity meter to stabilize productions of a reasonable intensity level. Habituate this level through words, phrases, paragraph readings, and conversational speech.

Rate

Seldom is the rate of a patient's speech deviant enough to cause laryngeal pathology. If rate becomes inappropriate enough to create a voice disorder, then, except in some neurologic disorders, it is typically because the rate is too fast. Speaking with too fast a rate may create vocal hyperfunction. A modification approach for reducing rate follows.

1. Make the patient aware of the problem by reviewing the voice on the diagnostic evaluation tape recording and comparing it to the rate of the voice pathologist. Use illustrations of vocal fold anatomy and discussion of physiology to explain how a fast rate creates vocal hyperfunction.

2. Many patients who attempt to slow down their rates of speech often attempt to accomplish this by pausing longer between words and phrases. While this is helpful, it is more effective to have the patient exaggerate vowel prolongations in words within moderately long phrases. This exercise is totally opposite their normal habit.

3. From deliberate vowel prolongations in phrases, you may move into reading song lyrics and poetry. The inherent

rhythms and inflectional patterns are ideal for indirectly teaching timing and melody, both of which are lacking.

4. When the patient has sufficiently mastered the reading of lyrics and poetry, begin paragraph readings of prose material. Monitor progress through tape recordings.

5. Begin negative practice. Listen to tape recordings of the same material read by the patient at an increased rate and at a normal rate.

6. Stabilize the new rate in structured conversational speech within the therapy setting. Use negative practice and expand the settings until the new rate is stabilized.

OTHER TREATMENT CONSIDERATIONS

Treatment of Laryngeal Area Muscle Tension

Vocal hyperfunction may be characterized by intermittent periods of laryngeal area tension, as may occur when someone shouts or clears the throat. It may also be a persistent general laryngeal area muscle tension. Several techniques that may be used to reduce persistent laryngeal area muscle tension are progressive relaxation, chewing exercises, digital massage, a yawn-sigh facilitator, and EMG biofeedback.

Progressive relaxation. Reduction of whole-body tension may serve as an indirect method of reducing laryngeal area tension. Progressive relaxation techniques presented by Jacobson (1938) are designed to teach patients to recognize the differences between muscles that feel tense and muscles that feel relaxed. The most popular exercise involves alternately tensing and relaxing all the muscles from the scalp to the toes. This technique may prove especially helpful in reducing tension in patients who may be anxious about therapy.

Chewing exercises. In 1952, Froeschels described the chewing method for laryngeal tension reduction. This method is based on the theory that phonating during vegetative chewing will relax all the structures involve in articulation, resonation, and phonation. Wilson (1979) described a six-step detailed approach in utilizing the chewing approach with children.

Digital massage. Aronson (1980) reported that all patients with voice disorders should be tested for musculoskeletal tension. If tension is an etiologic factor, then reducing it releases the capability of the larynx to produce normal voice. A seven-step program for decreasing laryngeal tension was suggested.

1. Encircle the hyoid bone with the thumb and middle finger, working them posteriorly until the tips of the major horns are felt.

2. Exert light pressure with the fingers in a circular motion over the tips of the hyoid bone and ask if the patient feels pain, not just pressure. It is important to watch facial expression for signs of discomfort or pain.

3. Repeat this procedure with the fingers in the thyrohyoid space, beginning from the thyroid notch and working posteriorly.

4. Find the posterior borders of the thyroid cartilage just medial to the sternocleidomastoid muscles and repeat the procedure.

5. With the fingers over the superior borders of the thyroid cartilage, begin to work the larynx gently downward, also moving it laterally at times. One should check for a lower laryngeal position by estimating the increased size of the thyrohyoid space.

6. Ask the patient to prolong vowels during these procedures, noting changes in quality or pitch. Clearer voice quality and lower pitch indicate relief of tension. Because these procedures are fatiguing, rest periods should be provided.

7. Once a voice change has taken place, the patient should be allowed to experiment with the voice, repeating vowels, words, and sentences. (pp. 200–201)

Aronson further stated that the rate of improvement varies depending upon the cause of the tension. Often change in voice quality may be expected within the first session. Aronson promotes this as a primary therapy approach.

Yawn-sigh approach. Another approach for reducing laryngeal area tension is the yawn-sigh facilitating technique as first described by Boone (1971). The action of the yawn tends to stretch and then relax the extrinsic muscles, lowering the larynx in the neck to a more neutral position. The subsequent sigh should then be more relaxed with less tension noted in the phonation of the tone. From the sigh phonation, the patient is taught to appreciate the sensation of relaxation. The yawn-sigh is then paired with various vowels and then stretched into words, phrases, and so on.

Biofeedback training. The basis of biofeedback is that self-control of physiological functions is possible with continuous, immediate information about the internal bodily state. Electromyographic biofeedback has been used successfully in the rehabilitation and treatment of a wide range of neuromuscular disorders. EMG feedback training permits patients to monitor electrical activities of their muscles and to exert some control over these areas. This form of biofeedback training has permitted patients to view the tension of the extrinsic laryngeal muscles and to reduce or increase these tension levels utilizing auditory and visual feedback. (Prosek, Montgomery, Walden, & Schwartz, 1978; Stemple, Weiler, Whitehead, & Komray, 1980). Stemple et al. (1980) demonstrated the successful use of EMG biofeedback in reducing laryngeal area tension and improving the vocal folds and voice production with a group of patients with vocal fold nodules.

Case Study 10: Ventricular Phonation

Occasionally patients increase laryngeal area muscle tension to such an extreme that they begin phonating on the false vocal folds. This may be a functional disorder or it may result from the patient's attempt to compensate for gross laryngeal pathology.

The patient was a 55-year-old lawyer who was referred for evaluation and treatment, with the diagnosis of ventricular phonation. The problem had begun 6 weeks prior to the evaluation, not coincidentally at about the same time that he was told he was being considered for a county judgeship. Voice quality was moderately dysphonic, characterized by harshness; however, the patient had gained a fair level of control and consistency of the voice. The major complaint was that the voice tired easily. He was not unduly concerned by the quality, which was puzzling to the voice pathologist. Results of the evaluation yielded no probable etiologic factors other than the patient's anxiety associated with the pending appointment. It appeared that the patient developed a voice disorder to satisfy a psychological need. He would us it as an excuse if he were not appointed judge.

Indirect therapy methods were first attempted utilizing general progressive relaxation and EMG biofeedback. The patient was readily able to reduce laryngeal tension levels, but this did not alter the production of ventricular phonation. Direct vocal manipulation was then employed. This followed the basic treatment approach presented by Boone (1977). This approach suggests that the voice pathologist use the following five steps:

1. Ask the patient to inhale and exhale in a prolonged manner with the mouth wide open. Do not attempt to phonate at this time.
2. Repeat the same procedure with the patient phonating on inhalation. Inhalation phonation is accomplished with the true vocal folds.
3. When true cord inhalation phonation is achieved, ask the patient to match this sound on exhalation phonation in the same breathing cycle. It is extremely important that the voice pathologist be persistent during this step in therapy. Boone (1977) suggested that failure to push long enough toward exhalation phonation with resistive patients is the major reason for failure in the approach.
4. When exhalation phonation is achieved, begin modifying this to a normal pitch level. This may be accomplished by singing down a musical scale in two- to three-note intervals on a vowel sound until the desired level is approximated.

5. Vary the vowel sounds and move on through syllables, words, phrases, and paragraphs and stabilize during conversational speech.

It may also prove helpful to utilize digital manipulation of the thyroid cartilage. The position of the larynx during ventricular phonation is high in the neck. Grasping the thyroid cartilage and holding or massaging it down during inhalation/exhalation phonation cycles may be effective.

Direct vocal manipulation proved effective in modifying this patient's voice, but only after he was appointed to the bench. Exercises to strengthen the laryngeal muscles were used to return the voice to a healthy condition.

TREATMENT STRATEGIES FOR PERSONALITY-RELATED ETIOLOGIES

Patients who develop pathologies as a result of personality disorders are among the more interesting in voice therapy. The major types of laryngeal pathologies caused by personality conflicts are conversion aphonia, conversion dysphonia, mutational falsetto, and juvenile voice. The management plans for all of these pathologies include four major stages. The first stage is the medical evaluation. As with all voice disorders, it is essential that the presence of organic pathology be ruled out prior to the initiation of therapy. The report of normal laryngeal structures will also confirm the diagnosis of a personality related disorder, in the presence of inappropriate and often unusual vocal symptoms.

The second treatment stage is the diagnostic evaluation. During the evaluation, the voice pathologist will develop the history of the pathology and will learn how the patient functions socially and physically within the environment. An impression of the patient's personality will evolve. The diagnostic time is also used to prepare the patient for vocal change. This is accomplished by explaining to the patient how the vocal mechanism works and by describing what is happening physiologically within the larynx to create the present voice. Although no attempt is yet made to explain why this is occurring, the physiological description provides the patient with a rationale for the vocal problems.

The third stage of vocal treatment is the direct manipulation of the voice. The type of manipulation will vary, depending on the non-speech phonation abilities demonstrated by the patient. Vocal manipulation most often begins during the diagnostic evaluation. The expected result is a dramatic change in the voice toward normal phonation. Greene (1972) and Boone (1977) both reported that these patients often attain normal voicing during the first treatment session. This has also been our experience.

The final stage of treatment involves counseling to determine why the disorder was present. Conversion voice disorders occur in patients who have undergone some physical or emotional trauma. It is the patient's subconscious effort to escape the unpleasant situation or the memory of the situation that promotes the reaction. Aronson (1980) suggested that the most appropriate professional to deal with this type of disorder is the voice pathologist, whose complete understanding of the vocal processes and counseling background provide the basic skills and abilities to remediate these pathologies. Once normal voicing has been achieved, it is a natural transition to begin examining why the problem existed. By this time the voice pathologist has gained an excellent trust and rapport with the patient. With interview questions that are structured in a nonthreatening manner, the voice pathologist can usually determine the cause of the problem. Patients frequently volunteer the necessary information, which often opens a floodgate of emotion.

Once the cause or causes have been identified and discussed, the voice pathologist needs to determine if further professional counseling is advisable. If so, the appropriate referral should be discussed with the patient and should be made with the patient's consent. Let us now examine each personality-related laryngeal pathology.

Conversion Aphonia

Conversion voice disorders, called hysteric, hysterical, nervous, functional, and psychosomatic aphonia, have been discussed in medical journals for scores of years. Many treatments have been advocated in the literature. Russell (1864) suggested that hysteric aphonia was a mental or moral ailment that required moral treatment. The method of cure was "to rouse the will, and thus rid the body of its thousand morbid things."

Ward (1877) advocated the application of an astringent to the vocal folds along with simultaneous electric shock. The pain of both procedures would influence the patient to talk. Goss (1878), Ingals (1890), and Bach (1890) also utilized painful "remedies" such as bitter tonics, iron, quinine, arsenic, and strychnia.

Two of the more imaginative remedies were described by Winslow (1919) and Howard (1923).

According to Winslow:

> My method of treatment is as follows: The patient is seated before me and a careful history of the case taken. Then with the laryngeal mirror I make a careful examination of the larynx, noting the movements of the vocal cords and the condition of the mucous membrane from the pharynx down as far as I can see. If I am satisfied that the case is

one of functional aphonia, I remove the mirror. The patient is then asked to take 10 or 12 deep breaths. He is next told to raise the arms above the head 10 or 12 times. Now looking the patient directly in the eye, I say to him that there is a little piece of cartilage in his throat which is slightly out of position and as soon as I put my finger down his throat and fix it, he will be able to use his voice. (This is to bring about the proper psychological attitude of the patient.) Then standing to his right with my left arm around his neck, the index finger of the left hand pushing in the cheek, between the upper and lower jaw (done to keep the patient from biting), the index finger of the right hand is shoved down the throat beyond the epiglottis and held there until the patient makes an attempt to get away. I continue to hold my finger there until it becomes quite uncomfortable. At this stage the patient will, as a rule, make a sound like a grunt and as soon as this happens I take my finger from the throat and begin to count fairly loud from one to five, at the same time urging the patient to count with me. If this does not work I repeat the count, from one to five, much louder than before. It may be necessary to yell while counting before the patient begins to use his voice. When the voice is restored, I keep it working for some time so that the patient will become accustomed to it. The attitude of the operator should be firm but gentle, and he must, by his demeanor, inspire the patient with the idea that he will restore the voice. (Winslow, 1919, pp. 1129–1130)

Howard described his case as follows:

Mrs. M.T., aged 51, whose nervous system has been below par since her husband committed suicide a year and a half ago, in January, 1922, contracted influenza. Prior to February 1, she enjoyed the full use of her voice, but that morning she found that she could not talk above a whisper. A diagnosis was made of functional aphonia, also known as hysterical nervous aphonia.

The patient was informed that there was no paralysis of the cords; that people affected in this way always recovered, and that the voice usually came back suddenly, just as it had left. The next day, she was told that we would put her to sleep and apply medicine to the parts, and that when she woke up she could talk. She was given ether, and, while she was under the anesthetic, the region was painted 1% silver nitrate as a local fillip to the parts. In coming out of the anesthetic, and while only partly conscious, she mumbles something above a whisper. She was encouraged to talk louder and asked to count out loud, and she did so. She has since then been talking normally. (Howard, 1923, p. 104)

Although these techniques are fun to review, the problem with all these so-called remedies is, of course, that their practitioners were not perfectly honest with the patients. Deceit is not necessary in modifying the vocal condition of conversion aphonic patients. Patients with this pathology have an unconscious need for the voice disorder and deserve an honest professional management approach. With this in mind, the following treatment strategies should be tried.

Strategy 1. By the time patients with conversion aphonia are referred to the voice pathologist, they are often truly seeking relief from the disorder and are subconsciously ready for change. Often, the event that precipitated the need for the conversion reaction has passed. Some patients may continue to receive secondary gains from the disorder and resist all therapeutic modifications, but the majority of patients will respond quickly to direct voice therapy.

Following the interview period of the diagnostic evaluation, the voice pathologist will present a physiological description of the vocal mechanism, utilizing simple line drawings. This will demonstrate how the adductor muscles are not pulling the vocal folds together, causing the voice to be whispered. This type of explanation may be given:

> For some reason, the muscles that pull the vocal folds together are simply not pulling the way that they should. Therefore the vocal folds are not closing all the way. When they don't close all the way, they can't vibrate and so all we can hear is a whisper. Our goal in therapy, therefore, is to manipulate the vocal muscle system in whatever way we need to encourage the vocal folds to come together.

With this approach, the voice pathologist has given the patient a non-threatening, reasonable explanation as to why phonation is not occurring. No comment is yet made regarding the patient's inherent ability to phonate. In fact, the "blame" for lack of phonation has been removed from the patient and placed squarely on the faulty laryngeal mechanism.

Traditional therapy approaches then examine the patient's ability to phonate during nonspeech phonatory behaviors such as coughing, throat clearing, laughing, crying, sighing, and gargling. When phonation is identified on one of these behaviors, it is then shaped into vowel sounds, nonsense syllables, words, and short phrases. The voice pathologist must demonstrate much patience at this time. Most patients have not phonated for several weeks. The possibility of proceeding too quickly and frightening the patient away from phonation is present. Once good, consistent phonation is established under practice conditions, the voice pathologist begins to gently insist that it be used during the therapy conversations. When voice is regained in this manner, it is seldom lost again, and patients do not substitute other conversion symptoms (Stevens, 1968).

Strategy 2. Another therapy technique utilizes the falsetto voice. The patient again is instructed in the physiology of the laryngeal mechanism and how it relates to the vocal difficulties. It is explained that we are going to manipulate the vocal mechanism in a manner that will force the muscles to pull the vocal folds together. The voice pathologist then produces the falsetto tone on the sound /aI/. The patient is told in a matter-of-fact manner that everyone can produce this tone, even those who are having vocal difficulties. The falsetto is again demonstrated by the voice pathologist, and the patient is instructed to produce the same sound. Some patients initially resist the falsetto production, but in our experience, with a little coaching, the majority of patients will eventually produce the tone. The falsetto is then stabilized briefly on vowels.

It is explained to the patient that we are going to use the muscle tension created by producing the falsetto tone to force the vocal folds to pull together normally. The patient is then given a list of two-syllable phrases and asked to read them in the falsetto voice. During this exercise, the patient is constantly encouraged to read swiftly and loudly. After the voice stabilizes in a relatively strong falsetto, the patient is halted and asked to match the clinician singing down the scale about three to four notes from the original falsetto tone. The patient is then asked to continue reading the phrases at this new pitch level. The same procedure is repeated two or three more times until the patient is fairly closely approximating a normal pitch level. The patient is continually encouraged to produce these phrases louder and faster until eventually the voice "breaks" into normal phonation.

Occasionally the patient will approximate normal phonation but then hesitate as if somewhat reluctant to produce normal voice. When this occurs, the patient is instructed to "drop way down" and produce a guttural voice quality while reading the phrases. This will "produce more tension." After a few minutes, the patient is taken back to the falsetto voice with the break into normal phonation usually occurring soon after.

Strategy 3.   Providing the patient with a reasonable physiologic explanation as to why the voice is whispered is an important part of encouraging the return to normal phonation. Another technique that we have found useful is the use of direct visual feedback using laryngeal videoendoscopy. While the patient is being scoped, either with rigid or flexible endoscopes, an explanation is given related to the positioning of the vocal folds and how that positioning relates to the present vocal problem. The patient is able to monitor the video over the voice pathologist's shoulder. The patient is then instructed in various manipulations of the vocal folds such as deep breathing, light throat clearing, and attempts to produce tones of various loudness levels and pitches. We have had surprising success in the quick return of normal voicing using this procedures.

It is extremely important that the voice pathologist be patient when utilizing any of these techniques. The normal time frame from aphonia to normal voice is approximately 30 to 45 minutes. The voice

pathologist must not only be patient but must also present a very matter-of-fact, confident manner. Voice pathologists are not cheerleaders.
They are simply presenting a technique that they know will work.

Why do these techniques work?

1. The patient is ready for change.
2. The voice pathologist has given a reasonable explanation for
   why the voice is gone.
3. The voice pathologist has demonstrated confidence in the
   therapeutic techniques.

Following return of voice, it is necessary to explore the actual
cause for the conversion reaction. It is desirable to do this in a direct
manner. For example , the voice pathologist may say:

> I'm very pleased that the muscles are all functioning well now and
> that your voice has returned to normal. It sounds very good. The
> thing that still puzzles me somewhat is why the muscles stopped
> closing the folds in the first place. I can tell you quite frankly that
> with many other patients that we have seen with the same problem,
> the cause is often related to an upsetting event or some form of emo-
> tional stress. Can you think of anything that has been going on lately
> that might have contributed to this kind of stress?

By this time the patient has developed strong confidence in the
voice pathologist and often freely provides information related to psychosocial problems that may be related to the development of the conversion reaction. In discussing these problems, the voice pathologist
attempts to accomplish two major objectives: (a) give the patient total
and final control over the laryngeal mechanism; and (b) determine the
patient's general emotional state to decide the need for further professional counseling. To this point, the voice pathologist has been manip-
ulating the voice. The patient now must understand that despite the
actual cause of the aphonia, he or she is in total control of the voice and
does not need to permit the problem to recur. If it does, the patient now
knows how to regain control of the voice (through whatever manipulations were used). The patient is in control. Finally, just because the
need for the conversion reaction may no longer be present, this does
not mean that formal family, psychiatric, or psychological counseling
would not be useful. If the voice pathologist feels that the psychosocial
problem has not resolved and further counseling is in order, the suggestion should be discussed with the patient and appropriate referrals
should be made.

Conversion Dysphonia

Aphonia is the most common conversion voice disorder, but many
other vocal symptoms with varying degrees of dysphonia may occur

as conversion voice disorders. The voice pathologist recognizes these vocal symptoms as a conversion disorder when the medical exam yields normal appearing vocal folds; when the history of the problem yields limited reason for the occurrence of a voice disorder; with the recognition of an atypical voice quality when compared to "normal" dysphonias; and in the patient's ability to produce normal phonation while producing nonspeech vocal behaviors.

Treatment for conversion dysphonia follows the same approach as that suggested for the aphonic patient with the major approach being, (a) explanation of what the vocal folds are doing physiologically, (b) direct vocal manipulation, and (c) follow-up counseling as required. It is important to note that some very bizarre sounding dysphonias can occur. Seldom, however, can a conversion voice disorder patient create a vocalization that the voice pathologist cannot also produce. True hoarseness is difficult to imitate. A helpful aid in determining exactly how the patient is producing voice and for confirming the conversion disorder diagnosis is to imitate the vocal behavior.

Functional Falsetto

Functional falsetto is the production of the preadolescent voice in the postadolescent male. The falsetto voice often draws unwanted attention to the postpubescent, physically mature patient. Whatever the reason for the development of this voicing behavior, most patients are ready and willing to modify the voice with direct therapy. It has been our experience that this diagnosis is often missed in the young postadolescent male because of the presence of a mild dysphonia which often accompanies the falsetto production. The dysphonia may result from strain placed on the laryngeal mechanism as the patient attempts to produce a more appropriate sounding voice. Voice pathologists working with males in this age group should be cognizant of this problem.

Treatment strategies.   Several therapy techniques are used to modify mutational falsetto voices. The first step of any technique is to offer the patient a reasonable explanation for the vocal difficulty. Consider, for example, an explanation similar to the following:

> Often, as we grow, our many muscles grow so fast that for a while we may experience a little lack of coordination or even clumsiness. I'm sure that you've known people whose legs have grown so fast in one year that it looks as if they are going to trip whenever they run. Well, our vocal folds are also made of muscles, and sometimes they grow so fast that we have to learn to use them correctly. That's why when voices begin to change, they crack and the voice breaks and sometimes sounds funny.
>
> In your case, all the muscles changed and grew physically just the way they're supposed to grow, but they are not yet functioning

properly. They need just a little bit of training to get them to work correctly. Our goal for today is to get the vocal folds to vibrate differently than they have vibrated before. I want you to do the things I ask you to do with your voice and do not be surprised by some of the changes that we're going to hear.

This simple, brief explanation has prepared the patient to accept the therapy procedure by providing a reasonable rationale for the problem. The second step is to utilize direct vocal manipulation. The following procedure is recommended.

1. Ask the patient to produce a hard glottal attack (HGA) on a vowel. Demonstrate how the vowel should be produced with effort closure. When the glottal attack is produced correctly, the pitch will break into the normal lower register as the falsetto positioning for the HGA cannot initiate this form of effort closure. If the pitch does not break, grasp the larynx with your thumb and index finger and hold it in a lowered position in the neck as the vowel is being produced. If, after several trials, this fails to elicit the desired sound, depress the tongue with a tongue depressor, again as the patient produces the glottal attack.
2. When the lower pitch is produced, identify it immediately as the appropriate voice sound. Have the patient repeat it several times using the glottal attack. Then produce several different vowel sounds while attempting to reduce and then extinguish the effort of the glottal attack. Stabilize the normal voice on vowel prolongations.
3. Immediately move from vowels into words and phrases while maintaining the lower voice register. Attempt to expand the phrases through paragraph reading and into conversational speech during the initial therapy session.

Using this approach, the voice change is expected to be sudden with the progress of therapy expected to be rapid. The best way of accomplishing this sudden improvement is for the voice pathologist to be aggressive with the therapy approach. It must be remembered that the voice is new to the patient. His auditory feedback system does not yet identify the new voice as belonging to him. Initially, the voice may want to shift back into the falsetto. Positive encouragement may be necessary.

Follow-up sessions may be utilized to stabilize the new voice. We often give the patient Vocal Function Exercises to build the strength and balance of the vocal mechanism. In addition, in our effort to aid the patient in developing total control of the voice, we will often use negative practice by having the patient shift back and forth between the two voices. Interestingly, the more the "new" voice is used, patients find it more difficult to produce the falsetto voice.

Most patients are somewhat excited by and proud of the new voice while some are embarrassed by the sudden voice quality change. When the latter is the case, the patient may require a gradual desensitization program as a part of the stabilization process. A desensitization program involves establishing with the patient a personal hierarchy of communication experiences from the least difficult to the most difficult speaking situation. A typical hierarchy may include:

1. talking to strangers in a fast food restaurant or a store
2. talking to family members
3. talking to selected friends
4. talking in the classroom.

We recently had a 17-year-old patient who developed normal voicing from falsetto over the Christmas holidays. This patient handled his drastic voice change in a humorous manner. He returned to school using the falsetto voice for half of the day in the classroom. During his afternoon math class, he began coughing and asked to be excused to get a drink of water. When he returned to class he exclaimed excitedly in his normal voice, "Mr._____, they must have put something in the water; listen to my voice!"

Other methods of initiating normal pitch levels include working from throat clearing and coughing and other nonspeech phonations. Vegetative sounds such as these are usually spontaneously produce in the modal range and can be used as a point of departure for voice therapy. It should also be noted that a female falsetto voice production may also be seen therapeutically. Our experience with these cases has been with older women who complain of a lack of power and strength in the voice. When examined stroboscopically, perceptually, and instrumentally, it becomes evident that they are producing voice in the falsetto register. In most cases, this form of voice production has been a lifelong habit and is more resistant to modification. The same therapy approaches utilized with the male are used with the female falsetto patient (Stemple, 1993).

The Juvenile Voice

The juvenile female voice is not often seen in voice therapy clinics in that the problem is more one of aesthetics than one which is considered a pathological problem. The voice quality of juvenile voice is characterized by an unusually high pitch with associated breathiness. The voice may be described as "childlike." Our experience has been with women who complain of laryngeal fatigue and latter day hoarseness. The vast majority of these individuals are involved in activities which require much voice use. When the patient seeks treatment, she is not aware of the functional ineffectiveness of her vocal habits. It is the role of the voice pathologist to describe the inappropriate voice components and to seek production of an improved voice. As with a *symptomatic voice therapy approach*, various facilitating techniques may be utilized in this exploration. One technique that we have found useful with the juvenile voice population is as follows:

1. Test the patient's entire singing pitch range. The juvenile voice patient's phonation for singing is often stronger and produced with improved respiratory support than is the speaking voice.
2. Ask the patient to produce a strong high note on the vowel /o/.
3. Gradually lower the note in two to three note steps. When the point has been reached where voice is produced in the lower one-third of the range, stabilize at this level by sustaining various vowel sounds. Use auditory feedback with a tape recorder and/or visual feedback with a pitch extraction device.
4. Progress from sustained vowels to words, phrases, paragraph reading, and conversational speech.
5. Introduce vocal function exercises to strengthen and balance the laryngeal and vocal mechanisms.

Unlike functional falsetto, modification of the juvenile voice is gradual and takes place over time. The desired voice quality demonstrates more mature vocal characteristics with a lower pitch, less breathiness, and overall improved timbre.

HOLISTIC VOICE THERAPY

Whenever a voice disorder is present, we may assume that its presence has caused a change in the functioning of the physiology responsible for voice production. These changes may interrupt airflow causing inappropriate subglottic air pressure (as with a mass lesion of the vocal folds) or they may cause airflow to be unimpeded by the normal glottal resistance (as with a unilateral vocal fold paralysis). Physiologic changes may take the form of a general laryngeal muscle weakness and imbalance (as in laryngeal myasthenia) , or increased laryngeal area muscle tension (as in vocal hyperfunction). Finally, the treatment of the glottal pulse may be restricted by supraglottic tension or an inappropriate coupling of the resonators. When any one or more of these voice subsystems is affected by pathology, the remaining subsystems must adjust to accommodate the change of the affected part.

Case Study 10: Laryngeal Muscle Weakness

The patient was a 35-year-old female who was referred for evaluation and treatment with a diagnosis of voice fatigue. Voice quality during the diagnostic evaluation was normal. The patient complained, however, of laryngeal fatigue when speaking and lately when singing and ineffective use of the lower range of her singing voice. While she could maintain a "reasonably good" singing quality if she "forced" the voice, she was sure that the forcing contributed to the fatigue. In addition, she reported feeling a "shortness of breath" as if she was "running out of air" before the end of a musical phrase. An operatic contralto, she was currently engaged to sing her first solo as a professional. She indicated that this particular aria, which she practiced many times a day, stretched her vocal range to its lower limit.

The evaluation yielded no significant etiologic factors or voice changes except for the symptoms described by the patient. Stroboscopic evaluation of vocal function revealed grossly normal appearing vocal folds bilaterally as the folds were free of any apparent edema or other visible pathology. The mucosal waves and amplitude of vibration were normal at comfort level. Glottic closure, however demonstrated an unusual anterior glottal chink which became larger as the pitch was reduced. The patient was able to sustain an upper range tone for 49 seconds and a lower tone for only 21 seconds. Her measured airflow rates were consistent, with a higher airflow rate measured at low pitch.

We felt that this imbalance between predominant cricothyroid muscle function and predominant thyroarytenoid muscle function was greater than normal, especially considering the expected increased stiffness of the folds at higher pitches. Electromyographic studies of the laryngeal muscle action potentials would have proven useful, but were not available. It was therefore our impression that this laryngeal muscle imbalance, most likely caused by voice strain, contributed to the fatigue in her speaking voice and the ineffectiveness of her lower singing range. The therapy focused on strengthening and balancing the muscle function and was successful in remediating her symptoms. Stroboscopic observation of the vocal folds following voice therapy demonstrated the anterior chink to be gone as glottic closure was complete at all pitch levels. It was speculated that this patient had spent so much time pushing her voice "to its lower limit" while practicing her aria that she fatigued the laryngeal musculature.

Stemple, Stanley, and Lee (in press), studied voice and vocal fold changes following prolonged voice use in a vocally normal group of subjects. Results of their investigation were consistent with the above example in that a significant number of subjects demonstrated the unusual anterior glottal chink following the voicing task. In addition, subjects experienced much difficulty in matching the lower limits of their pre-test voices. These authors speculated that laryngeal muscle strain contributed to these results.

This patient demonstrated that at least two parts of her vocal mechanism had been negatively affected by laryngeal muscle strain. When the muscular system became strained and imbalanced, the respiratory system was forced to adjust and, through increased air pressure and airflow could maintain a "reasonable" singing voice for a short period of time. For this elite vocal performer, "reasonable" was not good enough. Indeed, we would speculate that had she continued to force the voice that she would have developed a back-focused tone with the combination of all the faulty subsystems leading to more serious pathology.

The elderly population often complain of voice weakness, fatigue, and chronic hoarseness. As described in Chapter 2, several physiologic changes occur to the aging larynx which may account for voice quality changes such as loss of muscle fiber, stiffening of the vocal fold cover, and continued calcification of the laryngeal cartilages. Many geriatric patients present to otolaryngologists and voice pathologists complaining of various vocal symptoms. Often they have been told that this is part of the aging process and they would have to "live" with the problem.

Many elderly people are widowed and live alone, often with very little opportunity to talk for extended periods of time. Combine the natural physiologic changes with the lack of voice use and these individuals develop voice problems that interfere with their communication ability when they do have the need and desire to speak. Ramig, Horii, and Bonitati (1991) and Lowery (1993) demonstrated voice therapy techniques that proved successful in improving the voice quality of the elderly. Ramig et al. proved that voice therapy could improve the vocal functioning of elderly patients with Parkinson's disease. In Lowery's (1993) dissertation, the author tracked the improvement of voice qualities of geriatric women who engaged in regular aerobic exercise. In our clinic, geriatric patients have found great success using a systematic holistic exercise program as a means of strengthening and balancing respiration, phonation, and resonation of the glottal tone. All of these authors agree that regular, systematic voice use is essential in maintaining the healthy geriatric voice.

Imbalance of the voice subsystems may occur with any voice disorder. It is very common to have this occur in the post-surgical patient.

Case Study 11: The Postsurgical Patient

The patient, a 54-year-old insurance sales representative, was referred for evaluation and treatment following two surgeries for removal of bilateral vocal fold polyps. Voice quality during the evaluation was moderately dysphonic, characterized by low pitch and loudness and breathiness. He could not readily increase loudness to a shout. The patient was disturbed by the results of surgery, as it was his impression that his voice quality would be "normal." The evaluation indicated that the patient originally had a voice disorder due to several etiologic factors. These included

(a) excessive loud talking; (b) the use of a low-pitched telephone voice; (c) smoking 1¹/₂ packages of cigarettes per day; and (d) habitual throat clearing. Presurgical voice therapy had modified all factors except those for smoking which was reduced but not eliminated.

The presurgical vocal mechanism had adjusted the voice subsystems to accommodate the presence of the bilateral polyps. Once the polyps were removed, the subsystems were essentially in disarray and had not automatically rebalanced to provide the expected improved voice quality. Indeed, the patient had maintained the back-focused, strained voice production that had been required to produce voice prior to his surgeries. Direct, holistic voice therapy was used to accomplish the task of improving the voice.

As previously stated, a voice pathologist must develop a large armamentarium of treatment techniques. With experience, each clinician will choose techniques that feel comfortable; techniques that make sense and can be easily explained to the patient; techniques that work well for that clinician. In our clinic, we feel most comfortable with those treatment programs that integrate all of the voice subsystems into the rehabilitative effort. The following are examples of comprehensive therapy techniques that we feel may be applied to many patients with various pathologies of varying etiologic origins. The strength of each of these approaches is their comprehensive holistic nature in that each approach attends to all the subsystems of voice production. At once, they are symptomatic treatments, etiologic treatments, and physiologic treatments that address respiration, phonation, and supraglottic placement of the glottal tone. As seen from the previous discussion, their applications are many.

Vocal Function Exercises

The Vocal Function Exercise program is based on the assumption that the laryngeal mechanism is similar to other muscle systems and may become weakened, strained and, imbalanced through many etiologic factors. Indeed, the analogy that we often draw with patients is a comparison of the rehabilitation of the knee to rehabilitation of the voice. Both are comprised of muscle, cartilage, and connective tissue. When the knee is injured, rehabilitation includes a short period of immobilization for the purpose of reducing the effects of the acute injury. Immobilization is followed by assisted ambulation and then the primary rehabilitation begins in the form of systematic exercise. This exercise is designed to restrengthen and balance **all** of the supportive knee muscles for the purpose of returning the knee to as close its normal functioning as possible.

Rehabilitation of voice may also involve a short period of voice rest following acute injury or after surgery to permit healing of the mucosa to occur. The patient may then begin conservative voice use and follow through with all of the management approaches which seem necessary. Full voice use is then resumed very quickly and often the therapy program is successful in returning the patient to normal voice production. We would suggest, however, that on many occasions patients are not fully rehabilitated because one of the important rehabilitation steps was neglected. That step is the systematic exercise program that is often necessary to strengthen and balance the laryngeal muscle system and to regain the balance among airflow, to this muscular activity, to the supraglottic placement of the tone.

Vocal Function Exercises, as first described by Barnes (1977) and modified by Stemple (1984) strive to balance the subsystems of voice production. The exercise program has proven successful in improving and enhancing the vocal function of speakers with normal voices (Stemple, Lee, et al., in press). In addition Sabol, Lee, and Stemple (in press) demonstrated the effectiveness of Vocal Function Exercises in the exercise regimen of singers.

The program is rather simple to teach and, when presented appropriately, seems reasonable to the patients. Indeed many patients are enthusiastic to have a concrete program, similar in concept to physical therapy, during which they may plot the progress of their return to vocal efficiency. The program is as follows:

Describe the problem to the patient, using illustrations as needed or the patient's own stroboscopic evaluation video. The patient will then be taught a series of four exercises to be done at home, two times each, two times per day. These include:

1. Sustain the /i/ vowel for as long as possible on the musical note (F) above middle (C) for females and (F) below middle (C) for males.
   Goal: Based on airflow volume. In our clinic the goal is based on reaching 100 ml/sec of airflow. So if the volume is equal to 4000 ml, then the goal is 40 seconds. When airflow measures are not available, the goal is equal to the longest /s/ that the patient is able to sustain. Placement of the tone should be in an extreme forward focus, almost, but not quite, nasal. All exercises are produced as softly as possible, but not breathy. The subsystems must be "engaged." (This is considered a warm-up exercise.)

2. Glide from your lowest note to your highest note on the word "knoll."
   Goal: No voice breaks. (The glide forces the use of all laryngeal muscles. It stretches the vocal folds and encourages a systematic, slow engagement of the cricothyroid muscles. The word "knoll" encourages a forward placement of the tone. Voice breaks will typically occur in the transitions between low and

high tones. When breaks occur, the patient is encouraged to continue the glide without hesitation. When the voice breaks at the top of the present range and the patient typically has more range, the glide may be continued without voice as the folds will continue to stretch. Glides improve muscular control and flexibility.)

3. Glide from your highest note to your lowest note on the word "knoll."

    Goal: No voice breaks. (Some patients find it easier to initiate the tone and glide from one direction to another, depending on the stronger muscle groups. The downward glide encourages a slow, systematic engagement of the thyroarytenoid muscle.)

4. Sustain the musical notes (C-D-E-F-G) for as long as possible on the vowel /O/. (Middle (C) females, octave below middle (C) for males.)

    Goal: Remains the same as for exercise 1. The fourth exercise may be tailored to the patient's present vocal ability. While the basic range of middle (C), and an octave lower for males, is appropriate for most voices, the exercises may be customized up or down to fit the present vocal condition or a particular voice type.

Quality of the tone is also monitored for voice breaks, wavering, and breathiness. Quality improves as times increase and pathologies begin to resolve.

All exercises are done as softly as possible. It is much more diffi-cult to produce soft tones; therefore, the vocal subsystems will receive a better workout than if louder tones were produced. Extreme care is taken to teach the production of a forward tone that lacks tension. In addition, attention is paid to the glottal onset of the tone, and an easy, yet not breathy, onset is encouraged. It is explained to the patient that maximum phonation times increase as the efficiency of the vocal fold vibration improves. Times do not increase due to improved "lung capacity." Indeed, even aerobic exercise does not improve lung capac-ity, but rather the efficiency of oxygen exchange with the circulatory system, thus, giving the sense of more air.

The musical notes are matched to the notes produced by an inex-pensive pitch pipe that the patient purchases for use at home or a tape recording of live voice doing the exercises may be given to the patient for home use. Many patients find the taped voice easier to match than the pitch pipe. We have found that patients who complain of "tone deafness" can often be taught to approximate the correct notes quite well with practice and guidance from the voice pathologist. Finally, patients are given a graph on which to mark their times and to plot progress. Progress is monitored over time and, because of normal daily variability, patients are encouraged not to compare today to tomorrow and so on. Rather, weekly comparisons are encouraged. Estimated time of completion for the program is 6 to 8 weeks. Some patients experience minor laryngeal aching for the first day or two of the program similar to muscle aching that might occur with any new muscular exercise. As this discomfort will soon subside, they are encouraged to continue the program through the discomfort.

In short, Vocal Function Exercises provide a holistic vocal treatment program that attends to the three major subsystems of voice production. The program appears to work for the patient because it is reasonable in regards to time and effort; it is similar to other recognizable exercise programs; the concept of "physical therapy" for the vocal folds is understandable; progress may be easily plotted which is inherently motivating; and it appears to balance airflow , laryngeal activity, and supraglottic control.

Accent Method

Another holistic treatment approach is the Accent Method as described by Smith and Thyme (1976). This voice therapy approach is designed to (1) increase pulmonary output, (2) reduce glottic waste, (3) reduce excessive muscular tension, and (4) normalize the vibratory pattern during phonation. The technique is based on the principles of the myoelastic/aerodynamic theory of phonation. The originators state that because voice production is created by subglottal air pressure and transglottal airflow, stronger air pressures below the vocal folds result in an increased amplitude of vibration and a more stable closed phase of the vibratory cycle. The stronger closed phase improves the filtering process of the vocal tract as a result of a longer duration of the vocal fold contact within one period and a higher airflow through the glottis in the opening phase of the vibratory cycle, which together counteract the damping effect of the resonances in the vocal tract (Koschkee, 1993). The expected acoustic effects of treatment are (1) increased energy of the fundamental frequency, (2) increased energy in F_2 to F_3, (3) reduced irregular pitch perturbations, (4) optimal fundamental frequency, (5) increased frequency range, (6) increased dynamic range (Smith & Thyme, 1976).

The Accent Method procedures as described by Koschkee (1993) are as follow:

1. Facilitate diphragmal/abdominal breathing. Ideally the patient is placed in a recumbent position and normal diaphragm/abdominal breathing is elicited. The patient is instructed to place one hand on the stomach to monitor the abdominal movements while the clinician demonstrates abdominal breathing and upper body relaxation. A brief description of the lowering action of the diaphragm is given to demonstrate the appropriate increase in chest cavity size as air is inspired.

The patient is asked to gain a consciousness over the abdominal movements for both inhalation and exhalation. Abdominal muscle control is said to be important for achieving changes in pitch and loudness.

The patient is then instructed to watch the clinician as fricative-like sounds are demonstrated. The sounds are first sustained individually and then with a two-beat rhythm. The two-beat rhythm is accented, with the first sound being weak and the second sound produced with more force. A sample of this   sequenced breathing exercise would be:

Inhale /s/------------Inhale /sh/------------Inhale /f/------------

The two-beat accented rhythm would be:

s-S--

sh-SH--

f-F--   (The second sound is accented).

Throughout the Accent practice, changes in body position (sitting, standing, walking, swinging the arms) are used to encourage regulation and adaptation of the breathing patterns.

2. Utilize rhythmic vocal play. When the correct breathing pattern has been established, phonation is begun. Voice is initially introduced with a soft, breathy onset of the tone. Again, the clinician demonstrates the rhythm and the patient imitates the accent pattern. Each stressed beat (the second accented sound) is accompanied by a smooth abdominal contraction. Eventually, the exercises are carried out at three different speeds, largo, andante, and allegro (slow, moderate, and fast) tempos. In implementing the Accent Method, the clinician can utilize arm movements, tapping, or even beating on a drum to help establish the rhythm.

The largo tempo consists of one or two main stresses in a three beat rhythm in which breathy phonation and consonantal resistance are used at the lips and tongue. A sample of each rhythm sequence includes:

zh-ZH

zz-ZZ-ZZ

yoi-YOI

vv-VV-VV

In the andante tempo, phrases are increased in size to three main beats in a four beat rhythm and the breathiness of the voice is eliminated. This step introduces variability in pitch, intensity, timbre, and time. A sample sequence-andante tempo would be:

woo-WOO-WOO

yea-YEA-YEA-YEA

yee-YEE-YEE-YEE

In the allegro tempo, the voice exercises consist of an unstressed vowel followed by five stressed vowels. The speed is doubled and the main beats are divided into two faster beats. Phrase length, intensity, and a rich variety of sounds are incorporated into the practice as well as the other tempo patterns. This step encourages more variety to the voice and approaches the natural prosody used in conversation. A sample sequence of the allegro tempo would be:

yea-YEA-YEA-YEA-YEA-YEA-YEA

da-YA-YA-YA-YA-YA

ba-BA-BA-BA-BA-BA

no-NO-NO-NO-NO-NO

3. Transfer rhythms to articulated speech. The final stage of accent therapy involves transferring the rhythms to real speech. The transfer process includes (1) repetitions following the clinician's model, (2) reading aloud using passages marked for phrasing and stresses, (3) monologue, and (4) conversation.

The aim of both Vocal Function Exercises and the Accent Method is to develop reduced laryngeal effort, improved respiratory support, and an open vocal tract. By balancing these subsystems responsible for voice production, then the quality of voice and the effort to produce that voice should significantly improve. Voice pathologists are encouraged to view voice production from this holistic point of view.

REFERENCES

Andrews, M. (1993). Psychosocial aspects of children's behavior. Case study. In J. Stemple (Ed.), *Voice therapy: Clinical studies* (pp. 26–32). Saint Louis: Mosby Year Book.

Arnold, G. (1965). Physiology and pathology of speech and language. In R. Luchsinger, & G. Arnold (Eds.), Voice-speech-language. *Clinical communicology: Its physiology and pathology* (337–510). Belmont, CA: Wadsworth Publishing.

Aronson, A. (1980). *Clinical voice disorders: An interdisciplinary approach* (1st ed.). New York: Brian C. Decker.

Aronson, A. (1990). *Clinical voice disorders: An interdisciplinary approach* (2nd ed.). New York: Brian C. Decker.

Bach, J. (1890). Hysterical aphonia. *Medical News-Philadelphia, 57*, 263–264.

Barnes, J. (1977, September). *Voice therapy*. Paper presented at the Southwestern Ohio Speech and Hearing Association, Cincinnati, OH.

Boone, D. (1971). *The voice and voice therapy*. (1st ed.). Englewood Cliffs, NJ: Prentice-Hall.

Boone, D. (1977). *The voice and voice therapy*. (2nd ed.). Englewood Cliffs, NJ: Prentice-Hall.

Brodnitz, F. (1971). *Vocal rehabilitation* (4th ed.). Rochester, NY: American Academy of Ophthalmology and Otolaryngology.

Canfield, W. (1964). A phonetic approach to voice and speech improvement. *Speech Teacher, 8*, 42–46.

Case, J. (1984). *Clinical management of voice disorders*. Rockville, MD: Aspen.

Coleman, R. (1976) A comparison of the contributions of two voice quality characteristics to the perception of maleness and femaleness in the voice. *Journal of Speech and Hearing Research, 19*, 168–180.

Colton, R., & Casper, L. (1990). *Understanding voice problems: A physiological perspective for diagnosis and treatment*. Baltimore: Williams and Wilkins.

Cooper, M. (1973) *Modern techniques of vocal rehabilitation*. Springfield, IL: Charles C. Thomas.

Froeschel, E. (1952). Chewing method as therapy. *Archives of Otolaryngology, 56*, 427–434.

Froeschel, E., Kastein, S., & Weiss, D. (1955). A method of therapy for paralytic conditions of the mechanisms of phonation, respiration, and glutination. *Journal of Speech and Hearing Disorders, 20*, 365–370.

Goss, F. (1878). Hysterical aphonia. *Boston Medical and Surgical Journal, 99*, 215–222.

Greene, M. (1972). *The voice and its disorders* (3rd ed.). Philadelphia: J.P. Lippincott.

Herrington-Hall, B., Lee, L., Stemple, J., Niemi, K., & McHone, M. (1988). Description of laryngeal pathologies by age, sex, and occupation in a treatment seeking sample. *Journal of Speech and Hearing Disorders, 53*, 57–65.

Howard, C. (1923). Report of a case of functional aphonia cured under general anesthetic. *Journal of the American Medical Association, 80*, 104.

Ingals, E. (1890). Hysterical aphonia, or paralysis of the lateral crico-arytenoid muscles. *Journal of the American Medical Association, 15*, 92–95.

Jacobson, E. (1938). *Progressive relaxation* (2nd ed.). Chicago: University of Chicago Press.

Koschkee, D. (1993). Accent Method. Case study. In J. Stemple (Ed.), *Voice therapy: Clinical studies* (pp. 53–57). Saint Louis: Mosby Year Book.

Lee, L. (1993). Refocusing laryngeal tone. Case study. In J. Stemple (Ed.), *Voice therapy: Clinical studies* (pp. 49–53). Saint Louis: Mosby Year Book.

Lowery, D. (1993). *Aerobic exercise effects on the post-menopausal voice*. Unpublished doctoral dissertation, University of Wisconsin, Madison.

McWilliams, B. (1954). Some factors in the intelligibility of cleft palate speech. *Journal of Speech and Hearing Disorders, 19*, 524–527.

Murphy, A. (1964). *Functional voice disorders*. Englewood Cliffs, NJ: Prentice-Hall.

Nittrouer, S., McGowan, R., Milenkovic, P., & Beehler, D. (1990). Acoustic measurement of men's and women's voices: a study of context effects and covariations. *Journal of Speech and Hearing Research, 33*, 761–775.

Prosek, R., Montgomery, A., Walden, B., & Schwartz, D. (1978). EMG biofeedback in the treatment of hyperfunctional voice disorders. *Journal of Speech, and Hearing Disorders, 43*, 282–294.

Ramig, L., Horii, Y., & Bonitati, C. (1991). The efficacy of voice therapy for patients with Parkinson's disease. *National Center for Voice and Speech, Status Progress Report*, 61-86.

Russell, J. (1864). A case of hysterical aphonia. *British Medical Journal, 8*, 619–621.

Sabol, J., Lee, L., & Stemple, J. (in press). The value of vocal function exercises in the practice regimen of singers. *Journal of Voice*.

Smith, S., & Thyme, K. (1978). *Accent metoden: Special paedagogisk*. Forlag A-S. Herning, Denmark.

Spencer, L. (1988). Speech characteristics of male-to-female transsexuals: a perceptual and acoustic study. *Folia Phoniatrica, 40*, 31–42.

Stemple, J. (1984). *Clinical voice pathology: Theory and management*. Columbus, OH: Charles E. Merrill.

Stemple, J. (1993). *Voice therapy: Clinical studies*. St. Louis: Mosby Year Book.

Stemple, J., & Lehmann, D. (1980, November). *Throat clearing: The unconscious habit of vocal hyperfunction*. Paper presented at the American Speech-Language-Hearing Association National Convention, Detroit.

Stemple, J., Lee, L., D'Amico, B., & Pickup, B. (in press). Efficacy of vocal function exercises as a method of improving voice production. *Journal of Voice*.

Stemple, J., Stanley, J., & Lee, L. (in press). Objective measures of voice production following prolonged voice use. *Journal of Voice*.

Stemple, J., Weiler, E., Whitehead, W., & Komray, R. (1980). Electromyographic biofeedback training with patients exhibiting a hyperfunctional voice disorder. *Laryngoscope, 90*, 471–475.

Stevens, H. (1968). Conversion hysteria.: A neurologic emergency. *Mayo Clinic Proceedings, 43*, 54–64.

Terango, l. (1966). Pitch and duration characteristics of the oral reading of males on a masculinity-femininity dimension. *Journal of Speech and Hearing Research, 9*, 590–595.

Van Riper, C. (1939). *Speech correction principles and methods*. Englewood Cliffs, NJ: Prentice-Hall.

Ward, W. (1877). Hysterical aphonia. *Chicago Medical Journal and Examiner, 34*, 495–505.

West, R., Kennedy, L., & Carr, A. (1937). *The rehabilitation of speech*. New York: Harper and Brothers.

Wilson, D. (1979). *Voice problems of children*, (2nd ed.). Baltimore: William and Wilkins.

Wilson, D. (1987). *Voice problems of children*, (3rd ed.). Baltimore: William and Wilkins.

Winslow, P. (1919). Functional aphonia. *New York Medical Journal, 109*, 1129–1130.

Wolfe, V., Ratusnik, D., Smith, H., & Northrup, G. (1990). Intonation and fundamental frequency in male-to-female transsexuals. *Journal of Speech and Hearing Disorders, 55*, 43–50.

Zemlin, W. (1988). *Speech and hearing science: Anatomy and physiology* (3rd ed.). Englewood Cliffs, NJ: Prentice-Hall.

Zwitman , D., & Calcaterra, T. (1973). The "silent cough" method for vocal hyperfunction. *Journal of Speech and Hearing Disorders, 38*, 119–125.

8

MANAGEMENT OF MEDICAL PATHOLOGIES OF VOICE

Voice problems arise under many conditions and, as described in Chapter 3, numerous etiological factors may play a role. However, in general, three overriding categories prevail: medical or organic factors, voice use patterns and voice demands, and psychosocial or emotional contributors (Aronson, 1985; Damste, 1987; Rubin, 1987). Of course, there is considerable overlap between these three groupings. Inappropriate voice behaviors or excessive vocal demands may result in organic manifestations (e.g., polyps or nodules); psychological trauma or excessive emotional stress may trigger the onset of focal laryngeal dystonia. Treatment alternatives may include medical intervention (e.g., phonosurgery, pharmacologic treatment) or voice rehabilitation, or both. This chapter presents the diagnostic signs and management alternatives available for medical or organic pathologies of voice and considers the underlying contributions from medical/surgical, behavioral/rehabilitative, and psychosocial components.

The term phonosurgery refers to laryngeal surgeries that seek to improve voice quality as their primary goal. This definition is distinct from traditional concepts of laryngeal surgery, which seek to remove disease, with voice outcome as a secondary consideration. Recent advances in surgical instruments, bioimplant materials, and development of alternative surgical techniques have created a new awareness of the phonosurgical options that are available to enhance voice quality in patients with laryngeal pathology (Ford & Bless, 1991).

The voice pathologist plays a supportive role in this context by assisting in the correct diagnosis and prognosis for change based on the assessment of laryngeal anatomy, vocal fold vibratory pattern, vocal function measurement, and rehabilitative options for voice treatment. Collaboration between otolaryngologists and voice pathologists continues to expand through joint examination of the laryngeal image and vocal function, efficacious co-treatment alternatives that include both phonosurgery and voice rehabilitation, and clinical delivery models that encourage a team approach to voice disordered patients. More than ever, it is critical that the voice pathologist be aware of the medical pathologies in an otolaryngology patient population that affect the larynx and, specifically, voice productions.

SYSTEMIC INFLUENCES ON THE LARYNX

Focal or regional influences of the head, neck, upper back, and throat can influence laryngeal status. Musculoskeletal tension in the throat, temporomandibular joint problems, swallowing difficulties, blunt trauma to the neck, chin, or jaw are all examples of the possible local insults that may influence the larynx and, by extension, the voice. However, there is increasing evidence from both clinical and research settings that systemic or "whole body" influences may also affect the larynx and voice production. Endocrine, immunologic, and cardiac disorders, inflammatory and infectious diseases, and pharmacologic agents are all examples of systemic processes that may alter voice production.

RESEARCH EVIDENCE

To understand the relationship between body systems and the larynx, some researchers have examined normal and pathologic fluctuations of systems and measured vocal function as a dependent variable. Baer (1981) identified a relationship between single motor unit firing rates of the thyroarytenoid muscle and jitter (pitch perturbation) measurements. These findings were supported in a similar study by Larson and Kempster (1983). Orlikoff (1989, 1990) has examined acoustic perturbations as a function of cardiac status, including heartbeat, and suggested that stability of systemic blood flow may influence fine measures of laryngeal control.

Researchers have also used acoustic analysis to mark the varying time periods within the female hormonal cycle (Abitbol et al., 1989; Higgins & Saxman, 1989). Other studies addressing the relationship between hormonal levels and vocal function have supported the interpretation of a time-varying effect on voice performance based on fluctuations in hormone activity. This research finding supports a longstanding clinical impression among professional voice performers, notably singers, that range, quality, stability, and endurance of phonation can be affected by the hormonal cycle (Davis & Davis, 1993).

TREATMENT ALTERNATIVES

Treatment of systemic disorders is the domain of the medical physician who has diagnosed the disease, and effects on voice production are usually associated with the success or limits of that medical therapy. The role of the voice pathologist, then, is to support the voice disordered patient's optimal use of voice by providing information about the source and extent of systemic influences on voice and to offer behavioral compensatory strategies, if appropriate, to augment voice production and circumvent potential maladaptive vocal behaviors. Guidelines for voice conservation and hygiene strategies may also facilitate best voice production.

There are three basic treatment alternatives available for patients with medical pathologies affecting voice: medical (pharmacologic) therapy, phonosurgery, and voice rehabilitation. In many cases, although the primary therapy will be medical, some counsel in the area of voice rehabilitation, conservation, or hygiene will be appropriate as a second-order treatment.

PHARMACEUTICAL EFFECTS ON VOICE

The effects of medications on voice performance and vocal function have not been explored exhaustively. Martin (1988) reviewed some general characteristics of medications, and their predicted influence on the body, with possible applications to the larynx. Four drug actions that are common in medications that treat organic vocal pathologies are listed below. These include drugs that influence:

1. **airflow**, including **bronchodilators**, which expand the diameter of bronchioles in the lungs to increase the oxygen and carbon dioxide exchange during respiration. These medications are common for treatment of allergies, asthma, and other forms of upper respiratory compromise.
2. **fluid level in tissues**, especially **diuretics**, **corticosteroids**, and **decongestants**, which use separate chemical actions to reduce edema of tissues due to local inflammation.
3. **upper respiratory secretions**, through the use of agents that reduce secretions, such as **antihistamines**, **antitussives** (cough suppressants), and **antireflux** medications.
4. **vocal fold structure**, through long-term use of hormonal therapies, especially testosterone, which results in permanent deepening of the pitch of the voice.

This chapter describes some of the more common medical pathologies that can affect voice production.

ENDOCRINE DISORDERS

Because the endocrine glands secrete hormones which are responsible for body growth, certain **endocrine** disorders can alter or limit voice quality due to changes in vocal fold development. These disorders may become apparent at puberty, when expected body growth and associated changes in voice are most prominent. In females, cyclic changes in voice that fluctuate with puberty onset, pregnancy, menstrual cycle, and menopause may also affect voice production. The resulting edema may result in dysphonia, reduced pitch and loudness range, and loss of stability of phonation.

As a general rule, hormonal imbalances produce the greatest effect on vocal pitch, as has been seen with diagnoses of arrested or aberrant development of sexual and reproductive functions. **Virilization** is the abnormal secretion of androgenic hormones, resulting in male sex characteristics in females. The vocal effects are low pitch, hoarseness, and occasionally voice breaks (Aronson, 1985; Colton & Casper, 1990; Greene & Mathieson, 1989; Jafek & Esses, 1986). Treatment with estrogen or other hormonal therapy may improve voice quality, but pitch changes are usually permanent. Behavioral voice therapy can be used to augment the "feminine" quality of voice and speech.

Thyroid disorders affect the entire chemical and emotional balance of the body, so medical, intellectual, and affective influences are all possible. **Hyperthyroidism** results from excessive secretions of the thyroid gland, and either surgical excision or radioactive iodine treatment is used to slow production of the thyroid gland. **Hypothyroidism**, or reduced thyroxine production, may be treated medically using thyroid replacements. Thyroid function also affects voice production, but the predicted vocal outcomes are not clear. Aronson (1985), Jafek and Esses (1986), and Shemen (1988) have reported various physical signs and perceptual attributes associated with hypothyroidism, including hoarseness, low pitch, coarse and gravelly vocal symptoms due to thickened or edematous vocal folds. Perceptual features of hyperthyroidism include slight vocal instabilities, including "shaky" voice, breathy quality, and reduced loudness.

Immunologic disorders that create or exacerbate dysphonia include allergies, rheumatoid arthritis, and various infectious diseases (Pennover & Sheffer, 1988). **Allergies** can affect voice production because of the associated inflammation or irritation of the pharynx and nasal mucosa. Increased mucous production, nasal drainage, and congestion or edema of the respiratory mucosa may alter vocal function. Often, symptoms vary with the severity of the allergic response and may cycle with seasons, pollen counts, and specific exposures. Secondarily, the medications and treatments prescribed to treat allergies may also negatively influence voice production, through increased dehydration (antihistamines) and prolonged use of steroid inhalers, which has an uncertain effect on vocal folds.

Rheumatoid arthritis is a chronic inflammatory disorder that disrupts the normal structure and function of synovial joints, including the cricoarytenoid and cricothyroid joints of the larynx. When affected, laryngeal function for both respiration and voice production may be compromised, due to pain, swelling, and in the most severe form, mechanical fixation of the joints. Medical treatments include anti-inflammatory and corticosteroid drugs. Rarely, fixation of the arytenoid joint(s) creates an acute airway compromise, and results in the need for tracheotomy or unilateral arytenoidectomy for airway preservation (Bienenstock, Ehrlich, & Freyberg, 1963; Wolman, Darke, & Young, 1965).

Infectious disease, whether viral or bacterial in origin, can also create or aggravate voice problems due to chronic laryngitis, and occasionally, granulomas. Symptoms of chronic cough, irritation, edema, and eruptions of the mucous membranes of the larynx and pharynx, and the associated dysphonia generally resolve following antibacterial treatment of the microorganism (Shumrick & Shumrick, 1988). **Candida**, or yeast infection, occurs in the larynx, pharynx, and trachea, and can be particularly troublesome to treat, especially if the patient is immuno-compromised. Treatment is conducted using antifungal medications. In immunocompromised patients, a prolonged course (e.g., several months) may be required for full therapeutic effect. Candida is also a common finding in patients with human immunodeficiency virus (HIV) who exhibit symptoms of hoarseness, dry mouth, and mild chronic laryngitis due to a depressed immunologic system and repeated upper respiratory infections (Pennover & Sheffer, 1988).

Reflux esophagitis may result in both dysphonia and throat pain, especially if the irritation of the laryngeal mucosa is so great that granuloma tissue or contact ulcers have erupted (Koufman, Weiner, Wu, & Castell, 1988; Shumrick & Shumrick, 1988). Usually, the effects of reflux esophagitis are confined to the posterior larynx and may be indicated clinically by erythema or hyperplasia of the interarytenoid rim of the glottis. Formal assessment can be conducted using pH monitor over a 24 hour period (Jones, et al., 1990; Lumpkin, Bishop, & Katz, 1989). Pharmaceutic management with over-the-counter or prescription antacids, coupled with a behavioral anti-reflux protocol, can generally bring symptoms under control. The anti-reflux protocol may include recommendations for changes in diet, losing excess weight, elimination of caffeine, alcohol, and other substances that can aggravate or inhibit digestion, wearing loose clothing that does not bind the midriff, elevating the head of the bed at night, and avoiding unnecessary bending for activities such as bowling or gardening.

Respiratory disease, including **asthma**, **chronic obstructive pulmonary disease**, and **croup (acute laryngotracheobronchitis)** all result in acute or chronic symptoms of dyspnea, with audible inhalatory stridor and expiratory wheeze, and may include laryngeal edema. This latter symptom is most threatening for the pediatric airway, which is smaller in overall dimension. Although voice quality is clearly a secondary concern relative to ventilatory needs and airway preservation, any compromise of the respiratory power behind vocal fold vibration will have deleterious effects on phonation (Pillsbury & Postma, 1986). Treatment for these disorders usually includes bronchodilators and inhaled steroids, to suppress the symptoms of dyspnea and laryngeal edema, if present. As with other systemic disease, improvement in voice production is generally commensurate with overall return of respiratory function.

NEUROPATHIES

Vocal Fold Paralysis

Patients with unilateral vocal fold paralysis present with varied vocal symptoms, ranging from mild to severe dysphonias. Typically, voice is characterized by breathiness, low intensity, low pitch, and diplophonia. These vocal impairments result from irregular and incomplete valving of the pulmonary airstream through the glottis during the production of sound. Two physical dimensions account for this loss of vocal power and quality:

1. inadequate closure of the vocal folds at midline, as the paralyzed vocal fold remains lateral to the midline and cannot meet its contralateral pair
2. loss of vocal fold body and tonicity, resulting in bowing, flaccidity, and weakness of the paralyzed fold.

Both factors contribute to the asymmetric, aperiodic, and incomplete vibratory closure during phonation seen in patients with unilateral vocal fold paralysis.

The phonosurgical management alternatives for unilateral paralysis address both the midline glottic incompetence and the loss of vocal fold body. The traditional surgical treatment has been injection of a synthetic alloplastic, Teflon paste, into the lateral margin of the paralyzed fold. The paste forms a solid mass which displaces the paralyzed edge medially to improve midline competence. This technique has been used routinely for over twenty-five years (Ford, 1991), with good success. Occasional complications have been reported, due to migration of the Teflon material into other sites of the body. If injected too superficially, the Teflon may also impair the vibratory properties of the free edge of the paralyzed fold, due to excessive weight and stiffness.

Recently, the advent of new bioimplants have been explored as injectable alternatives to Teflon. A cross-linked bovine collagen has been developed for use in the skin and has been applied in clinical protocols for vocal fold injections (Ford, 1990; Ford & Bless, 1987; Ford, Bless, & Loftus, 1992). The bioimplant is injected superficially into the lamina propria of the vocal fold where it incorporates into the cellular structure of the vocal fold and reportedly enhances the vibratory properties in both paralyzed and scarred vocal folds.

A third injectable alternative to the management of paralyzed vocal fold is **autogenous fat**, a technique which has received variable review due to its frequent resorption rate, which limits its long-term success. The success of this technique can be improved by an initial overinjection of fat, to compensate for expected partial resorption (Brandenburg, Kirkham, & Koschkee, 1992). The autogenous fat technique has the obvious advantage of being a natural, soft, flexible material, which vibrates well and does not pose any risk for antibody or foreign body response.

Another surgical approach to medialization of the paralyzed fold is **laryngeal framework surgery**, or manipulation of the cartilaginous framework that houses the vocal folds. This procedure offers certain advantages over injection methods for the treatment of unilateral paralysis. First, it is completely noninvasive to the vocal fold body and mucosa; second, it is potentially reversible, barring excessive scarring of the surgical site. The Type I Thyroplasty utilizes a surgical implant (silastic block) inserted and locked into a small window of the thyroid lamina. This silastic implant will effectively "push" the paralyzed fold toward midline, to improve glottic closure. The exact size and placement of the implant is critical; if positioned too high or low, a vertical level mismatch will result, and voice quality will be suboptimal.

The concept of laryngeal framework surgery was introduced in 1974 by Isshiki and his colleagues. He and other otolaryngologists have continued to develop new types of framework surgery that manipulate the cartilage to alter the vocal fold configuration and restore voice in patients with unilateral paralysis, vocal fold bowing, and pitch disorders (Blaugrund, 1991; Isshiki, 1991; Koufman, 1986; Tucker, 1987). Laryngeal framework surgery is now being explored for use in managing pediatric laryngeal disorders (Smith & Gray, 1994).

REINNERVATION TECHNIQUES

Injection techniques and laryngeal framework surgery address the deficit of midline closure in their approach to management of unilateral vocal fold paralysis. Reinnervation techniques include **nerve muscle pedicle** (Tucker, 1987) and **nerve anastomosis** (synkinesis) (Crumley, 1991) and address the loss of vocal fold body and tonicity posed by atrophy and weakness of the denervated vocal fold. The principles behind neuromuscular reinnervation techniques have been described by Crumley (1991). Transplanted muscle blocks can provide innervation to a paralyzed muscle, and the contraction characteristics of the donor nerve or muscle will be imparted to the paralyzed muscle. Thus, selection of an appropriate **donor** nerve or muscle (i.e., one that is compatible with contraction properties of the original) is important. Neuromuscular pedicle reinnervation is limited to a single muscle, usually the lateral cricoarytenoid (LCA) or thyroarytenoid (TA), which are the main vocal fold adductors.

An alternative to the nerve to muscle reinnervation is nerve to nerve reinnervation. Recurrent laryngeal nerve (RLN) to RLN reinnervation is not consistently successful and does not always provide functional return of adductor and abductor activity. Furthermore, RLN to RLN anastomosis may result in dysphonia due to jerky movements and excessive synkinesis of adductor and abductor muscles simultaneously. Crumley (1991) has developed a nerve anastomosis procedure using the ansa cervicalis as a donor to the recurrent laryngeal nerve. Because the ansa nerve delivers a slower firing rate, no jerky movements or paradoxical vocal fold bulging result. Instead, a "quiet" tonicity of the vocal fold body is achieved, providing a better vibratory source for voice production.

Although reinnervation techniques increase the likelihood of vocal fold tonicity, they do not restore vocal fold mobility, and subsequent medialization procedures may still be necessary for an optimal result. Both surgical treatments can be used in combination with laryngeal framework surgery, and some otolaryngologists have advocated this combination approach, to decrease the glottic gap and improve the tonicity of the vocal fold body (Tucker, 1987).

VOICE THERAPY FOR UNILATERAL PARALYSIS

The goal of voice therapy with unilateral paralysis is to strengthen the normal vocal fold and encourage it to overadduct across the midline to better approximate the paralyzed fold. The most popular technique is the pushing exercise, which essentially combines the production of vowel sounds with isometric pushing. Using the arms in a pushing or pulling technique, the patient increases the muscular activity of laryngeal effort closure, forcing the normal vocal fold to adduct vigorously. When done systematically as a repeated exercise, pushing helps to strengthen muscles of adduction. Progression of exercises continues, utilizing vowels, syllables, words, and phrases.

Other exercises that have proved helpful are the use of hard glottal attack exercises, turning the head to one side or the other to increase tension on the paralyzed vocal fold, and digital manipulation of the thyroid cartilage (manual compression). The effect of these exercises is variable and often depends upon the degree of vocal fold gap (position of the paralyzed fold). To a certain extent, the prognosis for the success of rehabilitative therapy can be predicted following results of the videostroboscopic image. When light "touch" closure is achieved in glottic waveform, despite the position of the paralyzed fold, the likelihood of discrete benefits from behavioral therapy is greater than for vibratory patterns that display no touch closure whatsoever.

It is important to note that many patients with idiopathic etiologies for unilateral vocal fold paralysis have spontaneous return of function within the first year. For this reason, timing of surgical management is typically delayed at least 6 months to 1 year post-onset. Voice therapy may facilitate recovery of serviceable voice during the waiting period. Rehabilitation can also prevent the patient from adopting maladaptive compensatory strategies (e.g., extreme vocal strain and fatigue), which result in diplophonia or ventricular fold phonation. Finally, the effects of vocal fold paralysis may have a strong emotional impact on patients, and therapy may serve as a time to monitor progress and support the patient's need to adjust communicative demands at home, work, and in social settings to accommodate his disorder. Occasionally, referral to mental health professionals for additional support may be appropriate.

SPASMODIC DYSPHONIA

Spasmodic dysphonia (SD) is a focal dystonia of the central motor system believed to be extrapyramidal in origin. While the neural explanation for the etiology of spasmodic dysphonia has not been isolated definitively, a supranuclear lesion locus in proximity of the basal ganglia is generally cited as the likely source. This theory is supported by comparative examination of signs and symptoms of SD with the dysarthrias and brain imaging studies (Cannito, 1990) and brainstem conduction studies (Schaefer, Finitzo-Heiber, Gerling, & Freeman, 1987). As with other focal dystonias, SD is characterized by abnormal involuntary movements that are action-induced and task-specific. Thus, SD affects the movement patterns of the larynx during voicing, resulting in abnormal involuntary co-contraction of the vocalis muscle complex, despite normal laryngeal and vocal fold morphology (Blitzer & Brin, 1991).

There are two principle types of spasmodic dysphonia. **Adductor spasmodic dysphonia** results in a severely hyperfunctional voice, including a "strained-strangled" quality, multiple pitch or voice breaks and occasional voicing "blocks" of tension or effort that interrupt the continuity of phonation. Struggle is often a salient feature of voice onset patterns. **Abductor spasmodic dysphonia** is characterized by involuntary voice breaks and intermittent aphonia, with uncontrolled prolonged bursts of breathy phonation. Voice onset may appear normal, then loss of voice ensues with continued speaking. For both types of SD, these speech-related symptoms may co-exist with apparently undisrupted nonspeech laryngeal maneuvers, including singing, laughing, coughing, throat clearing, and humming. Symptoms may be exacerbated with psychosocial stress or increased speech demands, but persist regardless of the patient's emotional state (Aronson, 1985).

Because spasmodic dysphonia represents a complex of symptoms, rather than a specific diagnosis, determination of this disorder can be troublesome (Woodson, Zwirner, Murray, & Swenson, 1992). Perceptual attributes of SD may be similar to those of other organic, functional, or psychogenically based voice disorders. The history of onset does not provide differential clarification, as both SD and functional or conversion voice disorders may arise following excessive, prolonged, or extreme vocal demands, or following a period of unusual stress, trauma, or emotional upset. Thus, decisions about the presence and management of SD patients require careful examination of the individual's speech and voice symptoms across time, attending to the consistency, severity, and resistance to change following traditional treatment methods.

PHONOSURGICAL TREATMENT OPTIONS

Recurrent Laryngeal Nerve Resection

Dedo (1976) innovated the use of unilateral recurrent laryngeal nerve resection for the treatment of adductor spasmodic dysphonia. The treatment enjoyed early favorable reports, but long-term success has been disappointing due to relapse of symptoms within a few years of treatment (Aronson, 1985; Aronson & DeSanto, 1983).

BOTULINUM TOXIN INJECTION

Botulinum toxin (BOTOX) injections for treatment of spasmodic dysphonia have become a primary management option when symptoms persist and progress and are unresponsive to other behavioral treatment techniques (Blitzer & Brin, 1991; Blitzer, Brin, Fahn, & Lovelace, 1988; Ludlow, 1988). For adductor-type SD, a small amount of BOTOX is injected into the vocalis muscle, resulting in decreased spasm activity for a period ranging from 3 to 6 months. Individual responses vary, but the overall success of this treatment method in the management of adductor spasmodic dysphonia has been encouraging (Blitzer & Brin, 1991). Use of BOTOX for management of abductor SD has been less successful, in part due to the difficulty achieving consistent placement of the toxin in the posterior cricoarytenoid.

There are two techniques for injection of the BOTOX toxin in the vocal folds for adductor spasmodic dysphonia. An intraoral technique using a long curved syringe (Ford, Bless, & Lowery, 1990) has been reported successfully by Ford (1990). This procedure has advantage of visual inspection of the injection site, ensuring correct placement of the toxin in the vocalis muscle. It does require excellent patient compliance to tolerate the curved needle placement from an intraoral approach (Figures 8–1 and 8–2).

The alternative method, which can be used for adductor or abductor SD injections is "blind," using palpations of cartilage landmarks and percutaneous electromyography to discern correct locations in the intrinsic muscles (vocalis or posterior cricoarytenoid). This method usually requires the collaboration of the otolaryngologist, who inserts the needles and injects the toxin, and a neurologist, who assists in the set up and interpretation of the electromyographic feedback (Blitzer, Brin, Fahn, & Lovelace, 1988; Miller, 1992) (Figure 8–3). Placement of the EMG electrode in the correct muscle is verified using speech tasks designed to discriminate intrinsic laryngeal muscle activity. Both the timing and quality of the sound of muscle activity recording indicate when the needle edge is located in the muscle body.

VOICE THERAPY

The efficacy of rehabilitative voice therapy with spasmodic dysphonia is controversial, but many voice pathologists have reported good success with patients who are experiencing early or mild symptoms of SD or who use therapy in conjunction with BOTOX. Cooper (1977) reports a long history of success in treating SD with behavioral therapy only, beginning with a neutral "umhum" and expanding sequentially into vowels, syllables, words, and phrases. His success rates have not been replicated by others, however. Other techniques for treatment of adductor spasmodic dysphonia include the use of increased pitch, increased breathy quality, use of /h/ onset in

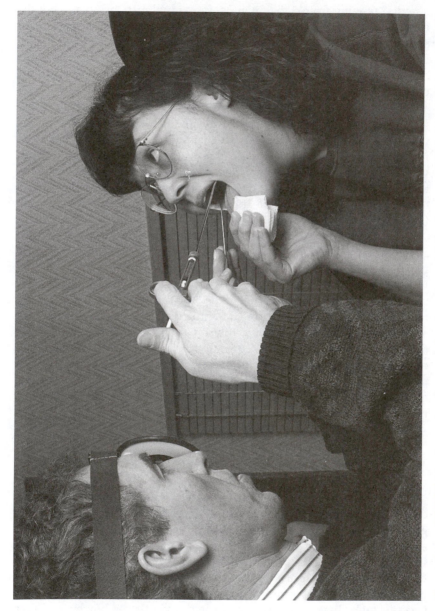

Figure 8–1. BOTOX injection using the curved syringe in an intraoral approach. (Photo by Rick Berkey, St. Elizabeth Medical Center, Dayton, Ohio.)

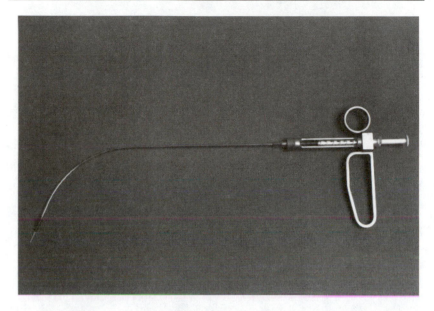

Figure 8–2. The curved syringe designed to inject the vocal folds through an intraoral approach. (Photo by Rick Berkey, St. Elizabeth Medical Center, Dayton, Ohio.)

phonation, and relaxation. Abductor SD is addressed through a "continuous voicing" technique, designed to turn the voice on and keep it on, avoiding the involuntary breaks in phonation characteristic of this disorder (Greene & Mathieson, 1989; Heuer, 1992).

OTHER NEUROLOGIC DISORDERS

Neurologic disorders that affect the larynx do not occur in isolation and, as such, other motor speech functions are often impaired, including respiration, articulation, resonance, and prosody. Indeed, many of the hallmark diagnostic signs and symptoms are based on clusters of perceptual attributes and deficits of the speech pattern (Aronson, 1985; Darley, Aronson, & Brown, 1975). The range and type of neurologic voice problems are as varied as the underlying dysarthrias, and detailed summaries of the associated vocal characteristics have been compiled by Aronson (1985), Sudarsky, Feudo, and Zubick (1988), Griffiths and Bough (1989), and Colton and Casper, (1990) (Table 8–1). In combination with findings from the neurologic examination and imaging studies, the classic audio-perceptual attributes of voice production in neurologic disease are often diagnostic.

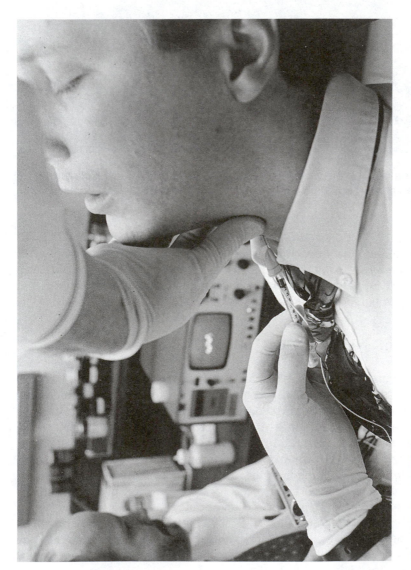

Figure 8–3. BOTOX injection using the percutaneous technique with electromyography guidance. (Photo by Peter Berglund, Minneapolis, Minnesota.)

Table 8–1.   Voice Deviations Associated with Dysarthrias

Flaccid:	vocal fold hypoadduction, resulting in weak, breathy phonation, reduced loudness
Spastic:	vocal fold hyperadduction, resulting in strained, effortful, and harsh phonation.
Ataxic:	irregular random variations in pitch and loudness, unusual or irregular speech rate, and occasional tremor.
Hyperkinetic:	
General:	voice and speech rigidity, with some dystonia, irregularities in respiration may influence aberrant breaks in vocal pitch and loudness
Quick:	sudden, irregular pitch breaks, loudness changes, intermittent aphonia, and strained phonation
Slow:	slower changes in pitch, loudness, and quality of phonation, monotone, aberrant intonational stress
Hypokinetic:	mono-pitch and loudness, hypernasal, imprecise articulation, weak phonation and limited vocal endurance,

Therapy for neurologic disorders that affect voice production is compensatory and will not reverse the underlying neuropathy, but may help maximize the patient's communicative skills. Ramig and Scherer (1991) presented a description of the range of laryngeal deficits that may present in association with neurologic disorders. These problems include vocal fold hypoadduction, hyperadduction, phonatory instability, and incoordination of both prosody and voice-voiceless contrasts. Thus, treatment may address both focal voicing behaviors (e.g., increasing loudness, reducing strained quality) or global speech targets (increasing respiratory support, increasing intelligibility). Following is a description of some neurologic pathologies that are more commonly referred to the voice pathologist.

Essential Vocal Tremor

The onset of this disorder is typically later than for spasmodic dysphonia, but it frequently occurs with SD. The principle perceptual features are regular wavering of pitch and intensity, measurable during sustained pitch productions at a range from three to five Hertz. In severe forms, voice breaks may be noticeable. In addition to the persistent perceptual features, the laryngeal tremor is visible during sustained phonation on indirect examination. This disorder is exclusive of other neurologic processes, such as Parkinson's and cerebellar disease. There is no successful treatment for essential vocal tremor. Patients with coexisting SD and essential vocal tremor who receive BOTOX commonly report relief from the focal dystonia, without any change in tremor activity.

Parkinson's Disease

Parkinson's disease is an extrapyramidal disorder that affects both speech and voice production. Phonation is characterized as monopitch and loudness, weak, breathy, with fading intensity and occasionally voice tremor. Speech intelligibility may be reduced. Diagnosis is made upon neurological examination, following exclusion of other neurologic processes, including laryngeal dystonia. Medical treatments are available to Parkinson's patients, with some degree of success. Recently, the use of behavioral treatment to increase the strength and intelligibility of speech in patient's with Parkinson's disease has been reported (Ramig, 1993). The central targets of this program are increased breath support, loudness, and endurance of steady state phonation in a rigorous exercise routine, conducted for multiple trials daily. Despite the focus on respiration and phonatory loudness, treatment effects generalize to increased articulatory strength, precision, and intelligibility, as well as improved vocal loudness and quality (Ramig, 1993).

Amyotrophic Lateral Sclerosis

Amyotrophic lateral sclerosis (ALS) is a degenerative neurological disorder with primary pathology of the motoneurons of the spinal cord, brainstem, and higher motor centers. Symptoms of ALS include weakness, fasciculation, and atrophy, as evidence of lower motor neuron involvement. Dysarthria and dysphagia occur frequently in persons with ALS (Kent et al., 1992). The dysarthria is described as a mixed spastic-flaccid type (Darley, Aronson, & Brown, 1975). Features of spastic dysarthria include slow speech rate, strained-strangled voice, and reduced stress and prosody. Features of flaccid dysarthria include hoarse, breathy voice, consonant distortions, and short phrases. Hypernasality may be a feature of both spastic and flaccid dysarthria. The voice of patients with ALS has sometimes been described as "wet" or "gurgly" or having a tremor or flutter on vowel prolongation (Aronson, 1985). Individual variability is great, however, and longitudinal assessment may be most useful for reliable description of perceptual features (Ramig, Scherer, Klasner, Titze, & Horii, 1990; Strand, Buder, Yorkston, & Ramig, 1993). Although voice therapy may address compensatory strategies, there is no successful medical or rehabilitative treatment identified for ALS.

PHONOSURGICAL MANAGEMENT OF BENIGN VOCAL FOLD LESIONS

Many benign vocal fold pathologies are the result of acute or chronic traumatic hyperfunctional voice and may respond readily to voice rehabilitation, as described in Chapter 7. When standard voice therapy fails, the otolaryngologist or voice pathologist may recommend surgery. Phonosurgery will be used to excise the lesion with a simultaneous goal of preserving the vocal fold mucosa and restoring the vocal fold edge. With assistance from the voice pathologist, post-surgical voice rehabilitation will be used to facilitate return of voice quality. Post-surgical rehabilitation is also critical to ensure establishment of voice behaviors that promote continued vocal fold health, and prevent recurrence of benign (hyperfunctional) lesions.

The differential diagnosis of benign lesions is made upon visual examination of the lesion appearance and frequently confirmed by the history of voice use. The audio-perceptual quality of voice in patients with benign lesions varies tremendously as a function of the lesion severity, the patient's habitual voice use pattern, and compensatory strategies (e.g., use of breath support, vocal tract tuning, loudness and pitch characteristics). Although certain perceptual attributes prevail across all types of vocal fold lesions, there are not distinctive audio profiles which discriminate differentially the type of vocal fold impairment. Typical voice complaints include dysphonia, including increased breathiness, roughness, and lowering of pitch, increased strain or effort with phonation, intermittent voice breaks or aphonia, loss of pitch and loudness range, and vocal fatigue. Following is a description of a variety of benign vocal fold lesions that may be treated with phonosurgery.

Vocal nodules and **polyps** are blister or callous type lesions that arise from acute traumatic or chronic hyperfunctional voice use. Occasionally, these etiologic factors will give rise to **vascular** vocal fold lesions, including **hemorrhage, varix** (mass of tortuous blood vessels), or **hematoma**, due to injury of the small blood vessels of the vocal fold (Bastian, 1986). The resulting effects on voice can be variable, depending upon the extent and length of time since the onset. If accompanied by laryngeal inflammation, these lesions may respond to a rapid course of oral steroids. Typically, however, nodules and polyps respond positively to voice therapy (Allen, Pettit, & Sherblom, 1991; Verdolini-Marston, Burke, Lessac, Glaze, & Caldwell, 1993), and phonosurgery is not usually needed unless the trauma has been longstanding and residual scarring is preventing full resolution of the vocal fold mucosa. In these cases, microexcision of the lesion with follow-up voice conservation and rehabilitation is recommended.

Epithelial hyperplasia is a general term that describes abnormal mucosal changes in the vocal folds. These changes usually occur in response to combinations of hyperfunctional voice use and chemical irritants, especially alcohol and tobacco use. Common pathologies are **hyperkeratosis** and **polypoid degeneration (Reinke's edema). Hyper-keratosis** is a pathologic diagnosis, and consists of a horny overgrowth of irregular margins on the vocal folds. **Polypoid degeneration** is a swelling of the interstitial space in the lamina propria of the vocal fold, increasing the mass and producing stiff irregular vocal fold edges due to multiple polyp-like lesions. **Leukoplakia** is a pre-diagnostic term that means "white plaque" and describes the appearance of a thick white substance that covers the vocal folds in diffuse patches. The pathology of leukoplakia is variable, and may include both benign and malignant lesions. All of these lesions are treated as cautionary signs for avoiding future exposure to tobacco smoke and other irritants. Occasionally, phonosurgery will be conducted to confirm the diagnosis with a small biopsy and to remove the hyperplasia from the vocal fold mucosa. Often, voice therapy is used to ensure that voice conservation strategies and vocal hygiene are in place and to assist in recovery of voice quality.

PHONOSURGICAL MANAGEMENT OF CONGENITAL LESIONS

Congenital Cyst

Congenital cysts are fluid filled, sessile cysts that can appear in the laryngeal ventricle, subglottis, or in the vocal fold. Diagnosis is made on visual inspection, which reveals a regular oval form just below the epithelial layer. Glottic closure pattern can appear similar to that of other benign mass lesions (e.g., polyps), but vibratory pattern upon video-stroboscopy will display a very stiff adynamic segment over the cyst, with no deformation of the vocal fold margin during collision of the contra-lateral vocal fold. Phonosurgery is the only treatment; the lesion is excised, usually from a superior approach to avoid scarring of the medial edge of the vocal fold (McGill, 1988).

Papilloma

One of the most common childhood tumors is papilloma. The cause of this pathology is thought to be viral infection. It first appears in children between the ages of 2 and 4 and occurs equally in males and females. Less frequently, the disorder can begin in adult years. The lesions appear wart-like, with a cellular composition of stratified squamous epithelium with connective tissue cores. They spread easily through the larynx, trachea, and bronchi, and pose risks for both voice disruption and more disturbingly, airway compromise. Because of the diffuse locations and rapid spread of the papilloma, medical treatments are aggressive, including interferon therapy, laser excision, and occasionally, tracheostomy. However, some risk of spread to the tracheostomy area has also been reported (Jones, Myers, & Barnes, 1988).

The role of voice therapy in treatment of papilloma is twofold. There is some evidence that papilloma spread and severity may be reduced in patients who avoid hyperfunctional voice use, including excessive medial compression of the vocal folds (Greene & Mathieson, 1989). Secondly, as papilloma tends to regress with age, and may eventually disappear following puberty, the resulting phonation may be impaired due to scarring from multiple surgical excisions. At this point, voice rehabilitation may be useful to maximize potential for optimal voice quality despite a compromised vocal fold mucosa.

Congenital Web

A congenital web occurs when the vocal folds fail to separate during the tenth week of embryonic development. Webbing may occur anywhere from the anterior to the posterior glottis. If the web is complete at birth, airway compromise is a threat. More commonly, webbing of the anterior glottis causes various degrees of dyspnea and stridor. Phonosurgery is conducted to separate the web, using a keel to maintain separation of the folds and to avoid reformation of the web due to postoperative scarring (McGill, 1988). Voice therapy may have a role in post-operative rehabilitation, to encourage proper development of voice pitch and quality.

SUMMARY

Medical or organic contributors play a significant role in the voice disordered patient population. The interaction between vocal function and laryngeal pathology, whether focal or systemic, has provided opportunity for development of new treatment approaches. Options for medical treatments, voice rehabilitation, and phonosurgery have enhanced the opportunity for voice pathologists and otolaryngologists to apply a combined team approach to diagnosis, treatment planning, and rehabilitation of voice disorders.

REFERENCES

Abitbol, J., de Brux, J., Millot, G., Masson, M. F., Mimoun, O. L., Pau, H., & Abithol, B. (1989). Does a hormonal vocal cord cycle exist in women? *Journal of Voice, 3*(2), 157–162.

Allen, M. S., Pettit, J. M., & Sherblom, J. C. (1991). Management of vocal nodules: A regional survey of otolaryngologists and speech-language pathologists. *Journal of Speech and Hearing Research, 34*(2), 229–235.

Aronson, A. (1985). *Clinical voice disorders: An interdisciplinary approach* (2nd ed.). New York: Thieme, Inc.

Aronson, A., & DeSanto, L. (1983). Adductor spastic dysphonia: Three years after recurrent laryngeal nerve resection. *Laryngoscope, 93*, 1–8.

Baer, T. (1981). Investigation of the phonatory mechanism. Proceedings of the Conference on the Assessment of Vocal Pathologies, *ASHA Reports, 11*, 38–47.

Bastian, R. W. (1986). Benign mucosal disorders. In C. W. Cummings, J. M. Frederickson, L. A. Harker, C. J. Krause, & D. E. Schuller (Eds.), *Otolaryngology-Head and Neck Surgery* (pp. 1965–1987). St. Louis: C. V. Mosby Co.

Bienenstock, H., Ehrlich, G. E., & Freyberg, R. H. (1963). Rheumatoid arthritis of the cricoarytenoid joint: A clinicopathologic study. *Arthritis and Rheumatism, 6*, 48–63.

Blaugrund, S. (1991). Laryngeal framework surgery. In C. N. Ford & D. M. Bless (Eds.), *Phonosurgery* (pp. 183–200). New York: Raven Press.

Blitzer, A., Brin, M. F., Fahn, S., & Lovelace, R. E. (1988). Localized injections of botulinum toxin for the treatment of focal laryngeal dystonia. *Laryngoscope, 98*, 193–197.

Blitzer, A., & Brin, M.F. (1991). Laryngeal dystonia: A series with botulinum toxin therapy. *Annals of Otology, Rhinology, and Laryngology, 100*, 85–89.

Brandenburg, J., Kirkham, W., & Koschkee, D. (1992). Vocal cord augmentation with autogenous fat. *Laryngoscope, 102*(5), 495–500.

Cannito, M. P. (1990). Neurobiological interpretations of spasmodic dysphonia. In D. Vogel & M. P. Cannito (Eds.), *Treating disordered speech motor control: For clinicians by clinicians* (pp. 275–317). Austin: Pro-Ed.

Colton, R., & Casper, J. (1990). *Understanding voice problems*, Baltimore: Williams and Wilkins.

Cooper, M. (1977). Direct vocal rehabilitation. In M. Cooper (Ed.), *Approaches to vocal rehabilitation.* Springfield, IL: Charles C. Thomas.

Crumley, R. (1991). Laryngeal reinnervation techniques. In C. N. Ford & D. M. Bless (Eds.), *Phonosurgery* (pp. 201–212). New York: Raven Press.

Damste, P. H. (1987). Diagnostic behavior patterns with communicative abilities. In D. M. Bless & J. Abbs (Eds.), *Vocal fold physiology* (pp. 435–444). San Diego: College-Hill Press.

Darley, F., Aronson, A. E., & Brown, J. (1975). *Motor speech disorders*. Philadelphia: W.B. Saunders.

Davis, C. B., & Davis, M. L. (1993). The effects of premenstrual syndrome on the female singer. *Journal of Voice, 7*(4), 337–353.

Dedo, H. (1976). Recurrent nerve section for spastic dysphonia. *Annals of Otology, Rhinology, and Laryngology, 85*, 451–459.

Ford, C. N., & Bless, D. M. (1987). Collagen injected in the scarred vocal fold. *Journal of Voice, 1*(1), 116–119.

Ford, C. N., Bless, D. M., & Lowery, J. D. (1990). Indirect laryngoscopic approach for injection of botulinum toxin in spasmodic dysphonia. *Otolaryngology-Head and Neck Surgery, 103*, 752–758.

Ford, C. N. (1990). A multipurpose laryngeal injector device. *Otolaryngology-Head and Neck Surgery, 103*, 135–137.

Ford, C. N. (1991). Laryngeal injection techniques. In C. N. Ford & D. M. Bless (Eds.), *Phonosurgery* (pp. 123–141). New York: Raven Press.

Ford, C. N., & Bless, D. M. (1991). Introduction. In C. N. Ford & D. M. Bless (Eds.), *Phonosurgery* (pp. 1–3). New York: Raven Press.

Ford, C. N., Bless, D. M., & Loftus, J. M. (1992). Role of injectable collagen in the treatment of glottic insufficiency: A study of 119 patients. *Annals of Otology, Rhinology, and Laryngology, 101*(3), 237–247.

Greene, M., & Mathieson, L. (1989). *The voice and its disorders* (5th Ed.). London: Whurr Publishers.

Griffiths, C., & Bough, Jr., I. D. (1989). Neurologic diseases and their effects on voice. *Journal of Voice, 3*(2), 148–156.

Heuer, R. (1992). Behavioral therapy for spasmodic dysphonia. *Journal of Voice, 6*(4), 352–354.

Higgins, M., & Saxman, J. (1989). Variations in vocal frequency perturbation across the menstrual cycle. *Journal of Voice, 3*(3), 233–243.

Isshiki, N. (1991). Laryngeal framework surgery. *Advances in Otolaryngology-Head and Neck Surgery, 5,* 37–56.

Jafek, B. W., & Esses, B. A. (1986). Manifestations of systemic disease. In C. W. Cummings, J. M. Frederickson, L.A. Harker, C. J. Krause, & D. E. Schuller (Eds.), *Otolaryngology-Head and Neck Surgery* (pp. 1933–1941). St. Louis: C. V. Mosby Co.

Jones, S., Myers, E., & Barnes, E. (1988). Benign neoplasms of the larynx. In M. Fried (Ed.), *The Larynx: A multidisciplinary approach* (pp. 401–420). Boston: Little Brown and Co.

Jones, N. S., Lannigan, F. J., McCullagh, M., Anggiansah, A., Owen, W., & Harris, T. W. (1990). Acid reflux and hoarseness. *Journal of Voice, 4*(4), 355–358.

Kent, J., Kent, R. D., Rosenbek, J., Weismer, G., Martin, R., Sufit, R., & Brooks, B. (1992). Quantitative description of the dysarthria in women with amyotrophic lateral sclerosis. *Journal of Speech and Hearing Research, 35*(4), 723–733.

Koufman, J. A. (1986). Thyroplasty for vocal fold medialization: An alternative to Teflon. *Laryngoscope, 96,* 726–731.

Koufman, J. A., Weiner, G. J., Wu, W. C., & Castell, D. O. (1988). Reflux laryngitis and its sequelae: The diagnostic role of ambulatory 24-hour pH monitoring. *Journal of Voice, 2*(1), 78–89.

Larson, C. R., & Kempster, G. B. (1983). Voice fundamental frequency changes following discharge of laryngeal motor units. In I. R. Titze & R. C. Scherer (Eds.), *Vocal fold physiology* (pp. 91–104). Denver, CO: Denver Center for the Performing Arts.

Ludlow, C. L., Naunton, R. F., Sedory, S. E., Schulz, G. M., & Hallett, M. (1988). Effects of botulinum toxin injections on speech in adductor spasmodic dysphonia. *Neurology, 38,* 1220–1225.

Lumpkin, S. M. M., Bishop, S. G., & Katz, P. O. (1989). Chronic dysphonia secondary to gastroesophageal reflux disease (GERD): Diagnosis using simultaneous dual-probe prolonged pH monitoring. *Journal of Voice, 3*(4), 351–355.

Martin, F. G. (1988) Drugs and vocal function. *Journal of Voice, 2*(4), 33–344.

McGill, T. (1988). Congenital abnormalities of the larynx. In M. Fried (Ed.), *The larynx: A multidisciplinary approach* (pp. 143–152). Boston: Little Brown and Co.

Miller, R. H. (1992). Technique of percutaneous EMG-guided botulinum toxin injection for treatment of spasmodic dysphonia. *Journal of Voice, 6*(4), 377–379.

Orlikoff, R. F. (1989). Vocal jitter at different fundamental frequencies: A cardiovascular-neuromuscular explanation. *Journal of Voice, 3*(2), 104–112.

Orlikoff, R. F. (1990). Heartbeat-related fundamental frequency and amplitude variation in healthy young and elderly male voices. *Journal of Voice, 4*(4), 322–328.

Pennover, D., & Shefer, A. (1988). Immunologic disorders of the larynx. In M. Fried (Ed.), *The larynx: A multidisciplinary approach* (pp. 279–290). Boston: Little Brown and Co.

Pillsbury, H. C., & Postma, D. S. (1986). Infections. In C. W. Cummings, J. M. Frederickson, L. A. Harker, C. J. Krause, & D. E. Schuller (Eds.), *Otolaryngology-Head and Neck Surgery* (pp. 1919–1931). St. Louis: C.V. Mosby Co.

Ramig, L. Scherer, R., Klasner, E., Titze, I. R., & Horii, Y. (1990). Acoustic analysis of voice in amyotrophic lateral sclerosis: A longitudinal case study. *Journal of Speech and Hearing Disorders, 55*(1), 2–14.

Ramig, L., & Scherer, R. C. (1991). Speech therapy for neurological disorders of the larynx. In I. R. Titze (Ed.), *Progress report 1* (pp. 167–190). Iowa City, IA: National Center for Voice and Speech.

Ramig, L. (1993). Speech therapy for patients with Parkinsons disease. In I. R. Titze (Ed.), *Progress report 5* (pp. 83–90). Iowa City, IA: National Center for Voice and Speech.

Rubin, W. (1987). Allergic, dietary, chemical, stress, and hormonal influences in voice abnormalities. *Journal of Voice, 1*(4), 378–385.

Schaefer, S. D., Finitzo-Heiber, T., Gerling, I. J., & Freeman, F. J. (1987). Brainstem conduction abnormalities in spasmodic dysphonia. In D. M. Bless & J. Abbs (Eds.), *Vocal fold physiology* (pp. 393-404). San Diego: College-Hill Press.

Shemen, L. (1988). Diseases of the thyroid as they affect the larynx. In M. Fried (Ed.), *The larynx: A multidisciplinary approach* (pp. 223–233). Boston: Little Brown and Co.

Shumrick, K., & Shumrick, D. (1988). Inflammatory diseases of the larynx. In M. Fried (Ed.), *The larynx: A multidisciplinary approach* (pp. 249–278). Boston: Little Brown and Co.

Smith, M., & Gray, S. (1994). Laryngeal framework surgery in children. In I. R. Titze (Ed.), *Progress report 5* (pp. 91–98). Iowa City, IA: National Center for Voice and Speech.

Strand, E., Buder, E., Yorkston, K., & Ramig, L. (1993). Differential phonatory characteristics of women with amyotrophic lateral sclerosis. In I. R. Titze (Ed.), *Progress report 4* (pp. 151–168). Iowa City, IA: National Center for Voice and Speech.

Sudarsky, L., Feudo, P., Zubick, H. (1988). Vocal aberrations in dysarthria. In M. Fried (Ed.), *The larynx: A multidisciplinary approach* (pp. 179–190). Boston: Little Brown and Co.

Tucker, H. M. (1987). *The larynx.* New York: Thieme Medical Publishers, Inc.

Verdolini-Marston, K., Burke, M. K., Lessac, A., Glaze, L. E., & Caldwell, E. (1993). A preliminary study on two methods of treatment for laryngeal nodules. In I. R. Titze (Ed.), *Progress report 4* (pp. 209–228). Iowa City, IA: National Center for Voice and Speech.

Wolman, L. Darke, C. S., & Young, A. (1965). The larynx in rheumatoid arthritis. *Journal of Laryngology and Otology, 79,* 403–434.

Woodson, G. E., Zwirner, P., Murry, T., & Swenson, M. R. (1992). Functional assessment of patients with spasmodic dysphonia. *Journal of Voice, 6*(4), 338–343.

9

COMMENTS ON THE PROFESSIONAL VOICE

We have described the laryngeal mechanism in terms of its physical structure and function and have discussed many etiologic factors that may lead to the development of various laryngeal pathologies. Management strategies were then presented that were designed to help patients return the laryngeal mechanism to as near a normal state as possible yielding improved or normal voice qualities.

Our discussion also focused on the motivations of patients in determining their personal needs and desires to modify the causes of their voice disorders for voice improvement. The personal impact of a voice disorder will vary with each patient. Some patients may recognize the problem and demonstrate a slight to moderate concern. With some patients, conditions may arise as a result of the voice disorder that could have a negative impact on their social lives, their emotional status, or their livelihoods. These patients may be deeply troubled by potentially serious consequences of a voice disorder.

A large group of individuals are, by the very nature of their occupations, at a greater risk of developing laryngeal pathology than the general population. This group consists of people who are directly dependent on vocal communication for their livelihood. These people are classified as users of a "professional" voice.

The impact of a voice disorder on this population is twofold. Not only does it cause vocal symptoms that are characteristics of the disorder, it also carries with it a high level of emotional strain and anxiety. This anxiety is caused by the disorder's potential impact on the person's reputation, the ability to meet professional commitments, or simply the ability to perform his or her job.

These concerns and anxieties, which sometimes border on emotional crises, add to the actual causes of the voice disorder and must also be dealt with in a positive manner within the vocal management program.

The management approach must go beyond the manipulation of inappropriate vocal properties and must involve all aspects of vocal hygiene counseling. The rehabilitation will often require the involvement of a team of professionals. The team may comprise the professional voice user, the otolaryngologist, the voice pathologist, and the professional voice user's vocal coach, producer, and manager. Successful voice rehabilitation may depend upon the abilities of these disciplines to compromise and work together with the patient's long-term vocal health as the primary consideration. Ideally, the professional voice user will ultimately become responsible for the well-being of his or her own laryngeal mechanism.

THE PROFESSIONAL VOICE USER

We are all dependent upon vocal communication in our everyday lives. Indeed, the loss of voice for even a brief time is viewed as a major inconvenience by most people. Those who rely directly upon their voices for their livelihoods in a public forum are likely to experience more than an inconvenience with the development of a voice disorder. Voice disorders, whether they are acute or chronic, may threaten, shorten, change, or even end some careers. For example, the singer who develops acute laryngitis on opening night places his or her livelihood and the livelihoods of a great many others in jeopardy or the stage actor who develops intermittent periods of dysphonia due to vocal misuse may develop a reputation of unreliability. The effectiveness of a political campaign may be diminished when the politician becomes dysphonic and is unable to project the desired image.

This chapter will focus primarily on the Elite Vocal Performer (Koufman & Isaccson, 1991) and highly visible professional voice users such as actors, singers, and politicians; but other professional voice users must also be considered. Many less "public" professionals are also "at risk" in the development of laryngeal disorders with the same levels of social, emotional, and job-threatening anxieties present. Some of these other professionals include teachers, ministers, lawyers, salespeople, auctioneers, and health care providers, to name a few. Dependency on their voices to function successfully in their occupations qualifies people as owners of a professional voice. For many, the care and proper use of the voice may never become an issue. For others, a voice disorder may create real or imagined personal threats. The psychodynamics of vocal management may dictate the success or failure these professionals experience within their professions.

THE "AT-RISK" STATUS

People who use their voices professionally are subject to the development of laryngeal pathologies due to any of the etiologic factors mentioned in previous chapters. It is not unusual to make the assumption that because of the intimate dependency and relationships these individuals have with their voices, they would not be as likely to develop disorders due to vocal abuse or misuse. We might also assume that the professional voice user's knowledge of the structure and function of the laryngeal mechanism is superior to that of people not as dependent upon their voices. Both assumptions, however, are not necessarily correct.

We find only a few professional voice owners who have even a vague awareness of the anatomy and physiology of the vocal mechanism. Also, although many people do indeed possess "trained" voices for acting, singing, and public speaking and excellent techniques for these functions, other vocal misuses and abuses are often present as primary causes of their vocal difficulties.

Khambato (1979) paralleled the experiences of singers and actors with those of athletes. He stated that because of the physical nature of their work, athletes are at a greater risk than most people in developing muscular and joint injuries. Likewise, because actors and singers are dependent upon their voices and, as a rule, demand more from them than the average person, they are at greater risk in developing laryngeal pathologies. Despite these similarities a major difference exists between the management approaches of athletes and professional voice users. The prized athlete generally rests the injury long enough for it to heal and for the possibility of permanent damage to be eliminated. Singers and actors, however, usually minimize the disability to avoid canceling an engagement. They continue using the voice, often risking permanent damage. After all, "The show must go on!"

The less "public" professional voice users behave in the same manner as singers and actors. Teachers continue to teach, speech-language pathologists continue to practice, salespeople continue to sell, and preachers continue to preach, rather than risk loss of income or damage to their reputations as reliable productive workers.

COMMON ETIOLOGIC FACTORS

We have stated that professional voice users are subject to developing laryngeal pathologies due to many etiologic factors. These frequently occurring causes are personality-related factors, vocal misuse, and chronic medical and health conditions.

Personality Factors

Intense, volatile, excitable, emotional, neurotic, anxious, temperamental, moody, intemperate, vain, and unstable are all terms that Punt (1979) used when describing the personalities of professional actors and singers. Although these personality attributes have also been described as necessary for the successful artist, a person's emotional or mental state will have an effect on vocal production. Weiner (1978) supported this view when he commented that the human voice is one of the most accurate and sensitive indicators of the state of a personality; it tends to mirror what is happening in a person's life.

Punt (1979) further indicated the direct relationship between emotions and voice quality by observing that in times of extreme stress, even the trained voice user will project emotional problems into the voice. The vocal mechanism may even be perfectly healthy and free of visible pathology, but its precision of movement may be adversely affected by the state of mind and the emotions of the owner of the voice.

Many of these personality factors are also present in many "unartistic" professional voice users. For example, salespeople are often described as hard driving, intense, and fast talking. Ministers may be subjected to great emotional strain due to the personal needs and problems of congregational members. Physicians may be under stress by the demands of patients and their families and the huge responsibility of controlling their health and well-being as well as in dealing closely with death. Teachers and lecturers may be intense or even anxious about the responsibility of educating their listeners. They may also be worried about receiving good evaluations on which their jobs or promotions may depend. In short, inherent personality characteristics, which are to some extent demanded of professional voice users, along with the anxieties and stresses created by the various professionals, may all contribute to the development of a voice disorder.

Vocal Misuse

Persons who use their voices professionally are subject to the same vocal misuses and abuses as those found in the general speaking public. The overall effect that vocal abuse has on the livelihood of the professional voice user is much more negative. For example, the laryngeal changes associated with shouting at a football game would be the same for the professional and nonprofessional voice users. Let us speculate that a mild edema and erythema developed resulting in a mild to moderate dysphonia. The nonprofessional voice user would certainly return to work the next day with no ill effect on job performance, whereas the professional voice user may suffer the consequences of a missed performance, a lost sale, an inadequate public appeal, or the like.

Another factor associated with vocal abuse and professional voice users is the life-style that they live. Inherent in the life-styles of many public "performers" are periods of nonperformance socializing and other activities that may contribute to vocal hyperfunction. These abusive activities may include talking over noise in the hustle and bustle of the backstage area following a performance; loud talking during post-performance dinners and parties; or unusual vocal demands created by frequent public appearances, usually in noisy public forums for promotional purposes.

Vocal misuse and abuse may also occur during performances. Many singers and actors have highly trained voices, but many others may be guilty of using inappropriate vocal techniques. These inappropriate uses of the vocal components may be present while singing musical parts not suited to the artist's voice; while utilizing inappropriate respiratory support for a particular role; or while singing or speaking with an improper tone focus. Although loud singing and stage shouting need not be vocally abusive, they often create vocal problems in the untrained voice. When these activities do cause vocal problems, the difficulties are usually the result of a lack of abdominal and diaphragmatic breath support, the use of hard glottal attacks, and a general constriction of the upper airway.

Another potential form of vocal abuse in singers is the use of a singing technique known as belting. The belted singing voice is produced at a high intensity level with strong vocal fold adduction. As long as the respiratory effort is adequate to support the voice and the supraglottic structures are not constricted, belting is not abusive. Vocal problems occur when the respiratory effort is inadequate for the high intensity level causing constriction of the entire upper airway. Numerous popular singers have constructed successful careers utilizing this form of singing, but many others have suffered harsh vocal consequences as a result of this form of laryngeal hyperfunction.

Vocal abuse may also be related to the environmental conditions in which the performer works. For example, the classical singer may be forced to compete with an overly enthusiastic and loud orchestra in a hall with limited or poor acoustics and a musty backstage area. Rock singers often compete with the high intensity levels of their own heavily amplified electronic instruments. Other entertainers sing or perform in small clubs, with dense ambient smoke and must compete with noisy patrons and poor amplification. Considering the environments in which many professionals are asked to perform, it is surprising that more voice disorders do not occur.

Other less "public" professional voice users have their forms of vocal abuse. Examples include teachers who shout during playground, cafeteria, or bus duty and salespeople who often hold business meetings or make sales presentations over lunch in noisy restaurants. Many salespeople also use a pseudo-authoritative voice for a greater vocal effect. Continued use of this hyperfunctional voice will often lead to laryngeal pathology. Voice pathologists may also be subjected to vocally abusive behaviors. Anyone who has taught vocal fold paralysis patients to use hard glottal attacks as an exercise must be aware of the negative vocal effects created in the normal laryngeal mechanism.

In concluding this section on vocal abuse and the professional voice user, it is strongly suggested that the voice pathologist not overlook the obvious when evaluating these patients. The obvious abusive behaviors are all common to all speakers, such as shouting at children, shouting during sporting events, talking loudly to a hard-of-hearing relative, constant throat clearing, and persistent coughing. These common vocally abusive behaviors are just as likely to occur in the professional and non-professional voice users.

Health and Health-Related Issues

People who utilize voices professionally have a special concern for the health of the laryngeal mechanism. The unfortunate aspect of this concern is that only a few people understand that the well-being of the mechanism is dependent on the well-being of the whole body. As stated earlier, the life-styles of many professional voice users are not compatible with the maintenance of a healthy larynx. Not only may these life-styles create vocal abuse and emotional stress, but they may also lead to less than adequate physical health.

Exhausting schedules, alcohol abuse, drug abuse, smoking, and improper dietary habits contribute to the development of poor physical health. Unfortunately, these conditions are not uncommon to many professional voice users. The health and health-related habits of this population must be examined in detail when attempting to discover the cause of a voice disorder.

The schedules of top performers who are in public demand are at times incredibly demanding. It is not unusual for every waking moment to be scheduled. A classical singer may perform in New York City, Houston, Denver, and Los Angeles in succession, completing one performance run and beginning rehearsals in the new city upon arrival the next day. Rehearsal days and nights are also filled with preperformance preparations, parties, and promotions. The schedule is typically nonstop with very little time set aside for rest and relaxation. A tired body will often yield a tired laryngeal mechanism. Efforts to phonate in a optimum manner may lead to vocal hyperfunction.

Exhausting schedules are certainly not limited to classical singers. Equally effective examples may be given for actors who perform daily and twice daily for matinees, circuit singing groups, and those groups that travel from city to city performing one-night stands. The professional voice user who is suffering with a voice disorder, must be made to understand the direct relationship between physical health and vocal health. Resolution of the voice problem may be dependent upon establishing a more reasonable daily schedule.

There are many reasons why people may turn to physically abusive habits. Habits such as excessive alcohol abuse, cigarette smoking, marijuana smoke inhalation, and cocaine snorting are not uncommon among professional voice users. All of these habits are irritating to the respiratory tract and larynx and may contribute to the development of voice disorders. Some of the reasons given by patients for utilizing these abusive agents include the stress and pressures of auditions and subsequent rejections; the stress of giving performances that will always please the audience; tight schedules that yield minimal time for relaxation; difficult personal relationships; and individual emotional conflicts. In addition to these reasons, it is fair to say that our culture has influenced the use of alcohol and "recreational" drugs not only in this population but in the general population.

Alcohol is abusive both as a local oral and laryngeal irritant and as a vasodilator of the mucosal lining of the larynx. The effect of vasodilatation is a drying of the mucous membrane that increases the likelihood of vocal fold hemorrhage during phonation. Excessive consumption of alcohol may lead to a chronic dysphonia, which has been commonly described as a "gin" or "whiskey" voice (Sataloff, 1991).

Caffeine is also a vasodilator. It's effect is drying of the mucosal membrane. Caffeine is found in products such as coffee, tea, soda, chocolate, prescription and non-prescription drugs. Excessive caffeine intake can lead to thick, sticky mucus that accumulates on the true vocal fold surface. Thick mucus on the vocal folds can lead to chronic throat clearing or coughing.

Cigarette and marijuana smoke are both irritants of the respiratory tract and larynx. Both types of smoke dry out the mucosal lining of the larynx causing mild edema and erythema. This laryngeal condition causes an increased sensitivity often creating excessive coughing, which is also vocally abusive. Cocaine is also a local irritant that produces changes in the nasal, pharyngeal, and laryngeal mucosal linings. (See Chapter 3 for a complete description of the effects of each of these substances on the vocal system.)

We have now stated several times that the health of the mucosal lining of the respiratory tract is important to the health of the laryngeal mechanism. The irritants of smoke and alcohol are most obviously recognized as damaging agents; we must also consider natural humidity when discussing vocal health. A low humidity level means that the air we breathe is dry. This dryness also causes the mucous lining of the larynx to become dry and irritated. Drying of the mucosa also interferes with the natural immune system (gamma globulin) contained within the lining. This interference may contribute to an increase in upper respiratory infections. Low humidity is often present in over-heated or air-conditioned homes, pressurized airplanes, and halls and theaters with stale air. Occasionally humidity levels may be too high. This condition tends to thin the mucus of the entire respiratory tract causing excessive drainage. This drainage will often cause excessive throat clearing. Drainage also exposes the respiratory cilia to irritation that leads to coughing.

Many professional voice users complain about the presence of mucus drainage. It is difficult for them to understand that "postnasal drip" as our commercial medicine industries have named it, is a normal and natural function. The normal mucus flow through the nasal system alone is approximately 1.5 quarts per day. This mucus flow is responsible for humidifying inhaled air as it travels through the respiratory tract.

Two factors must be considered when determining the professional voice user's preoccupation with mucus drainage. First, American advertising companies, in their zeal to sell products, have convinced the general population that "sinus drainage" is abnormal. Most of the over-the-counter "sinus" medicines dehydrate the mucosal lining causing the same laryngeal conditions that are present when relative humidity levels are too low. The second factor to be considered is that most professional voice users, because of their vocal dependencies, are hypersensitive to all laryngeal sensations. Therefore, normal mucus drainage may be perceived as an enemy to normal vocal fold function.

Many patients who complain of too much mucus drainage may actually have too little drainage or they may have mucus that is too thick and sticky. The most common reason for this condition is a lack of internal hydration. This problem may often be remedied simply by increasing the intake of nonalcoholic liquids, preferably 8 to 10 glasses of water per day. When the mucus is any color but clear or white, an infection may be present. The presence of a respiratory infection may require the use of antibiotics, anti inflammatory corticosteroids, steam inhalation, soothing syrups, and possibly nasal irrigation or nasal sprays for acute use. Patients with respiratory tract infections are advised to avoid aspirin products due to their anticoagulant effects that increase the likelihood of vocal fold hemorrhage. Occasionally expectorants are utilized to promote secretions of less viscous mucus (Sataloff, 1991).

As with the general population, professional voice users may suffer from airborne allergies and food allergies, which may increase the normal mucus flow. This condition often creates an edematous respiratory tract as a result of the reaction between the allergies and the antibody. Common allergic agents include pollens, dust, and molds as well as foods such as dairy products, chocolates, and yeast products such as beer and wine. Allergies require medical evaluation. Positive reactions to medical testing indicate that patients must either avoid the agent or submit to a long desensitization program.

Esophageal reflux, as described in Chapter 8, is also a common etiologic factor associated with voice disorders of professional voice users. Indeed, professional voice users may be even more likely to develop gastroesophageal reflux disease (GERD) as a result of several factors including poor diet, stress, and poor sleep habits. Reflux disease should be explored with this population and all precautions taken as described later in this chapter.

The general health of the professional voice user will have an effect on the laryngeal mechanism. The rested well-nourished individual who does not indulge in alcohol, cigarette, or drug abuse is less likely to develop a voice disorder than the person who maintains a schedule involving little sleep, poor nutrition, and abusive health habits. Although the health conditions mentioned in this chapter may be common to the professional voice population, they are not exclusive to this population. Likewise, the professional voice user may also suffer from any of the other chronic medical and health disorders.

COMMON PATHOLOGIES

The professional voice user may be susceptible to the development of all types of laryngeal pathologies, but functional pathologies are most likely to occur because of improper or excessive use of voice. These common pathologies include acute and chronic noninfective laryngitis, vocal nodules, contact ulcers, gastroesophageal reflux disease, and laryngeal muscle weakness

Acute and Chronic Noninfective Laryngitis

On examining the causes of all laryngeal pathologies in the professional voice user, it is most important to determine whether the cause is long-standing and frequently occurring or whether it is simply an acute occurrence. Acute noninfective laryngitis is usually the result of an unusual, short-term period of vocal misuse. It may result from a shouting argument, vocal enthusiasm at a sporting event, singing a song out of the optimum range, or consuming an unusual amount of alcohol, caffeine, and cigarettes in a short period of time.

During acute laryngitis, the vocal folds usually have a dull pink color or with a thickened, sticky mucus lining. The major symptoms may vary from a mild to a severe dysphonia characterized by hoarseness, lowered pitch, and impairment in the vocal range. Singers with acute laryngitis demonstrate difficulty in achieving the upper parts of their ranges, especially at low-intensity levels.

Treatments for acute laryngitis include elimination or modification of the causes, steam inhalation, and short-term voice rest when possible. Voice rest permits the laryngeal muscles and the mucosal lining to rebound from the acute abuse. Continued speaking or singing in the presence of the pathology may lead to more serious pathologies such as submucosal hemorrhages or nodules.

Chronic abuse or misuse of the laryngeal mechanism may lead to the development of chronic noninfective laryngitis. This laryngeal pathology is usually indicative of a long history of vocal difficulties. The vocal characteristics of the chronic condition are similar to acute laryngitis; the dysphonic quality is more permanent and resistive to change. The long-term voice misuse causes a drying of the mucous membrane and a more serious damage to the normal strength of the laryngeal musculature than does the acute condition.

Typical treatment for both acute and chronic laryngitis involves a short period of voice rest, if at all possible, followed by identification and modification of the causative factors. When a performance or presentation cannot be postponed, it is possible for the otolaryngologist to prepare the patient for the performance with the use of laryngeal spray solutions or corticosteroids that diminish laryngeal sensitivity and reduce congestion and edema. This treatment is usually considered if a period of vocal rest is available after the performance (Punt, 1979). Because of the high risk of more serious laryngeal damage, this treatment is only utilized when it is absolutely necessary that the patient perform.

The effects of a dysphonic voice quality caused by noninfective chronic laryngitis may have serious implications on the livelihoods of some individuals. Others, however, have used their voice disorders to their advantage by developing distinctive vocal characteristics. More often, the long-term vocal effects of chronic laryngitis lead to the premature end of a performance career or a reduction in earning capabilities.

Vocal Nodules

To the professional voice user, one of the most frightening of all laryngeal pathologies, and the bane of all professional singers, is vocal nodules. We suspect that this fear is present mainly because nodules are one of the most common and most discussed pathologies even among people with a relative naiveté regarding voice disorders. Indeed, it is not unusual for even the most trained professional singer to develop small bilateral nodules during particularly forceful singing.

The voice symptoms of vocal nodules are extremely variable depending on their size, duration of existence, and mechanical effects upon phonation. Efforts to produce normal phonation in the presence of nodules leads to forceful methods of phonation causing laryngeal muscle fatigue and often an inappropriate constriction of the supraglottic structures. Higher tones are most adversely affected, especially when produced at lower intensity levels. Phonation breaks, and obvious breathiness usually occur when nodules are of moderate size or larger.

The treatment of vocal nodules again involves identification and modification of their causes. Along with traditional vocal hygiene counseling, much emphasis is placed on patient education and counseling regarding the impact of nodules on the patient's career. Often, the anxiety level expressed by the patient as a result of the pathology is much higher than the pathology warrants. With the complete cooperation of the patient, nodules may often be resolved quickly and effectively with minimal career interruption. Frankly, it is often much easier modifying the causes of vocal nodules than attempting to modify the long-standing causes of chronic laryngitis.

The voice diagnostic examination may occasionally fail to identify any possible causes for the development of vocal nodules, especially in singers. When causes cannot be identified, evaluation of the singing technique by a competent vocal coach is appropriate. It is not the voice pathologist's role to evaluate artistic techniques or abilities. If the technique is found faulty by the vocal coach, then voice lessons designed to improve vocal technique may be advised.

Vocal nodules occur more often in the untrained singing voice than in the classically trained voice. Some pop and rock singers have capitalized on dysphonic voice qualities; others agonize over their inability to produce adequate phonation. Resolution of the nodules through traditional voice therapy along with vocal training becomes essential for many untrained singers who wish to continue their careers. Although voice therapy is not long term (usually lasting fewer than 3 months), the patient must often sacrifice some performance time in order to resolve the voice problem. However, it is much better to sacrifice a little time for concentrated voice training to resolve the problem than to continue the vocal struggles. A little time taken now may help to ensure a long career. The alternative may be no career at all.

Surgery is occasionally recommended for the excision of vocal nodules, but as a rule of thumb, surgery should be avoided on professionals' vocal folds, if at all possible. Although the physical risks of the surgery may be minimal, the psychological effects could be most damaging. Some patients become "vocal cripples" following vocal fold surgery. These patients are reluctant to return to full vocal use for fear of redeveloping the laryngeal pathology. Their fear is often so strong that even though the laryngeal mechanisms are normal, the patients will not use full voice. This fear, of course, jeopardizes their careers. Vocal fold surgery performed without strong counseling from the surgeon or voice pathologist is not advised. Even when surgery is performed, the causes of the pathology must be modified to reduce the possibility of recurrence, and the patient must also be prepared to return to normal phonation.

Contact Ulcers and Granulomas

Contact ulcers occur most commonly in male public speakers, teachers, sales representatives, politicians, and actors. Contact ulcers result from a grinding, hammering action of the vocal processes of the arytenoid cartilages. These actions occur during the repeated use of a loud, low-pitched, pseudo-authoritative voice, which is often used to project a desired masculine or authority image. The mild to moderate dysphonia that is a result of slowly developing ulcerations is characterized by a low pitch and huskiness. Other factors also associated with the development of contact ulcers involve cigarette smoking, excessive alcohol and caffeine consumption, and reflux of stomach acids into the laryngeal vestibule. Contact ulcers are most effectively treated through retraining the appropriate use of the vocal components of pitch and loudness. Reduction or elimination of alcohol, caffeine, and smoking is also strongly advised. If reflux is the cause of contact ulcers and granulomas, then an antireflux regimen is recommended with possible medications.

Gastroesophageal Reflux Disease (GERD)

Probably the most underdiagnosed and most common gastrointestinal problem that affects professional voice users is gastroesophageal reflux disease. Incidence of 7 to 10% of the population has been reported in the literature (Nebel, Forbes, & Castell, 1976). Professional and nonprofessional voice users are prone to many of the precipitating factors that promote reflux. Many singers or actors prefer to eat very minimally prior to a performance; however, after the performance is over, eating a larger meal may occur late into the evening. Overeating may take place and they may go to bed on a full stomach. Reclining after eating places the larynx and esophagus on the same plane as the stomach, making it easier for the acidic contents from the stomach to reflux into the pharynx. Foods that reportedly promote reflux include the following: coffee (with or without caffeine), chocolate, soda, high fat foods, citrus beverages, tomato products, spicy foods, and alcohol. Smoking and weight gain have also been shown to increase reflux.

Possible etiologies of gastroesophageal reflux include a hiatal hernia, lower esophageal sphincter dysfunction, and esophageal dysmotility. Individuals complain of heartburn and acid regurgitation with a report of a burning or bitter taste in the throat. Some patients will report a sensation of a "lump" in the throat feeling or may present with symptoms of chronic cough (nonproductive), hoarseness, chronic throat clearing with very little mucus, and chest pain or discomfort. Singers may not report any of the above symptoms but may be experiencing difficulty singing higher notes. Sometimes they will report chronic laryngitis.

Physical examination of the larynx may show erythematous arytenoids, small contact ulcerations in the vocal process area, but most commonly a thickening or mounding of tissue is noted in the interarytenoid space. Sometimes the true vocal folds appear erythematous and edematous. The true vocal folds may also appear very stiff in the amplitude of vibration as observed stroboscopically.

Treatment includes dietary restrictions (avoiding foods that cause heartburn), weight reduction (if necessary), avoidance of overeating or eating late at night (not within 3 hours of bedtime), cessation of smoking, and taking an antacid between meals and before bedtime. If a conservative approach is not effective in treatment, then the patient may need additional medical tests which may include an ambulatory 24-hour double-probe pH monitoring, a barium esophagram with fluoroscopy, or a direct endoscopy. There are several prescription medicines that are also available in the treatment of gastroesophageal reflux.

Laryngeal Myasthenia

The muscles of the larynx may be viewed as any other muscle group in the body. Like the arm, leg, or stomach muscles, the laryngeal muscles may become weakened or fatigued due to strain, overwork, or misuse. It is also probable that other pathological conditions of the larynx will lead to laryngeal myasthenia. The major characteristic of this condition in the speaker is voice fatigue within even a brief period of speaking time. The singer with laryngeal myasthenia will complain about a lack of consistency in the quality of the vocal output. Because of the muscle weakness, notes in one range, either high or low depending on the stronger muscle group, will be hard to achieve. In both the speaker and the singer, discomfort and muscular aching in the laryngeal area are often present.

Punt (1979) categorized this muscular disorder of the larynx into three groups: acute, subacute, and chronic myasthenia. Acute myasthenia was described as being caused by a brief period of severe vocal misuse and abuse. The myasthenia may also be accompanied by edema and erythema of the mucosal lining of the vocal folds.

Subacute myasthenia was described as having many causes. Punt (1979) suggested long-term vocal misuse, emotional difficulties, coughing, throat clearing, and overwork of the voice. He also suggested that the lack of preseason vocal training could lead to subacute myasthenia. This would be comparable to the football player who puts on the pads and equipment and takes part in a full-scale scrimmage the first day of training camp. More than likely the player would experience muscle strain, soreness, or even a pulled leg muscle. The larynx is also a muscular system. Attempting to sing or act without proper conditioning after an extended layoff will often cause a subacute weakness.

Chronic myasthenia was described by Punt (1979) as having the same causes as the subacute type. The difference was in the length of time that the causes were present. In chronic myasthenia, the voice user continues the same improper vocal habits over many years, creating a more permanent laryngeal muscle weakness, which is also more resistant to change.

Discussion of laryngeal pathologies typically focuses on what the eye can see. The presence or absence of mucosal change or growths is described. The discussion of laryngeal muscle function attempts to describe the changes to the muscular functions that cannot be observed by the eye. Evaluation of this disorder is therefore limited to the patient's history. Laryngeal videostroboscopy has added an additional diagnostic tool. Vibratory patterns of the vocal folds as observed through stroboscopy will often demonstrate underlying vocal muscle weaknesses through the observance of out of phase vibrations and incomplete glottic closure (Stemple, Stanley, & Lee, in press). In the case of laryngeal myasthenia, the underlying causes of the disorder, i.e. weakness and imbalance, not the apparent vocal symptoms, must be treated. The voice user must be made to understand that the larynx is a muscular system that requires care. It must be trained, warmed up, cooled down, and kept in shape, in much the same manner as the legs of a dancer or the arm of a baseball pitcher.

Punt (1979) prescribed a short period (24 hours) of voice rest for patients suffering with acute myasthenia and a longer period (1 to 8 weeks) of severely restricted voice use in chronic conditions. The use of long term voice rest is questionable because of the probable further weakening of the laryngeal muscles through inactivity that may in fact worsen the condition. Instead, as the underlying causes are identified and then modified or eliminated, the voice pathologist may choose to initiate direct Vocal Function Exercises for strengthening the laryngeal muscles (see Chapter 7). When significant progress has been made in the muscular condition, the patient should slowly and methodically be reintroduced to professional voice use.

PROFESSIONAL ROLES

The number of people who treat the professional voice user who is having vocal difficulties will depend on the profession itself. For the nonperformance professional, support is most often provided by the oto-laryngologist and the voice pathologist. The otolaryngologist evaluates the laryngeal condition and then treats the condition with rest, medication, surgery, or referral. The voice pathologist evaluates the causes of the laryngeal pathology and then establishes a program for the modification or elimination of these causes.

Professional voices used for stage and singing performances are often subjected to the concerns and influences of not only the otolaryngologist and voice pathologist, but also several other interested persons. These individuals may include the producer of the event, the agent or manager of the performer, and possibly the vocal teacher or coach. Let us examine the roles and pressures of each.

The Producer

The producer of a public event has the major responsibility of guaranteeing that the money investment placed in support of the event is secure. The producer is responsible for overseeing the operations of the event and for reacting quickly and positively to any situations that could threaten the event's success. These situations include dealing with the physical and emotional problems and needs of the performers. Keeping in mind that the producer's main concern is the financial success of the event, it is not difficult to understand that this pressure would possibly make the producer less than sympathetic with a performer suffering vocal problems. The inability to perform is a threat not only to the event's success but ultimately the producer's reputation, which is itself ultimately responsible for securing investors for future events. The producer may, therefore, apply great pressure on the performer or the performer's manager or agent to guarantee that the "show must go on."

The Agent or Manager

The agent or manager is responsible for the overall career development of the professional voice user. Career development involves selling the performer's services to producers, developing public relations strategies, deciding appropriate jobs to accept or reject, scheduling performances, and often handling business affairs.

There is huge competition among a great number of performers for a very limited number of parts. Those professionals who are good enough or lucky enough to find steady work in the performing arts are usually associated with top managers. These performers often sustain themselves as attractive employees through their own professional reliability. However, it is the manager's or agent's responsibility to guarantee that his or her clients remain as attractive as possible to those in the hiring positions. The success and the financial gain of the manager or agent are totally dependent on keeping clients working. The more clients that work, the more attractive is the manager to other potential clients. Producers will not hire performers who have developed reputations for unreliability. This reputation may be developed quickly, especially by performers in the nonstar category. Therefore, we may understand the pressure that the manager or agent may place on a client to perform even in the presence of vocal difficulties. This pressure to perform that is placed on the professional voice user is not an indictment of producers and managers or agents but is simply a statement of the pressures under which they operate.

The Otolaryngologist

The major role of the otolaryngologist in the treatment of the professional voice is in the physical diagnosis of the laryngeal mechanism to determine the condition and the function of the mechanism at that moment. Wise physicians will also attempt to tune into the psychodynamics of their patient's situation. Is fear contributing to the vocal difficulties? What is the overall health of the patient? Is he or she being pressured to perform with an unhealthy vocal mechanism? Several otolaryngologists associated with major stage and opera companies have become counselors, confidants, and advisors as well as physicians for many professional voice users.

When presented with a laryngeal pathology in a professional voice user, the otolaryngologist is often asked to "get me through this performance!" The physician must determine whether the voice problem is an acute or chronic condition. When faced with an important performance, such as a one-time audition, opening night, or a one-night stand, it is often possible for the otolaryngologist to administer anti-inflammatory agents that may make it possible for the patient to perform. In making the decision to help a patient make it through the one important performance, however, it is extremely important to balance the risk of further or more permanent damage against the need to perform. A short period of voice rest is often recommended after such performances. Chronic vocal disorders may often be treated with anti-inflammatory drugs for a period of time. Surgery is usually withheld as a last resort. When medication and vocal rest do not clear the disorder, then appropriate referrals are often made to competent voice pathologists.

The Voice Pathologist

The voice pathologist evaluates all aspects of voice production to determine the causes of the voice disorder. Two important points must be understood in dealing with the professional voice user. First, the technique used in the production of the performance voice is, more often than not, adequate and is not the cause of the vocal difficulties. Often the non-stage voicing habits are the primary etiologic factors. Therefore, our evaluation must focus on both the public and the nonpublic voicing habits. Second, if the public voicing techniques contain the primary causative factors of the voice disorder, then the causes will not be observed during the office evaluation. A sample of the "public" voices must be obtained. This need is especially critical with teachers, salespeople, preachers, politicians, and lecturers. Inappropriate vocal components that are not heard during the quiet conversational voice used throughout the diagnostic evaluation are often quite evident during public presentations.

Once the causes for the disorder have been identified, the impact these causes have on the vocal mechanism must be described in detail to the patient. Utilization of pictures, diagrams, and models describing the laryngeal mechanism and the pathology are extremely helpful for patient understanding. If a copy of the laryngeal videostroboscopic evaluation is available, the educational benefits are enormous. Many people who use their voices for their livelihoods have very little knowledge of the normal structure and function of the laryngeal mechanism. Providing this information is an important role of the voice pathologist. Issues regarding general vocal hygiene should then be discussed as they relate to the patient's specific voice disorder. A management plan is then tailored to the patient and is designed to modify or eliminate the causes of the voice disorder.

As the pathology begins to resolve, efforts are made to rebuild the patient's vocal confidence. The public voice is gradually reintroduced and tested by the patient for effectiveness. When the laryngeal mechanism is healthy and the patient's confidence has been renewed, the patient is discharged from therapy with occasional recheck times established.

At times, the diagnostic evaluation of a singer will yield no etiologic factors responsible for the development of the voice disorder. When this occurs, a competent vocal coach should be found who will evaluate the present singing techniques and modify them as needed to attain a healthy mechanism.

The final goal of voice therapy is not only the return of normal laryngeal structure and function, but also the development of an understanding that the ultimate responsibility for the well-being of the laryngeal mechanism rests with the professional voice user. The responsibility does not lie with the otolaryngologist, voice pathologist, the producer, agent, manager, or coach. In spite of the pressures to perform in the presence of vocal difficulties, the owner of the voice must take charge. Decisions regarding whether or not to perform may be made by honestly answering one question: "Will I compromise the rest of my career by performing tonight?"

SUMMARY

Voice evaluation and therapy for the professional voice user follows basically the same strategies as those used for the nonprofessional voice population. However, special considerations regarding career impact and emotional reactions must be made for the professional population. Although certain pathologies occur more often than others, professional voice users are susceptible to the development of any of the common pathological conditions. The focus of therapy remains in identification of the causes of the pathology and modification or elimination of these causes. The professional voice user must then develop the responsibility for his or her own vocal health.

REFERENCES

Khambato, A. (1979). Laryngeal disorders in singers and other voice users. In J. Ballantyne, & J. Groves (Eds.), *Scott Brown's diseases of the ear, nose, and throat*, vol. 4, throat (4th ed.). London: Butterworths.

Koufman, J., & Isaccson, G. (1991). The spectrum of vocal dysfunction. In J. Koufman, J. & G. Isaccson (Eds.), *The otolaryngologic clinics of North America: Voice disorders* (pp. 985–988). Philadelphia: W.B. Saunders.

Nebel, L., Forbes, M., & Castell, D. (1976). Symptomatic gastroesophageal reflux: Incidence and precipitating factors. *American Journal of Digestive Disease*, 21, 953–956.

Punt, N. (1979). *The singer's and actor's throat: The vocal mechanism of the professional voice user and its care and health in disease* (3rd ed.). London: William Heinemann Medical Books.

Sataloff, R. (1991). *Professional voice: The science and art of clinical care*. New York: Raven Press.

Stemple, J., Stanley, J., & Lee, L. (in press). Objective measures of voice production following prolonged voice use. *Journal of Voice*.

Weiner, H. (1978). Medical problems and treatment: Panel discussion. In Van Lawrence (Ed.), *Transcripts of the 7th symposium on care of the professional voice, part III: Medical/surgical therapy* (p. 67). New York: The Voice Foundation.

10

REHABILITATION OF THE LARYNGECTOMIZED PATIENT

Total rehabilitation of the laryngectomized patient involves interaction of a number of specialists from a multidisciplinary team. A primary participant on the team is the speech-language pathologist. The speech-language pathologist's role goes beyond basic speech retraining approaches to include both patient and family counseling. This chapter will discuss the methods of voice restoration for the laryngectomized patient and of the physical changes, emotional needs, and social adjustments that must also be considered for total rehabilitation.

SYMPTOMS OF LARYNGEAL CANCER

Cancer is the uncontrolled, rapid growth of malignant cells. Early identification of laryngeal carcinoma increases the chance that malignancy will remain localized, thus less difficult to treat. Hoarseness is one of the seven warning signals of possible cancer listed by the American Cancer Society (1987). Persistent hoarseness may motivate an individual to seek a medical examination because of a fear of "throat" cancer. The fear of cancer may also elicit the opposite reaction—refusal to seek medical evaluation. Fear of cancer may cause rational individuals to deny or ignore symptoms until the medical condition becomes more serious. Early recognition of the symptoms of laryngeal cancer is critical to successful treatment.

Hoarseness is the most common symptom of laryngeal cancer when a lesion involves the vocal folds. Vocal fold lesions can cause a change in vocal pitch and, if large enough, breathing problems or stridor. If the vocal folds are not involved, the lesion may progress with symptoms such as a feeling of a lump in the throat, throat clearing, coughing, a sense of discomfort in the throat, difficulty in breathing, a burning sensation when swallowing, or referred pain from the larynx to the ear. In later stages, the malignancy will cause difficulty in swallowing and breathing with the eventual appearance of hoarseness (DeWeese, Saunders, Schuller, & Schleuning, 1988). If the malignancy progresses beyond the confines of the larynx, it is likely to metastasize to the lymphatic system and appear as a lump on the neck. Pain is rarely reported until the later stages of the disease.

Most people experience periods of hoarseness and laryngeal discomfort due to acute laryngitis or vocal abuse during their lives. The important key in determining the seriousness of this condition is whether the symptoms are transient or persistent. Symptoms that persist for 4 weeks or more signal the need for medical evaluation. Examination by an otolaryngologist is strongly recommended if symptoms persist in spite of medication, voice rest, or other prescribed remedies.

INCIDENCE OF LARYNGEAL CANCER

Anyone is susceptible to the development of laryngeal cancer. The incidence of cancer increases markedly after age 50 (Rice & Spiro, 1989), although experience has shown that cancer of the larynx can occur from childhood through adulthood. Our clinics are seeing younger individuals in their 30s and 40s who have been diagnosed with laryngeal cancer. The American Cancer Society (1994) reported an estimated 12,500 new cases of laryngeal cancer (9,800 for males and 2,700 for females) in the United States. The estimated total number of deaths from laryngeal cancer in 1994 is given as 3,800.

The primary carcinogens appear to be inhaled cigarette, pipe, and cigar smoke (Levin, Devesa, Godwin, & Silverman, 1974) as well as heavy alcohol consumption and previous radiation therapy treatments. These agents have been consistently implicated as being carcinogenic, but laryngeal cancer may certainly develop in their absence.

MEDICAL EVALUATION

An indirect mirror laryngoscopy performed by an otolaryngologist is the first step in evaluating the presence of laryngeal cancer. If a malignant lesion is suspected based on this examination and the history the patient reports, then direct laryngoscopy is performed to take a biopsy of the lesion. A biopsy involves excising a small sample of tissue under suspicion and evaluating it microscopically to determine the cell type (squamous cell is the most common occurring type in the larynx). The otolaryngologist will also note the location and the extent of the lesion. The larynx and vocal folds may be viewed using indirect laryngoscopy, fiberoptic endoscopy, and stroboscopy. Laryngeal X rays utilizing a contrast dye to make the extent of the lesion visible are also taken. All microscopic, visual, and X-ray information is analyzed and the appropriate treatment is planned. Treatment may include radiation therapy, chemotherapy, surgery, or combination of these treatments.

RADIATION THERAPY

When a lesion is found isolated to a specific location, the treatment of choice may include conservative radiation therapy or a combination of treatments including chemotherapy and radiation. Radiation therapy usually involves 25 to 30 treatments of 6,000 cGy administered over a 6- to 7-week period. The extent of the lesion is identified topographically and mapped with dye on the skin surface of the patient's neck. The malignant cells as well as some of the surrounding normal tissue are irradiated and slowly destroyed during the treatments.

When surgery is required to excise a malignant lesion, the surgeon may choose to "shrink" the lesion with radiation therapy prior to surgery. Some surgeons prefer to withhold radiation therapy until after surgery. Radiation of the postsurgical region may eliminate the presence of any remaining cancer cells. The healing process following surgery appears to progress more rapidly when the patient has not undergone radiation therapy before surgery.

Most patients experience various side effects as a result of radiation therapy. These may include difficulty swallowing, diminished taste, skin irritation, tissue swelling, tissue hardening, decreased salivary flow, and nausea. These side effects may progressively worsen as the treatments progress and gradually subside when they are completed.

STAGING AND TNM CLASSIFICATION

Laryngeal cancer is classified using the TNM system. The clinical staging of cancer was developed with the underlying premise that cancers of similar histology or site of origin share similar patterns of growth and metastasis. The TNM staging is a clinical decision made by the physician after a physical examination and may be augmented by additional information obtained from radiographic and endoscopic examinations, surgical exploration and biopsy (American Joint Committee on Cancer, 1992; see Table 10–1). In describing the anatomic extent of the

Table 10–1.   The TNM classification system

Primary Tumor (T)

TX Primary tumor cannot be assessed
TO No evidence of primary tumor
Tis Carcinoma *in situ*

Supraglottis

T1 Tumor limited to one subsite of the supraglottis with normal vocal cord mobility
T2 Tumor invades more than one subsite of the supraglottis or glottis, with normal vocal cord mobility
T3 Tumor limited to the larynx with vocal cord fixation and/or invades the post cricoid area, medial wall of the pyriform sinus, or pre-epiglottic tissues
T4 Tumor invades through the thyroid cartilage and/or extends to other tissues beyond the larynx (e.g. to the oropharynx or soft tissues of the neck)

Glottis

T1 Tumor limited to the vocal cord(s) (may involve anterior or posterior commissures) with normal mobility
    T1a Tumor limited to one vocal cord
    T1b Tumor involves both vocal cords
T2 Tumor extends to the supraglottis and/or subglottis, and/or with impaired vocal cord mobility
T3 Tumor limited to the larynx with vocal cord fixation
T4 Tumor invades through the thyroid cartilage and/or extends to other tissues beyond the larynx (e.g., to the oropharynx or soft tissues of the neck)

Subglottis

T1 Tumor limited to the subglottis
T2 Tumor extends to the vocal cord(s) with normal or impaired mobility
T3 Tumor limited to the larynx with vocal cord fixation
T4 Tumor invades through the cricoid or thyroid cartilage and/or extends to other tissues beyond the larynx (e.g., to the oropharynx or soft tissues of the neck)

Regional Lymph Nodes (N)

NX Regional lymph nodes cannot be assessed
NO No regional lymph node metastasis
N1 Metastasis in single ipsilateral lymph node, 3 cm or less in greatest dimension
N2 Metastasis in a single ipsilateral lymph node, more than 3 cm but not more than 6 cm in greatest dimension; or in multiple ipsilateral lymph nodes, none more than 6 cm in greatest dimension; or in bilateral or contralateral lymph nodes, none more than 6 cm in greatest dimension
    N2a Metastasis in a single ipsilateral lymph node more than 3 cm but not more than 6 cm in greatest dimension
    N2b Metastasis in multiple ipsilateral lymph nodes, none more than 6 cm in greatest dimension
    N2c Metastasis in bilateral or contralateral lymph nodes, none more than 6 cm in greatest dimension
N3 Metastasis in a lymph node more than 6 cm in greatest dimension

(continued)

Table 10–1. *(Continued)*

Distant Metastasis (M)
MX Presence of distant metastasis cannot be assessed
MO No distant metastasis
M1 Distant metastasis

Stage Grouping

Stage O	Tis	NO	MO
Stage I	T1	NO	MO
Stage II	T2	NO	MO
Stage III	T3	NO	MO
	T1	N1	MO
	T2	N1	MO
	T3	N1	MO
Stage IV	T4	NO	MO
	T4	N1	MO
	Any T	N2	MO
	Any T	N3	MO
	Any T	Any N	M1

lesion, the "T" refers to the primary tumor size and extent, the "N" identifies the absence or presence and extent of the regional lymph node metastasis, and the "M" refers to the absence or presence of distant metastasis. The numbers assigned to the TNM classification system refer to the extent of the tumor. A patient with a clinical classification of T4 N1 MO has a large tumor with metastasis to the lymph nodes but no distant spread of the disease. This clinical classification system assists the physician in planning treatment, serves as a prognostic indicator, facilitates communication among treatment centers, and serves as a baseline to compare the results of treatment

TOTAL LARYNGECTOMY

Total laryngectomy involves the surgical excision of the entire cartilaginous larynx including the epiglottis, its inferior and superior muscular and membranous attachments, the hyoid bone, the extrinsic strap muscles, and may include the upper two to three tracheal rings. If the cancer cells have metastasized to the cervical lymph nodes, surgery will include a radical neck dissection and may be performed on the right, left, or both sides of the neck. A radical neck dissection involves excision of the lymph nodes, associated veins, the accessory nerve, and other involved neck muscles.

The biological function of the larynx serves as a valve to protect the trachea and lungs from aspiration of swallowed liquids and solids (Figure 10–1). After excision of the larynx, the original pulmonary airway cannot be maintained. Thus, the trachea is redirected and sutured to the external neck area just above the notch of the sternum. This opening in the neck is called a stoma. The stoma serves as the point of air exchange with the atmosphere. There no longer remains a connection between the trachea and the pharynx, nose, and mouth (Figure 10–2).

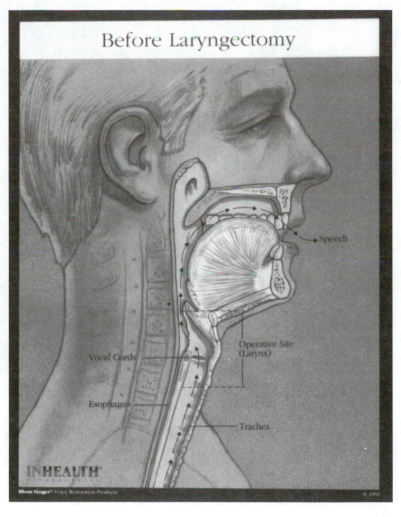

Figure 10–1. Larynx before laryngectomy. (Photo courtesy of InHealth Technologies.)

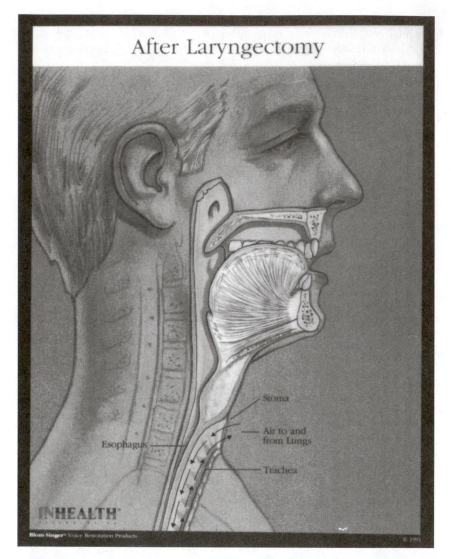

Figure 10–2. After laryngectomy. (Photo courtesy of InHealth Technologies.)

The esophagus remains intact during the total laryngectomy. Because of the previous attachment of the larynx and the pharynx, the anterior pharyngeal walls must be joined and sutured together with the hypopharynx and then sutured to the upper esophagus. When the pharynx is sutured to the base of the tongue, the oral-pharyngeal-esophageal track is completed. The passage of liquids and foods remains the same as before surgery.

REHABILITATION TEAM

Rehabilitation of the total laryngectomized individual involves many different professionals. A multidisciplinary team is essential to serve the medical, psychological, communication, and social needs of the patient and family. Indeed, in most medical settings where a number of total laryngectomies are performed each year, it is possible to form such a team from existing professional personnel. The interaction of the multidisciplinary team approach is ideal for evaluating the total needs of the patient and the family, including preconsultation and preparing the patient for surgery, providing support and educational training through the hospital stay, planning for discharge support, and planning actions to meet future needs. The primary goal of the multidisciplinary team and of the laryngectomee is to return to as normal a life-style as possible. The rehabilitation team includes the following people.

Surgeon. The surgeon serves as the primary patient manager and is responsible for diagnosis of the disease, treatment planning, and the entire medical management of the patient. The surgeon informs the patient of the medical condition and details the implications of the surgery and subsequent medical treatments. The surgeon also makes referrals to other appropriate team members, when necessary.

Speech-Language Pathologist. The speech-language pathologist is directly responsible for evaluating and providing for the patient's short-term and long-term communication needs. This involves both preoperative and postoperative consultations. Initial preoperative counseling with the patient as well as family and or friends is usually an informational-educational session discussing issues about the changes in speech and the alternate forms of communication. Postoperatively the patient is seen by the speech-language pathologist to address communication, swallowing issues, and voice restoration. (A complete description of the speech-language pathologist's role follows in the section "The Role of Speech Pathology.")

Oncology Nurse. This person is an essential member of the multidisciplinary team in the rehabilitation of the laryngectomized patient. Beyond the day-to-day care and moral support provided by the nurse, the nurse is responsible for teaching the patient and the family the skills necessary for independent stoma care. Breathing, coughing, and sneezing through the stoma are new and often uncomfortable experiences for the patient. Stoma hygiene is important and the tasks of caring for the respiratory system must be learned prior to hospital discharge.

Dietitian. Patients respond better to surgery and heal more rapidly when they are in good nutritional health. The dietitian is responsible for evaluating the nutritional needs of each patient. Because of the social habits of some patients and the presurgical swallowing problems experienced by others, many patients who undergo a total laryngectomy do not maintain adequate nutritional health. When possible, surgery is not scheduled until the patient's nutritional level can be improved. This improvement may involve supplementing food intake with high-nutrients which may be taken orally or in an intravenous solution. Following surgery, the dietitian monitors caloric intake and determines the nutritional requirements necessary for the patient to gain and maintain the appropriate weight. The patient and family are also advised of the proper eating habits necessary upon discharge. If the patient receives radiation, the dietitian also monitors the patient's weight and nutritional intake.

Radiologist. The radiologist interprets the results of the chest X ray, computerized tomography (CT), or magnetic resonance imaging (MRI) tests and aids the surgeon in planning the most appropriate treatment approach. The radiologist plans and conducts the radiation therapy program. Irradiation treatments may occur preoperatively or postoperatively depending on the size and extent of the tumor.

Social Worker. The medical social worker is involved in many aspects of patient and family support. This involvement may include family counseling, assistance with financial arrangements especially with insurance coverage for pre- or post-surgical needs, discharge planning to ensure patient care, arranging for special needs after discharge such as a suction machine or providing information about nutritional supplement, and arranging transportation for outpatient medical and therapy appointments.

Physical Therapist. Patients who undergo total laryngectomy along with radical neck dissection may require the services of a physical therapist. Surgical trauma and excision of neck and shoulder muscles and the accessory nerve will often limit the patient's ability to move the arm, shoulder, and neck of the dissected side freely. The physical therapist designs and implements therapy programs based upon the physical disabilities created by the surgery.

Psychologist. The psychologist provides extended patient and family counseling as needed. The laryngectomized patient is required to make many emotional and social adjustments. The psychologist may help the patient to deal with such issues as potential death, serious illness, disfigurement, anger, postoperative depression, changing family roles, self-image, and sexuality.

Audiologist. Hearing acuity and presbycusis may need to be addressed in this population. Hearing sensitivity may change following a laryngectomy (Campinelli, 1964). It is also possible that normal eustachian tube function may be impaired by the surgery or subsequent radiation therapy, or both, causing middle ear dysfunction. The audiologist is responsible for evaluating the auditory condition of the laryngectomized patient and recommending amplification when appropriate.

Hearing loss may impede the patient's speech monitoring during the rehabilitation process (Diedrich & Youngstrom, 1966; LaBorwit, 1980).

In addition to testing the patient, audiological evaluation of the spouse or companion is strongly recommended (Clark & Stemple, 1982). Successful rehabilitation may be hindered if the spouse is not able to hear the patient's speech efforts adequately.

The Laryngectomized Visitor. An important team member is the nonprofessional who has experienced the patient's situation and has adjusted to it well. The laryngectomized visitor who has learned to speak well may lift the patient's spirits and provide the motivation for success-ful recovery and rehabilitation. It is also recommended that the visitor's spouse meet with the patient's spouse. Spouse-to-spouse support is often just as valuable as patient-to-patient support.

SPECIAL CONCERNS OF THE LARYNGECTOMIZED PATIENT

The ultimate goal of a total laryngectomy is to "cure" the patient of cancer through surgical excision of the malignancy. Because of the ability to isolate and excise the cancer through laryngeal excision, cancer of the larynx is one of the most curable forms of cancer when the disease is identified early. The results of the surgery leave the patient with the major problem of reestablishing oral communication. There are several other physical, psychological, and social concerns with which the patient must also deal. If the patient is to live a quality life, the ability to make the appropriate adjustments are just as important as re-establishing speech. Let us consider some of these concerns.

Communication

Only one part of oral communication is missing following a total laryn-gectomy: a sound generator. The patient's language and cognitive abilities and ability to articulate remain intact. Although implications of the loss of voice have been explained well to the patient, the impact is often not fully realized until the patient awakens from the anesthesia and automatically tries to speak. The realization is even more dramatic later when the patient attempts to express his or her feelings and needs and is hindered by cum-bersome writing or unintelligible whispering. Many of us take our ability to speak for granted. Speaking is such an automatic act once it is learned in childhood. If the ability is withdrawn or impaired, we quickly realize the intimate relationships we have with this mode of communication.

The laryngectomized patient is soon confronted with communica-tion deprivation. There is a distinct difference in communicating to make one's needs known (such as, hungry, thirsty, yes, no, bathroom) and communicating thoughts, feelings, and actions. The initial forms of communication for the laryngectomized patient are usually writing and mouthing words. Writing is slow and laborious for both the patient and the reader, and, of course, not all patients can write. Mouthing words is effective only if the patient's articulation is excellent and if the listener has the ability to understand speech without sound. Often patients have many thoughts that they would like to express, but because of the effort to communicate do not try. If this situation were allowed to continue, the patient would soon become isolated.

It is, therefore, in the patient's best interest to reestablish some form of oral communication as soon as possible. This goal may be accomplished soon after surgery, even while the patient is an inpatient, with the use of an artificial larynx. If edema prevents neck placement of an artificial larynx, then intra-oral larynges may be used. We do not agree with the argument that with early use of an artificial larynx the patient will develop a dependency on the device and will therefore not be as likely to develop other forms of alaryngeal speech. Withholding an available means of communication is more likely to disrupt the rehabilitation process.

The early days following surgery are usually quite traumatic for the patient and the family. Providing an effective means of communication will ease this trauma. Other forms of communication will be explored as soon as the patient is physically healed and released by the physician.

Physical Concerns

Respiration

Another concern of the laryngectomized patient is adjustment to breathing through the stoma. Prior to surgery, normal respiratory exchange had the advantages of the nose. The nose is essentially an air treatment center. Before reaching the lungs, the air is filtered by the hairs in the nose, humidified by the mucous membrane of the nose and pharynx, and warmed along the entire upper respiratory tract. The laryngectomized patient no longer has advantages of a natural filtering, moistening, and warming air treatment system. Without a substitute, untreated air is inhaled directly into the trachea and lungs. The laryngectomee is subjected to the atmospheric conditions whether the air is dry or humidified. Dry air causes increased mucous buildup with thicker secretions and decrease ciliary function.

The Blom-Singer Humidifilter System (Figure 10–3) is a stoma air filtering system designed to be worn directly over the stoma. Air is exchanged through a foam filter. Inhaled air is therefore filtered by specially treated foam material, humidified by the natural moisture in the material created by the condensation from the exhalations, and warmed

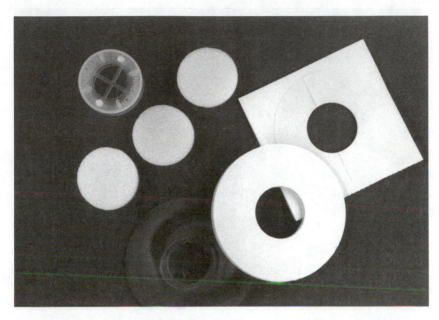

Figure 10–3. Blom-Singer Humidifilter. (Photo by Rick Berkey, St. Elizabeth Medical Center, Dayton, Ohio.)

by the warmth of the material. This warm, filtered, moist, air exchange reduces the amount of mucus and the likelihood for mucous encrustations to build up in the bronchial pathways and decreases coughing.

Stoma covers (Figure 10–4) are also designed to be worn directly over the stoma. A stoma cover is made of porous material, either cloth or foam. Stoma covers provide a protective function as well as improve the cosmetic appearance of the neck. The exchange of air through the material of the stoma cover aids to warm and add moisture when breathing. Stoma covers protect the airway by filtering out dust, fumes, insects, and other foreign matter. The laryngectomized patient should also consider wearing stoma covers for cosmetic reasons. The general population is likely to be more comfortable around laryngectomized patients when not required to view the stoma. This may be considered part of the patient's social adjustment and acceptance by others.

Covering the stoma is especially beneficial in cold weather and when the air is very dry. Use of a room humidifier is recommended following surgery, to lessen irritation of the lining of the trachea through drying (Keith, 1991).

Coughing and Sneezing

Breathing is only one of the respiratory functions of the stoma. Laryngectomized patients also cough and sneeze through the stoma.

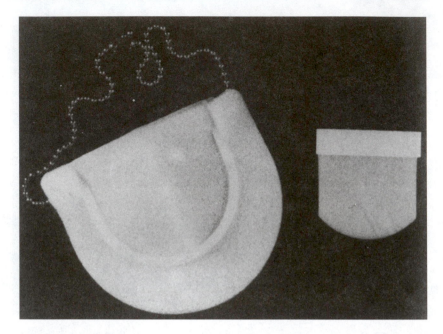

Figure 10–4.   Stoma covers.

These patients need to learn to cover the stoma instead of the mouth when coughing, otherwise the discharged mucus is expelled into the air or on others.

Another concern is the "running" nose. Posterior drainage and swallowing remain intact. However, because the respiratory connection between the nose and the lungs no longer exists, no mechanism prevents drainage through the nose. The laryngectomized patient must either wipe or use the small amount of intraoral pressure to blow the nose free of mucus. A tissue or handkerchief must be available at all times.

Tracheal Tubes and Tracheostoma Vents

Concerns regarding the stoma also include the use and care of the tracheal tubes and tracheostoma vents (Figure 10–5). At the time of surgery, a tracheal tube may be inserted in the stoma as a means of keeping it open and maintaining the air passage. As the tissue shrinks during the healing process, the tube maintains the integrity of the stoma, preventing a reduction in its size. Generally the patient does not need a tracheal tube; however, if after several days the stoma starts to shrink, the physician may insert a tracheostoma vent to prevent further stenosis of the stoma. Tracheostoma vents are manufactured in various diameter sizes and lengths.

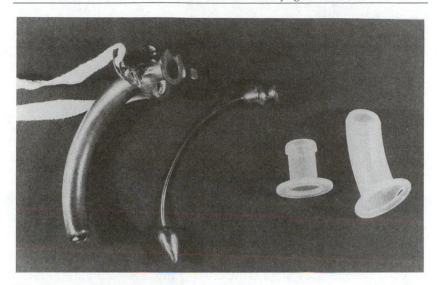

Figure 10–5.   Tracheal tube and stoma vents.

As mentioned previously, it is important for the patient to assume independent care of the stoma which includes cleaning the tracheal tube or vent. Following surgery, most patients secrete and cough thick mucus plugs. These plugs hinder air exchange, making breathing difficult. Care of the stoma and tracheal tube involves removing the inner tube (canula) for washing; removing dried mucus from the stoma with a long handle tweezers; and suctioning accumulated mucous secretions from the trachea with a suction machine (Gardner, 1971). Mild soap and water can be used to clean the tracheostoma vent. Patients are also taught to inhale a small amount of commercially prepared saline solution into the stoma to thin out thick secretions to make it easier to suction or expel. Regular stoma care maintains an open airway and prevents irritating mucous crusts from forming on the skin around the stoma.

As healing progresses, most patients are able to reduce gradually and eventually eliminate the use of a tracheal tube or stoma vent. Some patients are required to wear a tracheostoma vent 24 hours per day to prevent stoma stenosis; others maintain an adequate stoma size by wearing a vent only several hours per day. The tracheostoma vent can be fenestrated to accommodate the voice prosthesis for tracheoesophageal speech.

Swallowing

Generally swallowing is not affected following a total laryngectomy. If a tracheoesophageal puncture was performed as part of the primary procedure, the patient is fed through the catheter that is directed down the esophagus. Usually the patient is permitted by the otolaryngologist to start taking clear liquids orally on the seventh day following surgery. This is assuming normal healing has taken place. Sometimes patients will develop fistulas which will delay oral feeds.

Smell and Taste

Two other related physical changes with which the laryngectomized patient is concerned are changes in smell and taste. Since the patient can no longer inhale air through the nose, the ability to smell is impaired. There is actually no impairment in the olfactory organ itself. The odor is simply not able to reach the organ to be sensed. A patient who happens to be in an area with an intense odor such as fresh paint, gasoline, or smoke, may be aware of the odor as it permeates the nasal cavity. Otherwise, the inability to inhale air through the nose greatly limits this sense.

Diedrich and Youngstrom (1966) reported that 31% of the laryngectomized patients they studied reported a diminished ability to taste. Because taste is greatly influenced by the ability to smell (Pressman & Bailey, 1968), the act of eating may often be reduced to simply a necessary chore. Some patients report that, over time, the taste of food gradually improves. It is possible that this may be attributed to their adjustment to the loss of smell as this sense is related to taste.

Safety

Safety issues related to breathing through the stoma are real concerns of the laryngectomized patient and family. In the event of accident or illness, emergency medical personnel must be alerted that the patient is a neck breather so appropriate medical aid may be administered. This may include mouth-to-stoma resuscitation or administration of oxygen via the stoma. *First Aid For (Neck-Breathers) Laryngectomees* is a helpful pamphlet that provides explicit instructions for resuscitation. It is available from the International Association of Laryngectomees. Patients are strongly advised to wear medical alert bracelets, carry an emergency identification card, and place emergency identification cards on the windshields of their cars and in an obvious location in their homes (Figure 10–6) The laryngectomized patient should also inform the medical emergency personnel who service the area in which they live of the surgical alterations including first aid procedures for neck breathers.

Activities related to water, such as bathing, fishing, and swimming, are important to discuss with the patient. Because even a small amount of water entering the stoma may cause acute respiratory distress, safety around water is of the utmost importance Bathing and showering may, therefore, present special problems for the patient. A special rubber shower collar (Figure 10–7) is available as a safety aid for this purpose.

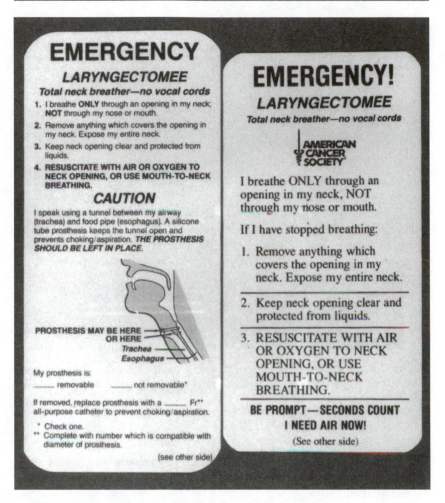

EMERGENCY

LARYNGECTOMEE

Total neck breather—no vocal cords

1. I breathe **ONLY** through an opening in my neck; **NOT** through my nose or mouth.
2. Remove anything which covers the opening in my neck. Expose my entire neck.
3. Keep neck opening clear and protected from liquids.
4. **RESUSCITATE WITH AIR OR OXYGEN TO NECK OPENING, OR USE MOUTH-TO-NECK BREATHING.**

CAUTION

I speak using a tunnel between my airway (trachea) and food pipe (esophagus). A silicone tube prosthesis keeps the tunnel open and prevents choking/aspiration. **THE PROSTHESIS SHOULD BE LEFT IN PLACE.**

PROSTHESIS MAY BE HERE
OR HERE
Trachea
Esophagus

My prosthesis is:
_____ removable   _____ not removable*

If removed, replace prosthesis with a _____ Fr** all-purpose catheter to prevent choking/aspiration.

* Check one.
** Complete with number which is compatible with diameter of prosthesis.

(see other side)

EMERGENCY!

LARYNGECTOMEE

Total neck breather—no vocal cords

AMERICAN CANCER SOCIETY

I breathe ONLY through an opening in my neck, NOT through my nose or mouth.

If I have stopped breathing:

1. Remove anything which covers the opening in my neck. Expose my entire neck.

2. Keep neck opening clear and protected from liquids.

3. RESUSCITATE WITH AIR OR OXYGEN TO NECK OPENING, OR USE MOUTH-TO-NECK BREATHING.

BE PROMPT—SECONDS COUNT
I NEED AIR NOW!

(See other side)

Figure 10–6. Safety cards. (Photo by Rick Berkey, St. Elizabeth Medical Center, Dayton, Ohio.)

The collar fits tightly around the neck to deflect water from entering the stoma. Holes on the underside of the collar permit safe air exchange. This device is recommended for patients who prefer to take showers (Lauder, 1989–1990).

Water sports require their own forms of caution and safety. Those who want to continue swimming as a hobby are advised to seek special training (Keith, 1991). This activity is extremely dangerous for the patient and is not advisable. Fishing from the bank requires caution. The patient should only fish where there is easy access to the water and where the footing is stable. Boating is also potentially dangerous. The laryngec-

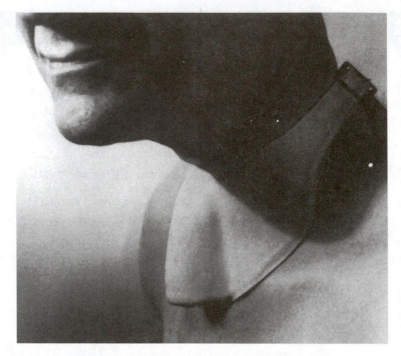

Figure 10-7. Shower collar. (From "Helping Words for the Laryngectomee," International Association of Laryngectomees.)

tomized patient should limit boating activities to stable crafts. A superior quality life vest should be worn, and extreme caution should be maintained at all times.

Lifting

One of the biological functions of the larynx is to allow pulmonary air to be trapped within the lungs when the vocal folds are held in complete adduction making it easier to lift objects. The laryngectomized patient can no longer regulate the larynx to build thoracic air pressure. Theoretically, lifting should be difficult for the laryngectomee. In Diedrich and Youngstrom's 1966 survey of patients, they found that 45% of their patients reported no difficulty lifting, 42% reported some difficulty, and 13% reported great difficulty. The majority of the surveyed patients had not experienced problems with lifting. Laryngectomees who usually have problems have undergone radical neck dissection and experience related neck, shoulder, and arm movement problems.

Psycho-Social Concerns

The laryngectomized patient may have many psychological adjustments to make. In an excellent review of the basic psychological stages of patients, Gardner (1971) described adjustments that were made preoperatively, immediately postoperatively, and upon reentering the familiar environment. These adjustments focused on the patient's reaction to the disease; the physical changes as a result of the surgery; self-concept based on the feeling of adequacy and appearance; and emotional reactions related to the physical and psychological changes.

When told that they have cancer of the larynx, it is not unusual for patients to be more concerned about the disease than about the ramifications of surgery. To many, cancer is synonymous with death (Snidecor, 1968). Upon hearing that they have cancer, patients often do not hear the complete explanation of the disease and its treatment as provided by the physician. Reality must eventually be dealt with and the patient must move forward toward understanding the surgery and its consequences.

The Laryngectomized Speaker's Source Book, published by the International Association of Laryngectomees (IAL), provides an excellent description of the fears and concerns of the patient. (The IAL is an international teaching and support group composed of and operated by laryngectomized people.) It describes fears related to the operation such as taking the anesthetic, fear of pain following surgery, fear of mutilation, and fear of not being able to speak.

The immediate postoperative period may be a time of considerable frustration. Many patients experience acute physical stress; worries about health, families and finances; and uncertainties about the future. The concept of being a "whole" person may also arise. The reaction of some patients is to resign themselves to being cared for by others, to become dependent. Those who make the appropriate adjustments work through these difficulties and maintain their presurgical independence. All of these concerns and frustrations are compounded by the inability to communicate feelings adequately because of limited nonverbal means.

As the patient returns to a normal environment, many family and social issues must be resolved. It is quite possible, especially in the typical age group, that temporary role reversals occur during the hospitalization and rehabilitation period. Husbands may take over the domestic roles of their wives, or wives may play the traditional male roles of the family. When role reversals take place, it is necessary for the family to evaluate relationships and either to maintain new role distributions or return to the previous roles.

Personal and sexual relationships may also be affected by the laryngectomy. Individuals with strong interpersonal relationships and positive self-images will seldom experience personal difficulties or sexual disorientation. Following surgery, however, some patients experience less than adequate self-images and often need psychological counseling to work through these problems.

Finally, laryngectomized patients returning to their previous work settings may experience various levels of success based on their own psychological adjustments and their abilities to communicate adequately.

Blood and Blood (1982) found that the laryngectomized patient who spoke openly and candidly about his or her disability and rehabilitation process was more socially accepted than the patient who was reticent or acted embarrassed about the situation. Therefore, the well-adjusted patient may find more success in attempting to return to the previous work setting. Indeed, many patients, even those who require skilled oral communication such as managers, business people, and salespeople, have successfully returned to their jobs and careers. When patients are not able to meet previous job requirements because of physical or communication deficits, job retraining or employment changes may be required. The various state rehabilitation commissions may be helpful in training patients for new employment opportunities. Some patients choose early retirement following laryngectomy surgery.

Attitudes that people have regarding cancer have become more sophisticated with increased understanding of the disease. However, we have experienced some patients, spouses, family members, and employers who have operated with the belief that "cancer is catching." If present, the serious misconception must be carefully dispelled in order for the rehabilitation program to be successful.

THE ROLE OF SPEECH PATHOLOGY

The speech-language pathologist plays an important role in the rehabilitation of the total laryngectomy patient. It is likely that no other professional of the multidisciplinary team will have as much contact with the patient and the family as will the speech-language pathologist. This contact includes formal preoperative and postoperative consultation sessions as well as informal hospital visits for supportive purposes. The speech-language pathologist evaluates the patient's communication needs and abilities and conducts the most appropriate management approaches.

Preoperative Consultation

After the surgeon has confirmed the diagnosis of laryngeal cancer, has counseled the patient regarding the surgery and its implications, and has scheduled surgery time, a referral is made for a preoperative speech consultation. The preoperative consultation serves as an information session for the patient and the family and introduces them to the speech-language pathologist who is likely to follow the patient throughout the rehabilitation program. The preoperative consultation may be easiest to schedule when the patient comes in for his or her preadmission workup.

All preoperative consultations should begin with the question "What has your doctor told you about your condition?" The answer will let you know the patient's emotional state and whether the surgeon's information has been understood. If the patient is vague about his or her condition or denies knowledge of the surgery and its consequences, it is best to take the patient's history of the symptoms and refer the patient back to the physician for further consultation. It is important to contact the physician to inform him of your meeting with the patient and provide reasons the patient is referred back. It is not the speech-language pathologist's role to inform patients of their medical condition and the implications of surgery.

Most patients have comprehended the surgeon's information and are able to tell you about the presence of laryngeal cancer and the subsequent surgery. The speech-language pathologist may then review and reinforce the surgeon's basic information about the surgery. In further preparing the patient and the family for surgery, it is helpful to provide them with a copy of *Looking Forward: A Guidebook for the Laryngectomee* (Keith, 1991). This manual briefly describes the surgical procedure, the immediate postsurgical hospital stay (including the presence of IVs, nasogastric tube, tracheal tube, drain tubes, and sutures) and a description of the typical rehabilitation process. The more information that the patient and family are able to comprehend prior to surgery, the less apprehension they will experience after surgery and the quicker the rehabilitation can begin. Patients and their families vary in their abilities to grasp and understand presurgical information.

The preoperative consultation time is used to assure patients that they will learn to talk again following surgery. The speech-language pathologist should describe the three methods of alaryngeal speech. Simplified explanations of these methods can be accomplished with the use of visual aids such as the *Post-Laryngectomy Training Aid* from InHealth Technologies.

The preoperative consultation is also used to plan for the patient's immediate postsurgical means of communication. Most patients write or gesture. A "magic slate," which should always be at arm's length to the patient, may be utilized for initial communication. Some patients may prefer to use paper and pencil. Patients who cannot write may be taught to use small hand-held communication boards. The board is personalized with family names and individual needs of patients. An intra-oral artificial larynx may also be introduced presurgically.

Finally, the preoperative consultation is a time to listen. It is the time to give the patient and the family the opportunity to ask questions and to verbalize thoughts and feelings about the surgery. It is also the time for the speech-language pathologist to determine whether the patient is mentally and emotionally ready for all that lies ahead.

Postoperative Consultation

The postoperative consultation is a time to begin moving the patient forward toward total rehabilitation. The speech-language pathologist will first make sure that the planned postsurgical method of communication is available and being used as effectively as possible. For example, patients often write long involved notes using complete sentences when two or three words might be adequate to get the point across. In this case, explaining the use of telegraphic writing may prove helpful.

A more complete explanation of the three types of alaryngeal speech typically used following a laryngectomy may be appropriate at this time. The patient is usually ready to understand this information and is eager to begin. A visit from a previously laryngectomized person is also recommended. The visitor will share personal experiences with the patient and will offer reassurance that things will get better. This visitor reassures the fact that the patient will learn to talk again.

During the postoperative consultation, the speech-language pathologist also evaluates the need for the patient to have immediate oral communication. This need may be based on the patient's inability to write, frustration level, family support on discharge, or simply an excellent adjustment to the surgery and the desire to get on with oral speech. When this need is present, attempts are made to use an artificial larynx. Often, because of edema, neck larynges cannot be used on the neck, but cheek placement will often direct the sound very well into the mouth. Intra-oral artificial larynges may also be used.

Plans are also made for outpatient speech rehabilitation during the postoperative consultation. Details involving finances and transportation are arranged so that there is no loss in continuity from the inpatient program to the patient's outpatient program.

Finally, the patient's physical and psychological recoveries are noted, and the patient and family are provided with more encouragement and support. It may also be helpful to meet with the spouse or family alone to determine if they are prepared for the patient's discharge. Some patients handle the whole surgical ordeal better than their family members. Preparation and encouragement for the family is an important part of the rehabilitation program.

The Speech Evaluation

When there are no postsurgical complications, the patient will be ready to begin outpatient speech restoration within 4 to 6 weeks after surgery. The speech-language pathologist will attempt to accomplish several things in the initial evaluation session.

The first goal is to review the patient's knowledge of the surgery and to clarify any misconceptions. All questions the patient or family members may have should be answered at this time. The speech-language pathologist will find that some patients remember very little of their hospital experience.

The second step of the evaluation involves teaching the patient the differences between the presurgical anatomy and the postsurgical anatomy. Diagrams are used to explain the new respiratory route and to demonstrate that the "food pipe" has not changed. The major anatomical point that the patient must understand is that there is now no connection between the areas of the mouth and nose and those of the windpipe and lungs. If the patient underwent a tracheoesophageal puncture, then an explanation of the lumen that connects the esophagus and trachea should be given. Understanding the anatomy will make it easier for the patient to comprehend the various methods of speech rehabilitation to be discussed.

When the patient understands the anatomical changes, much of the information contained in the section of this chapter entitled "Special Concerns of the Laryngectomized Patient" should be reviewed. This information includes air filter changes, coughing, taste and smell concerns, and safety considerations. Information regarding these matters is invaluable to the patient in making the appropriate adjustments.

The speech evaluation is the final goal of the evaluation process. All three methods of speech communication following a total laryngectomy are explained. These include the use of various types of artificial larynges, the development of esophageal voice, and the use of surgical prostheses. If the patient is using an artificial larynx, the speech-language pathologist evaluates the success of using the device to communicate. Suggestions are made to increase speech intelligibility.

The patient who has undergone a tracheoesophageal puncture may be ready for the voice prosthesis sizing and fitting. Most patients are quite eager to have the catheter removed and look forward to this session. A complete description of the tracheoesophageal method of speaking is provided for the patient and family. The procedures for the voice prosthesis sizing and fitting are described in the "Speech Rehabilitation" section of this chapter.

Advantages and Disadvantages of Alaryngeal Speech Methods

Artificial Larynx

All three forms of communication have both inherent advantages and disadvantages. The artificial larynx provides immediate communication for the patient. These devices can be demonstrated to the patient and family preoperatively and used shortly following surgery with little effort to communicate (Casper & Colton, 1993).

There are numerous manufacturers of artificial larynges. The artificial larynx is the most available and easiest means of communication to learn for the laryngectomized patient. Some of the devices offer a limited ability to vary the pitch and volume of the speech. The artificial larynx is equal in intelligibility to esophageal speech (Kalb & Carpenter, 1981) and is more easily discriminated in noise than is esophageal speech (Clark & Stemple, 1982). An oral connector can be purchased to fit over the head of many of the neck-type artificial larynges thus creating an intraoral device. Casper and Colton (1993) indicate the intraoral device as an effective instrument to use immediately after surgery regardless of which type of alaryngeal speech the patient will end up predominantly using. Artificial larynges provide immediate communication and serve as an adjunct form of communication while the patient is learning esophageal speech or waiting to be fitted for a voice prosthesis. The relative expense of purchasing and learning to use an artificial larynx is favorable compared to other methods.

Disadvantages associated with the use of an artificial larynx as a primary means of communication include a dislike for the mechanical sound. Although patients can be taught to speak utilizing appropriate phrasing, pauses, pseudoinflections, and facial expressions to eliminate a "robot-like" sound, the mechanical quality is a reality.

Another disadvantage is that it requires the use of one hand for operational use. This limitation is a problem primarily for those who work with their hands and need or want to talk simultaneously. This is also a problem when patients talk on the telephone and need to write at the same time. It would be advantageous to the patient to use a telephone with a speakerphone in this case.

Being mechanical, the artificial larynx has the potential of failure through mechanical breakdown or battery failure, leaving the patient without speech. Immediate service and repair is not always accessible.

Finally, even though some of the artificial larynges have frequency control buttons to alter pitch, using this feature is ackward and requires intensive practice to add infection and intonation to the patient's speech. Lerman (1991) reported that elderly patients have greater difficulty with the pitch manipulation buttons.

Esophageal Speech

The major advantage of esophageal speech is that it does not require the use of any mechanical or prosthetic devices for its production. Both hands are free while talking and there are no mechanical devices that could break down and need replaced or repaired. It is a voice produced by the patient with his or her own remaining anatomical structures. The voice is viewed as the patient's "own" voice, which provides a great sense of independence. Esophageal voice is produced in a more natural manner than artificial laryngeal speech, as the vibration of the upper esophagus more closely approximates the sound of laryngeal vibration even through the fundamental frequency is usually lower. Good esophageal speakers may be complimented when a stranger asks, "Do you have a cold?"

The major disadvantage of developing esophageal speech as a primary means of communication is in the time that is required for its development. Four to six months is not an unreasonable amount of time to expect that it will take the patient to learn this method of speaking. Learning esophageal speech is often a long and arduous task requiring much patience and dedication on the part of the patient. Although the majority of laryngectomized patients can be taught to produce esophageal sounds, only about 30% of the total laryngectomy patients are able to develop and use esophageal voice as their primary means of communication (Gates, Ryan, Cooper, et al., 1982).

Surgical Prosthetics

The major advantage of this form of communication is the use of pulmonary air as the driving force for the esophageal pseudoglottis. Since lung air was used to vibrate the vocal folds prior to surgery, this method provides a more natural speech-breathing action for the patient. Because more air pressure is available to drive the pseudoglottis, the acoustic characteristics of voice, including intensity, frequency, and rate, more closely approximate the same measures for laryngeal speakers than does esophageal speech (Robbins, Dudley, Blom, Singer, Fisher, & Logemann, 1980). In other words, the use of pulmonary air enables production of a superior pharyngeal-esophageal voice.

Another advantage of the use of surgical prosthetics is that it requires a shorter training period, which has the secondary practical advantage of making this method cost effective. The average amount of time the speech-language pathologist spends with a prosthesis patient is 10 hours, ranging from 15- to 30-minute sessions. This time includes evaluating patient suitability for the prosthesis, fitting the prosthesis, and training the patient in its care and use.

One of the greatest advantages of surgical prosthetics is the high success rate it yields in providing patients with speech. Complications experienced by those who are not successful include esophageal spasms, failure of the fistula to heal due to diabetes, and patient unreliability to care for the prosthesis due to chronic alcoholism.

A disadvantage associated with the use of surgical prosthetics is the necessity of a second surgical procedure if the surgery is not done as part of the primary procedure. Although the surgery is relatively simple, many patients fear surgery and may choose to forego another hospitalization.

Another disadvantage may be required fitting and care of the prosthetic device. This disadvantage depends on the patient and how the patient feels about having to perform these tasks. When done as a part of the regular stoma care, most patients do not find care of the prosthesis to be a chore. Sometimes poor manual dexterity and visual acuity interfere with prosthetic care. A significant other may be trained to accept the responsibility of stoma and prosthesis care.

Candida colonization on the voice prosthesis is a problem for some individuals. This requires frequent cleaning to prolong the device's lifetime.

The final disadvantage is the required use of the hand to occlude the stoma when producing voice. The tracheostoma valve (Singer & Blom, 1980) has eliminated this need for many. However, patients with sunken stomas or very uneven tissue around their stomas may not be able to use this device. Some individuals are not able to wear the valve because of skin breakdown secondary to the adhesive required to affix the housing around the stoma.

Once the advantages and disadvantages of each method of communication have been discussed, the patient is encouraged to think about each and to discuss them with his or her family. Even before the final decision is made, the speech-language pathologist may choose to proceed on two fronts. First, it is recommended that all patients learn to use an artificial larynx. No matter what form of communication is ultimately used, an artificial larynx provides the patient with immediate communication. If the patient chooses this method as the primary means of communication, no time has been wasted. If not, the artificial larynx is always available as a backup means of speaking.

Let us now discuss in detail specific management approaches for the development of each method of alaryngeal speech.

SPEECH REHABILITATION

The ultimate goal of the speech rehabilitation program following total laryngectomy is to achieve the most effective speech possible, that is, speech that reflects the speaker in terms of age, sex, and dialect. As we have discussed, there are three options available to the laryngectomized patient: an artificial larynx, esophageal speech, and surgical prosthetics. No categorical statements concerning the "best" approach can be made. Each option must be weighed and evaluated against each patient's own set of circumstances. The deciding factor is based on which method is the most effective for the individual patient.

Artificial Larynges

Keith and Shanks (1986) provided an excellent historical review of artificial larynges. There are two major types of artificial larynges, pneumatic and electronic. The pneumatic larynx (Figure 10–8) utilizes pul-

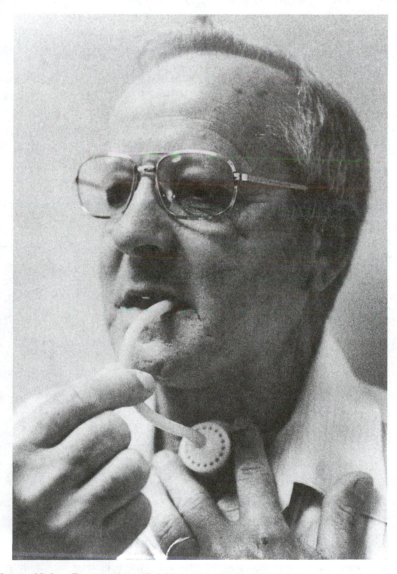

Figure 10-8.   Pneumatic artificial larynx.

monary air as its power source. A cuff that contains a reed or a membrane fits over the stoma. As the patient expels air for speech, the vibration from the membrane is transmitted by a flexible rubber or plastic tube into the patient's mouth. The patient articulates as the sound is produced. Loudness variations occur as the air pressure levels change during breathing for speech. Sound quality from the pneumatic larynges may be more pleasing than the electromechanical devices. There is no electronic noise or buzzing sound with the pneumatic device. The major disadvantage of the pneumatic instruments is the presence of the tube in the mouth that may interfere with articulation and collect saliva. The cuff, as well, may become clogged with mucus. It does require the use of one hand for placement of the cuff over the stoma.

There are two types of electronic artificial larynges, intra-oral devices (Figure 10–9) and neck-type devices (Figure 10-a-b). Electronic larynges are essentially battery-powered sound generators. There are a number of battery-operated electronic artificial larynges that are commercially available. These devices may differ in size, weight, quality of sound, ability to

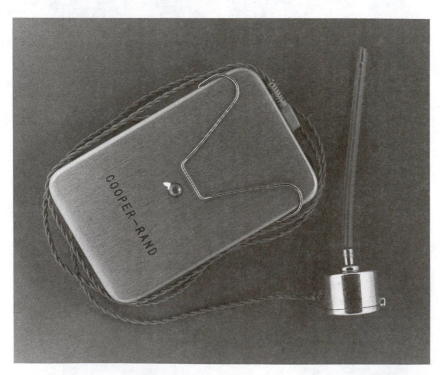

Figure 10-9.   Cooper-Rand intra-oral artificial larynx. (Photo by Rick Berkey, St. Elizabeth Medical Center, Dayton, Ohio.)

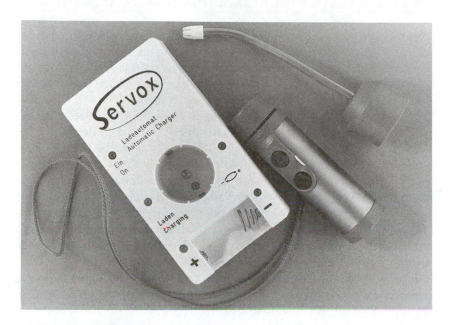

Figure 10–10a. Servox artificial larynges. (Photo by Rick Berkey, St. Elizabeth Medical Center, Dayton, Ohio.)

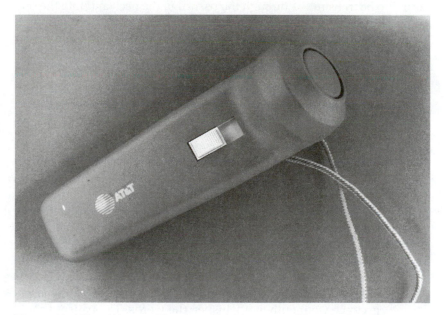

Figure 10–10b. Western Electric artificial larynges. (Photo by Rick Berkey, St. Elizabeth Medical Center, Dayton, Ohio.)

control pitch and volume, appearance, type of batteries needed, and durability. The intra-oral device, such as a Cooper-Rand artificial larynx, generates sound in a small transducer and transmits this sound through a plastic tube and into the patient's mouth. The plastic tube is attached to the tone generator with a small button to activate the device. This type of device is ideal for patients who experience extensive scar tissue or edema of the neck. The patient can also effectively use the intra-oral device immediately following surgery to communicate with the hospital staff and family members even though they may pursue another type of alaryngeal speech. As with the pneumatic larynx, the disadvantage involves the oral tube's interference with articulation and collection of saliva.

The intra-oral artificial larynx does require some instruction. The patient should place the plastic tube approximately one to one and a half inches in the mouth on top of the tongue. The plastic tube can either enter the mouth at midline or from the corner of the mouth with the tube entering at a diagonal. The patient must be taught to coordinate the sound generator when speaking. Practice should incorporate the use of natural pauses and reducing the rate of speech.

The neck-type artificial larynges are the most popular devices. These devices are relatively easy to learn to use providing almost immediate speech restoration. The patient operates the neck-type artificial larynges by placing the head of the device firmly against the neck allowing for the sound to be transmitted through the tissues of the neck and into the oral cavity. The sound from these devices comes from a vibrating diaphragm (Figure 10–11). They currently range in cost and relative quality from around $230 for a Western Electric to about $600 for a Servox artificial larynx. The electronic devices afford variations in volume and pitch through manipulation of switch controls.

Teaching a patient to use an artificial larynx will follow several steps, which may include the following:

1. Following surgery, the laryngectomized patient breathes through the stoma. If air is forced through the stoma, either during inhalation or exhalation, a noise can be heard which is referred to as "stoma noise". This stoma noise can interfere with the patient's intelligibility of speech and become annoying for the listener. Rapid muscular contraction of the thoracic or abdominal muscles may result in increased air turbulence at the level of the stoma. If you ask the patient to whisper or speak with increased loudness, much stoma noise will be produced. To help eliminate or reduce the amount of stoma noise, teach the laryngectomee to mouth, not whisper, the words. The patient should practice reading phrases by just mouthing the words and at the same time monitoring the amount of stoma noise being heard.

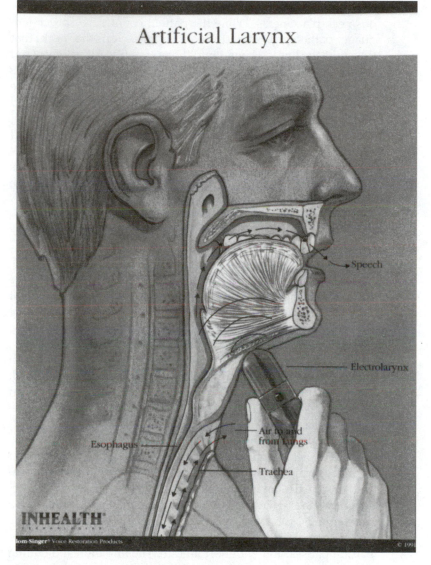

Figure 10–11.   Representaton of speech being produced with a neck-type artificial larynx. (Photo courtesy of InHealth Technologies.)

2. Instruct the patient to slightly overarticulate words without overexaggerating oral movements. Patients who articulate with little oral movement are difficult to understand. Teaching patients to overarticulate slightly will help to open the cavities to improve resonance of the sound.

3. The speech-language pathologist should experiment with various neck placements. While the patient counts, the speech-language pathologist should find the place on the neck that transmits the loudest sound into the oral cavity. All patients (and speech-language pathologists) have a particular site that serves to transmit the sound with the greatest amount of energy into the mouth. The difference in sound between this placement and other placement sites should be demonstrated for the patient. The best placement site is usually under the mandible and slightly off midline of the neck. The vibrating head of the artificial larynx should be directed toward the oral cavity. Sometimes the best placement site is the patient's cheek, especially if the neck tissue is dense or hardened from radiation treatments.

4. Teach the patient to vibrate the artificial larynx against his or her hand. Important for the successful use of the neck device is making sure the vibrating head is completely sealed and making contact with the skin. Training the patient to seal the device on the hand will make it easier when the artificial larynx is used on the neck. Using the device on the hand will also teach the patient how to manipulate the sound generator control. If the head of the artificial larynx is not in full contact with the skin on the neck, noise from the device will interfere with speech intelligibility.

5. Practice neck placement. Permit the patient to experiment with various neck placements until the appropriate one is identified. Allowing the patient to view the placement site in a mirror can be helpful as well as marking the site with a piece of tape. Practice placing and removing the artificial larynx while counting and saying short phrases.

6. Expand quickly into conversational speech. As the patient becomes consistent with placement and appropriate sound generation, practice saying phrases and sentences and then conversational speech. Patients will have a tendency to talk in a monotonous, robot-like speech. Demonstrate and insist on the use of normal phrasing, with appropriate cessation of sound for natural pauses, and with normal rate. The initiation and ending of speech must be coordinated with the activation and deactivation of the sound generator respectively.

7. Teach the patient to remove the artificial larynx from the neck when not speaking. Patients are likely to fall into the habit of leaving the artificial larynx positioned on the neck during conversational speech. The flow of the conversation can be much improved if the patient places the artificial larynx on the neck only when he or she wants to talk. This serves as a natural signal to the other speakers, much as when we take a deep breath prior

to speaking during conversation, that the patient has something to say.

8. Teach the patients to enhance their articulation by instructing them to use the intraoral air for the articulation of voiceless consonants.

The patient who has mastered these steps should be encouraged to discontinue whatever nonoral means of communication were being used. This discontinuation of nonoral speech is usually accomplished with little argument because oral communication is much more flexible and expansive. The patient will continue to improve simply by using the artificial larynx in all speaking situations. As a final means of demonstrating its effectiveness, the speech-language pathologist should consider talking to the patient on the telephone during a therapy session. The 60-80 Hz tone generated by the artificial larynx is carried well over the telephone. Using the artificial larynx on the telephone reopens another avenue of communication for the patient.

Esophageal Speech

An artificial larynx provides the patient with a new, external source of sound vibration. Esophageal voice utilizes the patient's remaining anatomical structures to provide a new, internal source for sound generation. These vibrating structures are the cricopharyngeus muscle of the upper esophagus and the middle and inferior pharyngeal constrictor muscles. When used for sound generation, these structures collectively are termed the pharyngo-esophageal, or PE segment. The PE segment lies approximately at the level of C-5 (Figure 10–12).

To generate sound, this segment needs a power source. Because the patient can no longer inhale air into the nose and mouth, another air source must be used. This source is simply the residual or atmospheric air that is always present in the oral and nasal cavities. With training, patients can be taught to place this ambient air into the upper esophagus, which serves as an air reservoir, and then expel this air vibrating the PE segment and surrounding tissues. When the patient articulates using this sound for voice, esophageal speech is produced. Fluent esophageal speech depends on the rapid intake and release of air from the esophagus.

The first step in developing esophageal speech is learning how to place air into the upper esophagus. The two major methods of air intake: the inhalation and injection (includes glossopharyngeal press and plosive injection) methods are described by a number of individuals (Casper & Colton, 1993; Diedrich & Youngstrom, 1966; Duguay, 1991; Salmon, 1986). These techniques of esophageal speech production are based on how the PE segment opens to allow for air intake and then expels the air during voicing.

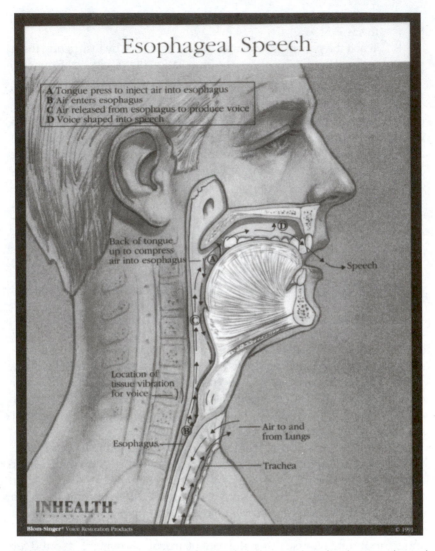

Figure 10–12. Representation of speech being produced using esophageal speech. (Photo courtesy of InHealth Technologies.)

Inhalation

The inhalation method involves creating negative pressure in the thoracic cavity, which helps draw residual air into the esophagus. The esophagus is also in a state of negative pressure and as air is inhaled into the lungs, air also enters the esophagus. Air pressure in these two areas become equalized (Salmon, 1986). This is accomplished when the patient inhales quickly through the stoma. Upon inhalation, the diaphragm drops, enlarging the thoracic cavity, thus creating negative thoracic cavity pressure. Although the inhaled air through the stoma has nothing to do with the PE segment vibration, it does draw the air to be used for this purpose into the esophagus. Instructions to the patient may include the following:

1. Demonstrate the expansion of the thoracic cavity, utilizing a diagram. This demonstration will make the patient aware of how the normal respiratory system works. As the cavity expands, air is drawn into the lungs; as it contracts, the air is expelled.

2. Explain to the patient that as the cavity expands, so, too, does the diameter of the esophagus. As the esophagus expands, the increased area is filled with ambient air. This air can then be expelled to produce vibration of the PE segment.

3. The patient is then asked to close his or her mouth and to take air into the stoma through a quick, sharp inhalation. This inhalation may be enhanced by momentarily covering the stoma with the hand. It may be helpful to have the patient imagine that he or she is sniffing through the nose (Diedrich & Youngstrom, 1966). The patient should then attempt to expel the air by saying "ah." The subsequent decrease in thoracic size will force the air out of the esophagus if esophageal insufflation has occurred. Continue this procedure until sound is produced.

Injection

The injection method of air intake is achieved by compressing the intraoral air into the esophagus with assistance from the tongue or lips and sometimes the cheeks. There are two types of injection. The first type is air injection by tongue pumping which is also referred to as a glossopharyngeal press or a glossal press (Diedrich & Youngstrom, 1966). Instructions to the patient for teaching this method may include the following:

1. Tell the patient to open his or her mouth and "bite off" a piece of air. This action and imagery helps the patient feel the ambient air from one point to another. It also helps to increase the air pressure in the back of the oral cavity.

2. At the end of the "bite" the patient is instructed to close the lips to seal the oral cavity. At the same time, with the tongue tip pushing against the alveolus, the middle section of the tongue should pump the air against both the hard and soft palates. This action will cause the base of the tongue to move backward in a rocking motion, pushing the air into the upper esophagus. In using the glossopharyngeal press, the patient may feel the tongue moving posteriorly and actually making contact with the pharyngeal wall. Once the patient learns this method of air intake the lips

can either be slightly open or closed since the tongue serves to pump the air into the esophagus.

3. The patient should feel and perhaps hear the air as it is forced past the PE segment and into the esophagus. When the air passes the segment, an attempt should be made to expel the air by saying "ah."

The consonant injection method of air intake is the second type of injection. This method uses the natural intra-oral air pressures created by plosive and fricative sounds to inject air into the esophagus. Instructions to the patient for teaching this method may include the following:

1. Ask the patient to produce voiceless consonants such as t, k, p, and sk one at a time in quick succession. The consonants should be made firmly with exaggerated oral movement to encourage airflow into the esophagus. This rapid repetition of the consonants, especially a tongue-tip alveolar stop, fricative or a bilabial, as well as tongue positioning facilitates buildup of air pressure in the esophagus. Production of the consonants forces the air into the esophagus with the result of almost immediate expulsion and sound production. Discourage any stoma noise or sounds made by the tongue and palatal-pharyngeal contact.

2. When the esophageal sound is produced consistently utilizing the consonants, add consonant-vowel combinations to the practice regimen. This will force a lengthening of the esophageal sound.

3. Constantly add new consonant-vowel combinations, expanding the patient's repertoire of sounds on which injection can take place.

4. Finally, attempt to drop the consonant and have the patient inject the air using the tongue for production of the vowel only.

Although the inhalation and injection methods are of primary interest, a swallow method has also been advocated (Morrison, 1981). Using this method, the patient is asked simply to open and close the mouth and to swallow air. The underlying theory of this method is that a normal swallow produces esophageal relaxation of the cricopharyngeus thus allowing air to enter the esophagus. In the swallow method the laryngectomee is encouraged to swallow air and trap the air within the esophagus and immediately expel the air to produce voice. This method of air injection is the least efficient and may be taught as the last resort. One of the problems with this method is that if the swallowed air reaches the stomach, it cannot be readily expelled.

A final word on air injection is to encourage the speech-language pathologist to adopt the method easiest for the patient. Often the most effective approach is a combination of these procedures. Indeed, Isshiki and Snidecor (1965) report that most esophageal speakers actually do use a combination of injection techniques. Perhaps the most simple approach is to ask the patient, "Can you burp on purpose?" You will be surprised how many patients can inject air and burp before the therapy program begins. Therefore, before you go into the long explanation of air injection, just ask!

Once the patient can place air consistently into the upper esophagus, by whatever method, much time should be spent practicing single-syllable words. A solid foundation for conversational esophageal speech must be laid at the single-syllable level. All vowel-consonant and consonant-vowel combinations should be practiced and drilled until the percentage of successful intelligible productions is at least at a 90% level. Lengthening the vowels in the single-syllable productions will prepare the patient to move on to two-syllable words.

From two-syllable words it is possible to start building phrases. Phrase work may continue from two-syllable phrases through eight syllable phrases produced on one air injection. The average length of a conversational phrase is approximately seven syllables.

It is important for the patient to inject the air into the esophagus as smoothly as possible and to expel the air producing voicing with minimal effort. Berlin (1963, 1965) listed four objectives in establishing proficient esophageal speech during the training period. These four objectives may be used by the patient and clinician to quantify progress when learning esophageal speech. The first skill is the ability to phonate reliably on demand. Proficient esophageal speakers are able to produce phonation 100% of the time. The second skill is to maintain a short latency between air injection into the esophagus and phonation. A stopwatch is used to measure the latency period. When the patient signals the clinician that he or she initiated the air injection into the esophagus the clinician starts the stopwatch and then stops the stopwatch when the clinician hears vocalization. Proficient esophageal speakers are able to maintain a short latency, ranging between 0.2 to 0.6 seconds between air injection and phonation. Since the laryngectomee's esophageal air capacity ranges from 40 to 80 cubic centimeters (cc) of air (Van den Berg & Moolenaar-Bijl, 1959), which is much less than the vital capacity of lungs in healthy adults, frequent reinflation of the esophagus must take place while the patient is talking. Thus it is important for the patient to quickly inflate the esophagus and expel the air during conversational speech. The third skill is to maintain an adequate duration of phonation. A stopwatch is also used to record the maximum sustained duration of the vowel /a/ on one air intake. Good esophageal speakers are able to sustain /a/ for 2.4 to 3.6 seconds. The fourth skill is the ability to sustain phonation during articulation. This skill refers to the number of times the syllable /da/ can be repeated on one air intake without consciously reinjecting air into the esophagus. Proficient esophageal speakers are able to phonate 8 to 10 plosive syllables per air intake.

Several factors are monitored and modified throughout the phrase building process. These include stoma noise, air "klunking," eye blinking, and other unnecessary facial expressions. Loudness and inflection manipulations are also practiced throughout the process.

Proficient esophageal speech is a learned process that requires much work and dedication to be mastered. Motivation, desire, and vigor are essential factors that must be present for successful development to occur (Gates, Ryan, Canta, & Hearne, 1982). Patients who do not make a positive commitment or who are unwilling to devote sufficient time to the process are not likely to do well. Other factors that may have a negative influence on the successful development of esophageal voice include post radiation fibrosis, pharyngeal scarring, esophageal stenosis, recurring suture line fistulas, and defects in neural innervation (Aronson 1980). Sloane, Griffin, and O'Dwyer (1991) found that anatomic differences in the reconstructed PE segment had a profound affect in the acquisition of esophageal speech. They used the Blom-Singer esophageal insufflation test combined with videofluoroscopy to assess the PE segment during esophageal speech and found hypotonicity, hypertonicity, PE spasm, and stricture of the reconstructed pharynx to affect the dynamics of esophageal speech.

Surgical Prosthetics

Another option of speech rehabilitation following a total laryngectomy is the use of a surgical prosthesis. The possible reestablishment of voice through laryngeal reconstruction and prosthetic surgery has long been recognized. Reports dating as far back as 1874 detail the results of voicing achieved either through the spontaneous creation of a tracheoesophageal (TE) fistula or through the creation of planned TE shunts (Gussenbauer, 1874; Guttman, 1932; Kolson & Glasgold, 1967). In their excellent article, Blom and Singer (1979), detail the history of the attempts to restore voicing through various laryngeal reconstruction techniques, shunt surgeries, and surgical prostheses (also see Amatsu, Matsui, Maki, & Kanagawa, 1977; Arslan & Serafini, 1972; Asai, 1972; Conley, DeAmesti, & Pierce, 1958; Shedd, Schaaf, & Weinberg, 1976; Singer & Blom, 1980; Staffieri, 1973; Taub, 1975).

The primary goal of all the shunt-type surgeries was to effectively channel pulmonary air into the esophagus where the air could set the pharyngo-esophageal segment into vibration for the production of voice. Although several of these procedures were very successful in meeting this goal, two major problems seemed to persist with these techniques. These problems were aspiration of saliva, liquids, and foods into the trachea through the fistula and breakdown or stenosis of the shunts (Conley et al., 1958).

Singer and Blom (1980) developed the tracheoesophageal puncture (TEP) voice restoration technique to solve these problems. In this 15- to 20-minute surgical procedure, a fistula is created between the trachea and the esophagus in the superior border of the stoma. The tracheoesophageal puncture can be performed as a primary or secondary surgical voice restoration procedure. Following the puncture, a No. 14 French [Fr.] balloon catheter is directed downward through the incision from the trachea and into the esophagus (Hamaker, Singer, Blom, & Daniels, 1985). Approximately 5 cc of water is injected into the catheter balloon to weight it down. The other end of the catheter is capped and secured to the neck with tape. The catheter can serve as a feeding tube following a primary laryngectomy or a myotomy at the time of the tracheoesophageal puncture.

The tracheoesophageal puncture creates a fistula for the insertion of a voice prosthesis. The voice prosthesis, also called a duckbill, is a one-way valve made of high-grade silicone. The Blom-Singer voice prosthesis is radiopaque and will show on an X ray. Once inserted into the tracheoesophageal puncture the voice prosthesis prevents aspiration during swallowing and fistula stenosis. This one-way valve permits pulmonary air to enter the esophagus when the stoma is occluded while the patient exhales. The valve opens under positive pressure as the air enters the esophagus and closes by elastic recoil. It does not permit a reverse flow of saliva or liquids into the trachea. The voice prosthesis is cylindrical in shape with a neck strap(s) that is taped to the skin of the neck to keep it in place. A slit or hinged valve is in the esophageal end, and an anterior opening allows pulmonary air to flow through the voice prosthesis and permits internal cleaning. The prosthesis is securely retained in the fistula by a flexible "retention collar" that holds the prosthesis in place by gripping the inside of the esophageal wall preventing dislodgment (Figure 10–13)

The length of the voice prosthesis ranges in size from 1.4 to 3.6 cm. The most commonly used diameter of voice prostheses is a 16 Fr, however, a 20 Fr. is also available. InHealth Technologies manufactures the duckbill voice prosthesis, low pressure voice prosthesis, and the indwelling low pressure voice prosthesis (Figure 10–14a-c). Bivona Medical Technologies manufactures an economy voice prosthesis, a duckbill voice prosthesis, and an ultra low resistance voice prosthesis (see Figure 10–15a-b)

When a patient is using a voice prosthesis, the stoma may be occluded manually with a thumb or a finger, or it may be occluded by a tracheostoma valve. The tracheostoma valve has component parts. A housing collar is taped and glued around the stoma. A valve is inserted into the housing collar. When the patient produces sufficient pulmonary air pressure to produce speech, the valve will close, thus occluding the stoma and directing the air into the voice prosthesis.

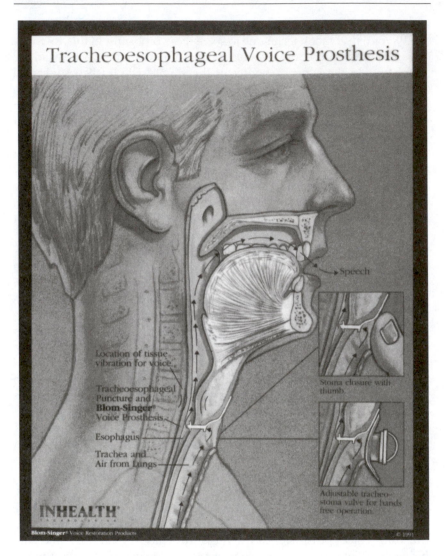

Figure 10–13. Representation of speech being produced using a tracheoesophageal voice prosthesis. (Photo courtesy of InHealth Technologies.)

The success rate for achieving tracheoesophageal speech is quite high, although Donegan, Gluckman, and Singh (1981) and Andrews, Mickel, Hanson, Monahan, and Ward (1987) pointed out the possibility of long-term problems and complications. It has been our experience, however, that if patients are prepared well and properly trained, most total laryngectomy patients can be successful users of this form of communication. Let us examine the speech-language pathologist's role with surgical prosthetics.

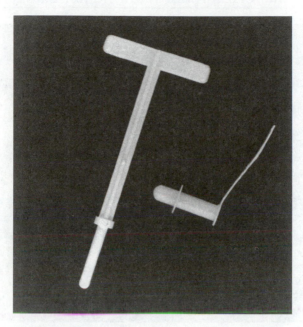

Figure 10–14a. Blom-Singer duckbill voice prosthesis. (Photo by Rick Berkey, St. Elizabeth Medical Center, Dayton, Ohio.)

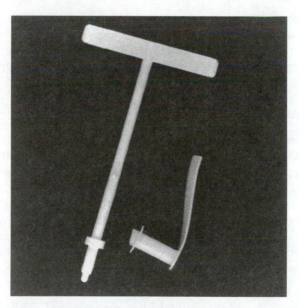

Figure 10–14b. Blom-Singer low pressure voice prosthesis. (Photo by Rick Berkey, St. Elizabeth Medical Center, Dayton, Ohio.)

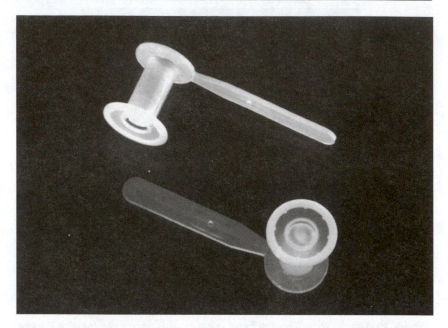

Figure 10–14c.   Blom-Singer InDwelling low pressure voice prosthesis. (Photo courtesy of InHealth Technologies.)

The speech-language pathologist is responsible for (a) aiding the surgeon in evaluating the patient's suitability to use this form of communication; (b) sizing and fitting the prosthesis; (c) teaching the patient to fit and care for the prosthesis; (d) maximizing the patient's ability to communicate while using the prosthesis; and (e) fitting the tracheostoma valve.

Patient Evaluation

Although most laryngectomized patients may be candidates for surgical prosthetics, certain social situations and medical and physical conditions may decrease the chances for long-term successful use.

For example, patient motivation is important. At times, the family may be more motivated than the patient for the patient to attempt this form of communication. In most cases, however, the patient must be capable of and interested in caring for the prosthesis. Andrews et al. (1987) listed a number of characteristics necessary for patient selection. These include the following:

1.   motivation and mental stability,
2.   adequate understanding of the anatomy and the mechanics of the prosthesis,

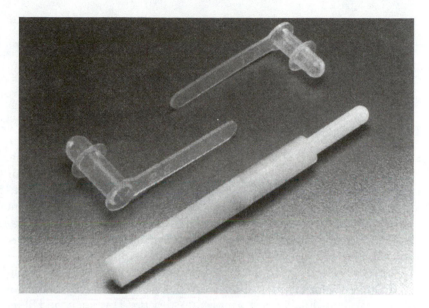

Figure 10–15a. Bivona duckbill voice prosthesis. (Photo courtesy of Bivona Medical Technologies.)

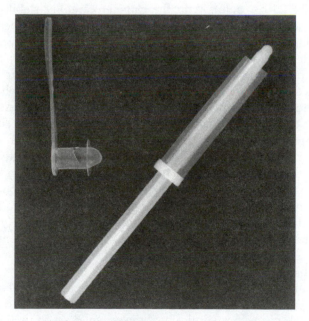

Figure 10–15b. Bivona ultra low™ resistance voice prosthesis. (Photo by Rick Berkey, St. Elizabeth Medical Center, Dayton, Ohio.)

3. adequate manual dexterity and visual acuity to care for the stoma and the prosthesis,
4. no significant hypopharyngeal stenosis,
5. speech production with esophageal insufflation via a properly positioned esophageal catheter,
6. adequate pulmonary reserve, and
7. stoma of adequate depth and diameter to accept the prosthesis without airway compromise

Singer and Blom (1980) reported that chronic pulmonary disease, diabetes, and alcoholism have not presented significant problems. Our experience has not been positive with patients who have chronic drinking problems. Alcohol abuse has also been found to be a major deterrent in the production of efficient voice as well as personal care of the tracheoesophageal puncture (Donegan, Gluckman, & Singh, 1981; Johns & Cantrell, 1981; Schuller, Jarrow, Kelly, & Miglets, 1983).

Cricopharyngeal spasm and pharyngeal constrictor have been implicated as reasons for failure to utilize the voice prosthesis successfully. An esophageal air insufflation test, a procedure described by Singer and Blom (1980), informs the speech-language pathologist, surgeon, or both of the ability of the PE segment to vibrate prior to surgery. In this procedure a 14 Fr. catheter is inserted transnasally into the upper esophagus to approximately the 25 cm point. With the catheter carefully stabilized at this length, the examiner instructs the patient to open and relax the jaw for the production of the vowel /a/. The examiner blows air gently into the esophagus to elicit an esophageal sound. The catheter may need to be slightly pulled forward to produce an oral escape of air or sound. Martinkosky (1991) monitors the pressure changes in the esophagus using a Bird Pressure Manometer. The Blom-Singer insufflation test kit is also available containing a tracheostoma adapter and housing. The housing and adapter are affixed to the stomal area and the 14 Fr. catheter is inserted transnasally to the 25 cm mark. The patient is instructed to inhale, covering the stoma adapter with his or her thumb or finger and self-insufflate the esophagus. The patient should be able to sustain phonation without interruption of the sound for 10 to 15 seconds and produce fluent speech when counting or saying sentences. If the patient's sound production is strained or experiences esophageal spasms, the patient may be a candidate for a pharyngeal myotomy or a pharyngeal plexus neurectomy (Singer, Blom, & Hamaker, 1986) at the time of the TEP.

The air insufflation test is valuable for successful patient selection. It may well indicate in advance those patients who are likely to experience esophageal spasms postsurgically. If the spasm does occur, the patient is prepared for this possibility. If not, we can all be happily surprised and pleased with the results.

Patient Fitting

To prevent the risk of disease transmission from blood-borne pathogens, the speech-language pathologist must follow Universal Precautions when fitting a voice prosthesis. These precautions can be reviewed in the "Centers for Disease Control Morbidity and Mortality Weekly Report" (1988) or in ASHA's "Aids/HIV Update" (1990). The American Speech-Language-Hearing Association also publishes guidelines for "Evaluation and Treatment for Tracheoesophageal Fistulization/Puncture" (1992).

When the tracheoesophageal puncture is surgically created, the surgeon will place a size 14 Fr balloon catheter through the puncture and direct it into the distal esophagus. If the tracheoesophageal puncture is created as a secondary procedure, prosthesis sizing and fitting may take place approximately 36–48 hours after the fistulization. The fistula site must be healed before the voice prosthesis is inserted, otherwise there may be a delay in fitting the patient. If the patient undergoes a tracheoesophageal puncture as part of the primary laryngectomy, prosthesis sizing and fitting may be delayed for three weeks or until the patient's surgical incisions show adequate healing.

The Blom-Singer duckbill voice prosthesis is available in six sizes ranging in length from 1.8 cm to 3.6 cm and seven lengths in the low pressure voice prosthesis ranging from 1.4 cm to 3.6 cm. The Bivona duckbill voice prosthesis ranges in length from 1.4 cm through 3.3 cm and the ultra low resistance in sizes 1.4 cm to 3.0 cm. At the time of fitting the speech-language pathologist will measure for the size most appropriate for the patient. It is important for the speech-language pathologist to give an overview of the entire fitting process and then explain each step in detail so that no surprises are incurred. The following steps may be taken during the initial voice prosthesis fitting process:

1. Clean the stoma area of mucus and any encrusted material using hydrogen peroxide applied with cotton applicators and 4 × 4 gauze.
2. Remove any sutures that are holding the catheter in place.
3. Slowly but deliberately remove the catheter from the puncture. In case of an inflated balloon catheter, the residual air or water must be withdrawn using a standard 10-cc syringe before the catheter is removed. Before removing the catheter, instruct the patient to refrain from swallowing to prevent saliva from flowing through the TEP.
4. Replace the catheter with another size 16 Fr. soft red rubber catheter (when using a catheter make sure the larger end is knotted or capped to prevent leaking of fluids through the catheter) or a Blom-Singer tracheoesophageal puncture dilator (Figure 10–16). Either device can be used by the patient to plug the punc-

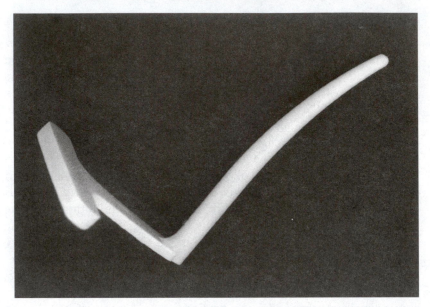

Figure 10–16.   Blom-Singer tracheoesophageal puncture dilator. (Photo by Rick Berkey, St. Elizabeth

ture when cleaning. It is strongly recommended to teach the patient to always keep the puncture stented with either a catheter, dilator, or voice prosthesis. Teach the patient to insert the catheter in the unlikely event the voice prosthesis would ever come out.

5. Control any mucus from the stoma and/or from the oral cavity and nose that was produced when the catheter was removed.

6. With the catheter removed and the puncture unstented, the phonatory mechanism can be tested with the least resistance to airflow. Ask the patient to take a breath. Occlude the stoma with your thumb or finger while the patient slowly exhales saying the vowel /a/. This gives the speech-language pathologist a subjective idea of the ease or difficulty with which the patient can produce voice. If the patient demonstrates much difficulty, then it is possible that internal edema is still present. It may also be an indication of esophageal spasm. If no voicing is produced, one should continue with the sizing and fitting procedure and have the patient return to your office in a week to try voice again.

7. Place a sizing device into the puncture as far as it will go. The sizing device is essentially a dummy voice prosthesis that has incremental markings and numbers that correspond to the var-

ious lengths of manufactured prostheses. When the sizing device is completely inserted you may feel the duckbill end touch the posterior pharyngeal wall. Gently pull the prosthesis back out until the retention collar grasps the inside of the anterior wall of the esophagus. Look at the number on the prosthesis that can be seen on the outside of the puncture. Choose the size prosthesis that corresponds to that number. If the size is between numbers, choose the longer prosthesis. It is best to oversize initially. If the prosthesis is sized too short, the fistula will start to stenose, preventing airflow through the prosthesis. The speech-language pathologist should allow for a small amount of "play" (forward/backward movement) when the patient swallows.

8. Remove the sizing device and insert the voice prosthesis you have sized into the puncture using the insertion tool. Make sure you follow the angle of the puncture and firmly push the prosthesis until you feel or hear the retention collar "pop" into the esophagus. Hold the outer flange and gently remove the insertion tool by rotating and pulling it forward. When the insertion tool has been removed, check the seating of the prosthesis by tugging gently on the flange. Tape the flange to the neck. After the prosthesis is fitted, ask the patient to inhale. Occlude the stoma with your thumb or finger while the patient exhales gently sustaining the vowel /a/. If the prosthesis is sized correctly, the diverted air will cause the PE segment to vibrate. The patient must, however, increase the air pressure greater than when voice was produced without the prosthesis in place.

9. Check to make sure there is no leaking of fluids either around or through the voice prosthesis by having the patient drink water. If leaking is noted around the prosthesis, allow more time for the fistula to seal around the prosthesis. A new or different prosthesis should be inserted if leaking is noted through the prosthesis.

10. The patient should be taught to occlude the stoma with his or her own thumb or finger and to produce voice independently. Start with sustained vowels then words such as counting. Speech material should be provided and the patient encouraged to practice frequently throughout the day.

11. Teach the patient or significant other to clean the voice prosthesis without removing it. Mucus and crust can be removed by using cotton applicators and hydrogen peroxide. Usually the patient is scheduled back to the office in a few days after the initial voice prosthesis fitting to learn independent care.

Independent Care

Usually when the patient is seen for the second time, the speech-language pathologist begins to teach the patient and/or significant other to remove, clean, and reinsert the prosthesis. The prosthesis should be removed for cleaning as needed. Some patients may choose to do so weekly, and others may choose to leave the prosthesis in place for several weeks. Cleaning is preferably accomplished at the same time the patient does the stoma care using adequate lighting and in front of a mirror. To remove the prosthesis, the patient is instructed to firmly grasp the flange and pull forward. When the prosthesis is removed, the size 16 Fr. catheter or a tracheoesophageal puncture dilator is immediately inserted into the fistula to prevent aspiration and stenosis. The prosthesis is cleaned according to the instructions given by the manufacturer. Care should be taken not to violate the slit valve end of the tube. Solvents or petroleum-based cleaning products should not be used as they might damage the silicone.

Patients may also clean the voice prosthesis without removing the device from the tracheoesophageal puncture by using the Blom-Singer Flushing Pipette. The Blom-Singer Flushing Pipette is a plastic tapered tube with a bulb on one end. The patient is instructed to fill the pipette with water and position the device into the voice prosthesis until it abuts against the stopper on the stem of the pipette. Once properly positioned, the patient squeezes the bulb on the pipette to inject the water through the prosthesis flushing out any debris which may have accumulated inside the prosthesis. The debris is flushed into the esophagus. Removal of the prosthesis for cleaning is recommended if a large mucous plug is contained within the prosthesis.

Instructions for fitting the prosthesis would then include

1. Check the slit valve or flapper valve to make sure the edges are not stuck together. Place the tip of the insertion tool into the open end of the voice prosthesis. Avoid squeezing or damaging the slit valve at the tip of the prosthesis.
2. Place a small amount of oil-free water-soluble lubricant such as Surgi-Lube on the tip of the prosthesis. Place the tip of the voice prosthesis in the fistula with the neck strap pointed upwards. Firmly insert until the circular retention collar can be felt to "snap" open within the esophagus. (Insertion or removal of the prosthesis occasionally causes slight bleeding at the fistula. Persistent bleeding should be brought to the attention of the physician.)
3. Place a finger against the flange and gently withdraw the insertion tool from the fully inserted prosthesis.
4. Apply a small strip of hypoallergenic adhesive tape over the flange to prevent movement or accidental dislodgment

The low-pressure voice prosthesis differs from the duckbill prosthesis. The low-pressure prosthesis has a recessed valve and a low profile tip making it slightly more difficult to insert into the fistula. The patient is instructed to insert an 18 Fr. catheter or tracheoesophageal dilator for a few minutes to dilate the lumen. An alternative method of insertion for the Blom-Singer Low Pressure Voice Prosthesis is using the Blom-Singer Gel Cap Insertion System (Figure 10–17a-b). The gel cap provides a smooth, rounded shape to the tip by folding the retention collar in a forward position inside the cap making insertion of the prosthesis less traumatic to the surrounding tissue. The gel cap is designed to dissolve inside the esophagus within minutes after insertion. It is important for the patient to hold the prosthesis in place with the inserter for at least 3 minutes allowing time for the gel cap to dissolve and the retention collar to unfold. Explicit instructions in applying the gel cap are provided by the manufacturer.

The Blom-Singer InDwelling Low Pressure Voice Prosthesis (see Figure 10–14c) is a new device that was designed for patients who are unable or resisted changing the Low Pressure Voice Prosthesis every two to three days as recommended. The Blom-Singer InDwelling Low Pressure Voice Prosthesis should be inserted and removed by a physcian or a trained speech-language pathologist. Inserting the prosthesis requires using the gel cap (described above). A Fr. 22 tracheoesophageal puncture dilator is inserted into the fistula to slightly dilate the opening. The dilator is removed and the voice prosthesis is inserted with the neck strap pointed upwards. The voice prosthesis should be held into position for at least 3 minutes allowing the gel cap to dissolve and the retention collar to unfold within the esophagus. Check to make sure the prosthesis is secured by rotating the prosthesis 360°. Once the prosthesis is correctly placed, the voice prosthesis strap is detached from the safety peg on the inserter. If the prosthesis does not rotate freely, an A-P radiographic examination of the tracheostoma is recommended to confirm if the retention collar is positioned within the esophagus. The InDwelling Voice Prosthesis may be worn until it ceases to function correctly or begins to leak. A hemostat is used to remove the prosthesis by grasping the outer rim of the device pulling gently and firmly until the prosthesis is completely removed. Once removed, insert a Fr. 22 tracheostoma dilator. Keep the dilator in the fistula for at least five minutes before inserting a new prosthesis. The InDwelling Low Pressure Voice Prosthesis can be cleaned without removal by using the flushing pipette.

The Blom-Singer voice prosthesis is available from International Healthcare Technologies (1110 Mark Avenue, Carpinteria, CA 93013-2918, 805-684-9337 or 800-477-5969). The Bivona voice prosthesis is available from Bivona Medical Technologies (5700 W. 23rd Ave., Gary, IN 46406, 219-989-9150 or 800-348-6064).

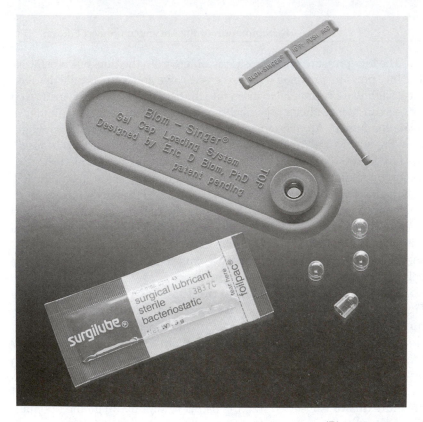

Figure 10–17a. Blom-Singer gel cap insertion system. (Photo courtesy of InHealth Technologies.)

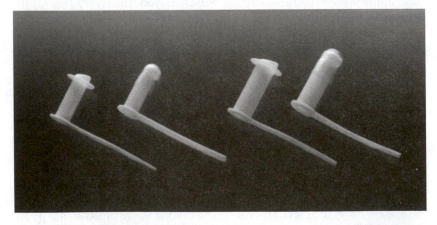

Figure 10–17b. Example of gel cap on low pressure voice prosthesis. (Photo courtesy of InHealth Technologies.)

Maximizing Communication

Once fit with the prosthesis, some patients readily occlude the stoma and speak with excellent phrasing and inflection, similar to their prelaryngectomy speech patterns. Other patients may need instruction in occluding the stoma and in proper breath control, phrasing, and articulation. Patients who have used esophageal voice prior to surgical prosthetics often must be broken of the habit of injecting air. The result of the use of a surgical prosthesis is a superior esophageal voice.

Tracheostoma Valve

The tracheostoma valve is a device designed for laryngectomees who have undergone a tracheoesophageal puncture and communicate with various types of voice prosthesis. The use of this valve negates the need to manually occlude the stoma for speech production, thus freeing both hands. The Blom-Singer Adjustable Tracheoesophageal Valve (Figure 10–18) is available from InHealth Technologies and the Bivona Tracheostoma Valve (Figure 10–19) and Bivona Tracheostoma Valve II (Figure 10–20) are available from Bivona Medical Technologies. In evaluating patient use of the tracheostoma valve, the speech-language pathologist focuses on the topography of the stoma and surrounding tissue.

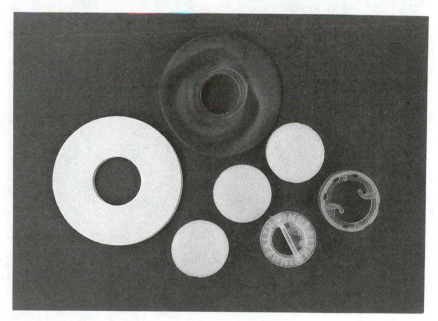

Figure 10–18.   Blom-Singer adjustable tracheostoma valve with Humidifilter. (Photo by Rick Berkey, St. Elizabeth Medical Center, Dayton, Ohio.)

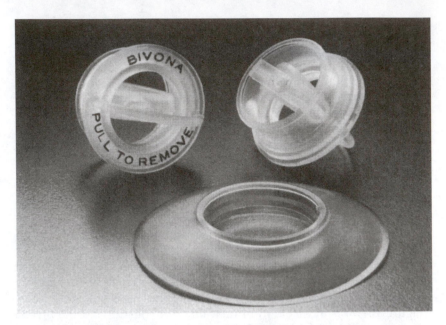

Figure 10–19. Bivona tracheostoma valve. (Photo courtesy of Bivona Medical Tehnologies.)

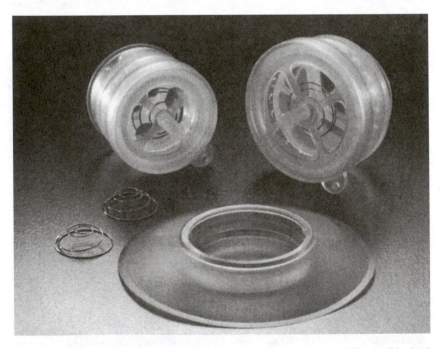

Figure 10–20. Bivona tracheostoma valve II. (Photo courtesy of Bivona Medical Tehnologies.)

Successful use of the breathing valve is dependent upon the ability to tape and glue the valve collar to a sufficient amount of tissue surrounding the stoma to prevent it from being dislodged by the pulmonary air pressure. Patients with sunken stomas or uneven skin tissue surrounding the stoma may not have an adequate skin surface for collar adhesion.

The first step in evaluating patient use is to attach the housing collar using a special skin adherent and double-sided tape discs or double-sided foam discs provided in the fitting kit. Once the housing collar is in place, the tracheostoma valve is fitted. The Blom-Singer tracheostoma valve has an internal adjustment sensitivity which allows the patient to adjust the valve from ultra light to medium sensitivity by rotating the face plate. A proper valve weight must be chosen for the Bivona tracheostoma valve. The proper valve weight (ultra light, light, medium, or firm) is the weight that does not close during heavy respiratory effort, but will close when sufficient air pressure is exhaled to produce speech. The Bivona tracheostoma valve II has a set of four interchangeable springs designed to provide different degrees of sensitivity.

A simple way to determine the degree of valve closure or proper valve weight (depending on the type of valve) is to have the patient walk up and down steps. Begin with the ultra-light setting or valve in place. If the valve closes when the patient is breathing heavily, turn the valve slightly or if using a valve or spring move up to the next weight. Continue this process until a valve that does not close during heavy breathing is found. Rotating the face plate to adjust the valve sensitivity is an advantage when using the Blom-Singer adjustable tracheostoma valve. The valve must be removed from the housing collar to make the proper valve or spring sensitivity adjustments for the Bivona tracheostoma valve or tracheostoma valve II, respectively.

Use of the tracheostoma valve has been beneficial for many patients, especially those who are required to use both hands while working. A Humidifilter can be placed on the Blom-Singer adjustable tracheostoma valve to moisten, warm, and filter inspired air. Some patients report a decrease in coughing with the use of the Humidifilter.

Coughing can present a problem for all tracheostoma valve users. The increased air pressure that is produced when coughing will close the valve requiring the valve to be completely removed. Sometimes repeated coughing will cause strain on the adhesive discs that hold the housing collar in place causing premature leaking of air around the housing. Increased mucus will also work the adhesive free from the skin. Another complication is skin irritation from the adhesive. We have found that even with a commercial skin preparation that is brushed on the skin prior to the adherent, some patients still experience skin irritation.

SUMMARY

Total rehabilitation of the laryngectomized patient is challenging for the patient, the patient's family, and for all professionals involved in this process. Rehabilitation included physical, psychological, and social adjustments as well as learning a new method of oral communication. The speech-language pathologist's role in working with the cancer patient and family involves both counseling and management of all communication needs. Our interactions with the cancer patient and family may, at times, be mentally taxing and personally stressful, but most often the results of our efforts are both satisfying and rewarding. No other group of communicatively impaired patients has the potential to progress from very limited communication to functional oral communication as rapidly as the laryngectomized patient.

The patient who undergoes a total laryngectomy now has several communication options from which to choose. The speech-language pathologist is encouraged to become familiar with all these options and, for the sake of the patient, to show no biases against any. As research continues to expand and improve these options, so, too, will the role of the speech-language pathologist also expand.

REFERENCES

Amatsu, M., Matsui, T., Maki, T., & Kanagawa, K. (1977). Vocal reconstruction after total laryngectomy: A new one-stage surgical technique. *Journal of Otolaryngology, Japan, 80*, 779–785.

American Cancer Society. (1987). *Facts on cancer of the larynx*. Atlanta, GA: Author.

American Cancer Society. (1994). *Cancer facts and figures*. Atlanta, GA: Author.

American Joint Committee on Cancer, Manual for Staging of Cancer. (1992). Larynx (4th ed.). Philadelphia: J. B. Lippincott Company.

American Speech-Language Hearing Association. (1990). AIDS/HIV: Implications for speech-language pathologists and audiologists. *ASHA, 32*, 46–48.

American Speech-Language Hearing Association. (1992). Position statement and guidelines: Evaluation and treatment for tracheoesophageal fistulization/puncture. *ASHA, 34*, 17–21.

Andrews, J. C., Mickel, R. A., Hanson, D. G., Monahan, G. P., & Ward, P. H. (1987). Major complications following tracheo-esophageal puncture for voice rehabilitation. *Laryngoscope, 97*, 562–567.

Aronson, A. (1980). *Clinical voice disorders: An interdisciplinary approach*. New York: Brian C. Decker.

Arslan, M., & Serafini, I. (1972). Reconstructive laryngectomy: Report of the first 35 cases. *Annals of Otology Rhinology and Laryngology, 81*, 479–486.

Asai, R. (1972). Laryngoplasty after total laryngectomy. *Archives of Otolaryngology, 95*, 114–119.

Berlin, C. I. (1963). Clinical measurement of esophageal speech. I. Methodology and curves of skill acquisition. *Journal of Speech and Hearing Disorders, 28,* 42–51.

Berlin, C. I. (1965). Clinical measurement of esophageal speech: III. Performance of nonbiases groups. *Journal of Speech and Hearing Disorders, 30,* 174–183.

Blom, E., & Singer, M. (1979). Surgical-prosthetic approaches for post-laryngectomy voice restoration. In R. L. Keith & F. L. Darley (Eds.), *Laryngectomy rehabilitation.* Austin, TX: Pro-Ed.

Blood, G., & Blood, I. (1982). A tactic for facilitating social interaction with laryngectomees. *Journal of Speech and Hearing Disorders, 47,* 416–418.

Campinelli, P. A. (1964). Audiological considerations in achieving esophageal voice. *Eye, Ear, Nose, and Throat Montly, 43,* 76–80.

Casper, J., & Colton, R. (1993). *Clinical manual for laryngectomy and head/neck cancer rehabilitation,* San Diego, CA: Singular Publishing Group, Inc.

Centers for Disease Control. (1988). *Perspectives in Disease Prevention and Health Promotion, 37,* 377–388.

Clark, J., & Stemple, J. (1982). Assessment of three modes of alaryngeal speech with a synthetic sentence identification (SSI) task in varying message-to-competition ratios. *Journal of Speech and Hearing Research, 25,* 333–338.

Conley, J., DeAmesti, F., & Pierce, M. (1958). A new surgical technique for the vocal rehabilitation of the laryngectomized patient. *Annals of Otology Rhinology and Laryngology, 67,* 655–664.

DeWeese, D. D., Saunders, W. H., Schuller, D. E., & Schleuning, A. J. (1988). *Otolaryngology-head and neck surgery* (7th ed.). St. Louis: C.V. Mosby.

Diedrich, W., & Youngstrom. (1966). *Alaryngeal speech.* Springfield, IL: Charles C. Thomas.

Donegan, J., Gluckman, J., & Singh, J. (1981). Limitiations of the Blom-Singer technique for voice restoration. *Annals of Otology Rhinology and Laryngology, 90,* 495–497.

Duguay, M. J. (1991). Esophageal speech training: the initial phase. In S. J. Solmon & K. H. Mount (Eds.), *Alaryngeal speech rehabilitation, for clinicians by clinicians* (pp. 47–78). Austin, TX: Pro-Ed.

Gardner, W. (1971). *Laryngectomee speech rehabilitation.* Springfield, IL: Charles C. Thomas.

Gates, G., Ryan, W., Cooper, Jr., J., Lawlis, G., Cantu, E., Hayashi, T., Lauder, E., Welch, R., & Hearne, E. (1982). Current status of laryngectomee rehabilitation: I. Result of therapy. *American Journal of Otolaryngology, 3*(1), 1–7.

Gates, G., Ryan, W., Cantu, E., & Hearne, E., (1982). Current status of laryngectomy rehabilitation: Causes of failure. *American Journal of Otolaryngology, 3*(2), 8–14.

Gussenbauer, C. (1874). Ueber die erste durch Th Billroth am Menschen ausgefuhrte Kehlkopf-Exstirpation und die Anwendung eines kunstlichen Kokokopfes. *Arch. f Klin. Chir, 17,* 343–356.

Guttman, M. R. (1932). Rehabilitation of the voice in laryngectomized patients. *Archives of Otolaryngology, 15,* 478–479.

Hamaker, R. C., Singer, M. I., Blom, E. D., & Daniels, H. A. (1985). Primary voice restoration at laryngectomy. *Archives of Otolaryngology, 111,* 182–186.

International Association of Laryngectomees, *First aid for (Neck-Breathers) laryngectomees* (No. 4522). New York: National Office of the American Cancer Society.

International Association of Laryngectomees. *Laryngectomized speaker's source book* (No. 4521). New York: National Office of the American Cancer Society

Isshiki, N., & Snidecor, J. (1965). Air intake and usage in esophageal speech. *Acta Oto-Laryngologica, 59*, 559–574.

Johns, M. E., & Cantrell, R. W. (1981). Voice restoration of the total laryngectomy patient: The Singer-Blom technique. *Otolaryngology, Head and Neck Surgery, 89*, 82–86.

Kalb, M., & Carpenter, M. (1981). Individual speaker influence on relative intelligibility of esophageal speech and artificial larynx. *Journal of Speech and Hearing Disorders, 46*, 77–80.

Keith, R. (1991). *Looking forward A guidebook for the laryngectomee* (2nd ed.). New York: Thieme Medical Publishers, Inc.

Keith R. L., & Shanks, J. C. (1986). Historical highlights: Laryngectomy rehabilitation. In R. L. Keith & F. L. Darley (Eds.), *Laryngectomee rehabilitation* (2nd ed, pp. 3–53). Austin, TX: Pro-Ed.

Kolson, H., & Glasgold, A. (1967). Tracheo-esophageal speech following laryngectomy. *Transactions of the American Academy of Ophthalmology and Otolaryngology, 71*, 421–425.

LaBorwit, L. (1980). Speech rehabilitation for laryngectomized patients. *Ear, Nose, and Throat Journal, 59*, 82–89.

Lauder, E. (1989–1990). *Self-help for the laryngectomee.* Unpublished manuscript. (Available from 11115 Whisper Hollow, San Antonio, TX 78230.)

Lerman, J. W. (1991). The artificial larynx. In S. J. Solmon & K. H. Mount (Eds.) *Alaryngeal speech rehabilitation, for clinicians by clinicians* (pp. 27–45). Austin, TX: Pro-Ed.

Levin, D., Devesa, S., Godwin, H. J., & Silverman, D. (1974). *Cancer rates and risks* (2nd Ed.). (Department of Health, Education and Welfare Publication, No. 75–691.) Washington, DC: U.S. Government Printing Office.

Martinkosky, S. J. (1991). Tracheoeophageal puncture: General considerations. In S. J. Solmon & K. H. Mount (Eds.), *Alaryngeal speech rehabilitation, for clinicians by clinicians* (pp. 107–138). Austin, TX: Pro-Ed.

Morrison, W. (1981). The production of voice following total laryngectomy. *Archives of Otolaryngology, 14*, 413–431.

Post-laryngectomy training aid. (1994). Carpinteria, CA: InHealth Technologies.

Pressman, J., & Bailey, B. (1968). The survey of cancer of the larynx with special reference to subtotal laryngectomy. In J. Snidecor (Ed.), *Speech rehabilitation of the laryngectomized.* Springfield, IL: Charles C. Thomas.

Rice, D. H., & Spiro, R. H. (1989). *Current concepts in head and neck cancer.* Atlanta, GA: The American Cancer Society.

Robbins, J., Dudley, B., Blom, E., Singer, M., Fisher, H., & Logemann, J. (1980). *Acoustic characteristics of voice restoration following tracheo-esophageal puncture.* Paper presented at the American Speech-Language-Hearing Association Annual Convention, Detroit.

Salmon, S. (1986). Methods of air intake for esophageal speech and their associated problems. In R. L. Keith & F. L. Darley (Eds.), *Laryngectomee rehabilitation* (2nd ed., pp. 55–69). Austin, TX: Pro-Ed.

Schuller, D. E., Jarrow, J. E., Kelly, D. R. & Miglets, A. W. (1983). Prognostic factors affecting the success of duckbill vocal restoration. *Otolaryngology, Head and Neck Surgery, 91*, 396–398.

Shedd, D., Schaaf, N., & Weinberg, B. (1976). Technical aspects of reed-fistula speech following pharyngolaryngectomy. *Journal of Surgical Oncology, 8,* 305–310.

Sindecor, J. (1968). *Speech rehabilitation of the laryngectomized* (2nd ed.). Springfield, IL: Charles C. Thomas.

Singer, M. I., & Blom, E. (1980). An endoscopic technique for restoration of voice after laryngectomy. *Annals of Otology, Rhinology and Laryngology, 89*(6), 529–533.

Singer, M. I., Blom, E. D., & Hamaker, R. C. (1986). Pharyngeal plexus neurectomy for alaryngeal speech rehabilitation. *Laryngoscope, 96,* 50–53.

Sloane, P., Griffin, J., & O'Dwyer, T. (1991). Esophageal insufflation and videofluoroscopy for evaluation of esophageal speech in laryngectomy patients: Clinical implications. *Radiology, 181,* 433–438.

Staffieri, M. (1973). Laryngectomie totale avec reconstitution de la glotte phonatoire. *Revue de Laryngologie, Otologie, Rhinologie, 95,* 63–68.

Taub, S. (1975). Air by-pass voice prosthesis for vocal rehabilitation of laryngectomees. *Annals of Otology, Rhinology and Laryngology, 84,* 45–48.

Van den Berg, J., & Moolenaar-Bijl, A. J. (1959). Cricopharyngeal sphincter, pitch, intensity, and fluency in oesophageal speech. *Practica Oto-rhino-laryngologica, 21,* 298–315.

INDEX

A

Accent method, 224–226
Acoustic measurements, 120, 124–132
  normative data, 149–154
Acoustic recording routines, 132
Aerodynamic measurement, 120
  normative data, 149–154
Aerodynamic myoelastic theory, 40
Aerodynamic recording routines, 139
Airflow rate, 151, 152
Alaryngeal speech, 291–294
  artificial larynx, 291–292, 295–301
  esophageal speech, 292–293,
    301–306
  surgical prosthetics, 293–294,
    306–321
Alcohol abuse, 56–57, 258
Allergies, 55, 232–233, 259
Amplification, 122
Amyotrophic lateral sclerosis (ALS),
  244
Anemometer, 137
Antihistamines, 54
Aristotle, 4
Arthritis, 56, 233
Aryeppiglotic folds, 16
Arytenoid, cartilage, 27–28, 77
Asthma, 54
Assimilative nasality, 50
Audiometric examination, 113, 278
Autogenous fat, 235

B

Basement membrane zone (BMZ), 38
Blood supply, 22
Botulinum toxin (Botox®), 239,
  242–243
Breathiness, 193–194
Bronchodilators, 55

C

Caffeine, 57, 258
Cancer
  laryngeal, 81–82, 270–276
  lung, 54, 55
Cardiac disorders, 56
Central nervous system, 24
Cerebral palsy, 58
Chronic illness, 54–57
Chronic obstructive pulmonary disease
  (COPD), 54, 55, 234
Circulatory disorders, 56
Classification of pathologies, 66–67
Cleft pal,ate, 57–58
Cohen, J. Dobs, 10
Congenital web, 67–68, 247
Conversion disorders, 60, 91–92
  treatment of, 210–218
Corniculate cartilage, 27–28
Corticosteroids, 55
Coughing, 48, 54, 174, 175, 258
  laryngectomy, after, 281–282, 321
Cricoid cartilage, 24–27
Cricothyroid muscle, 29
Croup, 234
Cul-de-sac nasality, 51
Cuneiform cartilage, 27–28
Cysts, congenital, 68, 76–77, 246
Czermak, Johann, 10

D

da Vinci, Leonardo, 6
Deafness, 58
Denasality, 50
  therapy for, 196–197
Diagnostic evaluation, 97–118
  audiometric examination, 113
  components of, 98–99
  impressions, 112, 174
  medical examination, 101–103
  medical history, 172